Cold War, Deadly Fevers

Cold War, Deadly Fevers

Malaria Eradication in Mexico, 1955–1975

Marcos Cueto

Woodrow Wilson Center Press
Washington, D.C.

Johns Hopkins University Press
Baltimore

EDITORIAL OFFICES

Woodrow Wilson Center Press
Woodrow Wilson International Center for Scholars
One Woodrow Wilson Plaza
1300 Pennsylvania Avenue, NW
Washington, DC 20004-3027
www.wilsoncenter.org

ORDER FROM

Johns Hopkins University Press
Hopkins Fulfillment Services
P.O. Box 50370
Baltimore, MD 21211-4370
Telephone: 1-800-537-5487
www.press.jhu.edu/books/

2 4 6 8 9 7 5 3 1

The Library of Congress has cataloged the hardcover edition of this book as follows:

Cueto, Marcos
    Cold war, deadly fevers : malaria eradication in Mexico, 1955–1975 / Marcos Cueto.
    p. ; cm
    Includes bibliographical references and index.
    ISBN: 978-0-8018-8645-4 (cloth : alk. paper)
    1. Malaria—Mexico—History. 2. Social medicine—Mexico—History. I. Title.
[DNLM: 1. Malaria—history—Mexico. 2. Health Policy—history—Mexico.
3. Health Promotion—history—Mexico. 4. History, 20th Century—Mexico.
5. Malaria—prevention & control—Mexico. WC 750 C965c 2007]
RC162.M6C8448 2007
614.5′3200972—dc22   2007004959

    ISBN: 978-1-4214-1556-7 (paperback : alk. paper)

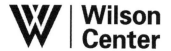

The Wilson Center, chartered by Congress as the official memorial to President Woodrow Wilson, is the nation's key nonpartisan policy forum for tackling global issues through independent research and open dialogue to inform actionable ideas for Congress, the Administration, and the broader policy community.

Conclusions or opinions expressed in Center publications and programs are those of the authors and speakers and do not necessarily reflect the views of the Center staff, fellows, trustees, advisory groups, or any individuals or organizations that provide financial support to the Center.

Please visit us online at www.wilsoncenter.org.

Jane Harman, Director, President, and CEO

Contents

Figures and Tables   ix

Preface and Acknowledgments   xi

A Note on Sources   xv

1   Introduction: The Burden of an Infection   1
The Origins and Development of Malaria Control Efforts   2
Organizing Principles for This Volume   7
Plan of the Book   11

2   Global Designs   15
Foreign Aid and the Cold War   17
International Health Cooperation   33
The Encounter of International Health and Politics   49
Concluding Thoughts   67

3   National Decisions   70
Mexican Politics and Medicine   71
Mexican Malaria Control   82
Organizing Malaria Eradication   86
The Mexicanization of the Campaign   100

4   Local Responses   112
Intercultural Challenges   112
Anthropological Critique   120
A Provincial Doctor Rebels   128
Indigenous Resistance   136
A Campaign in Decline   139

5   Conclusions: The Return of Malaria and the
    Culture of Survival   159
    Mexico's Recent Experience with Malaria   159
    The Lessons of Malaria Eradication:
        Patterns of Vertical Health Programs   163

Notes   167

Bibliography   225

Index   253

Figures and Tables

Figures

2.1 The face of malaria: A Mexican woman shakes with the all-too-familiar fever (1968).   64

3.1 In the mountains, a pony is better than a jeep. This man looks at home in the saddle, his spraying equipment beside him (1968).   106

3.2 A teacher in the village of Calotmal explains malaria to his class, showing how blood samples are taken and then examined in the laboratory (1962).   110

4.1 A little Mexican girl gives a sample of her blood for a test (1962).   116

Tables

2.1 Comparison of Malaria Control and Malaria Eradication Programs   47

3.1 Fourteen Working Areas of the Comisión Nacional de Erradicación del Paludismo   92

Preface and Acknowledgments

The idea for this book emerged from my direct experience with public health education and my indirect experience with public health practice. For the past ten years, I have been a university professor of the history of public health in a School of Public Health. Most of my students have worked, are working, or will work in public health. There is one question that they usually ask again and again: "What are the main lessons of the stories we are analyzing?" Initially, I rejected this question under the assumption that they were trying to simplify complex historical investigations.

However, in the past few years, I have been resorting to the following response: "We need more historical research." I truly believe that the best way to answer my students' question is to make a strong plea for considering the lessons of history in public health thinking and practice. I am convinced that poor and unsophisticated historical knowledge among public health scholars and officers, especially in developing countries, is related to inconsistent, fragmented, and discontinued health policies and programs. Moreover, a lack of historical knowledge contributes to the low prestige of public health work and to the absence of long-term sanitary perspectives in many developing countries.

I am aware that the history of public health will not dictate what should be done. But it can illuminate the recurrent patterns of sanitary backwardness and suggest what might be done to make a real difference from the past. That is why historians of public health can contribute not only by enriching social history—by revealing dimensions not usually studied by mainstream historians, such as the perception and impact of sickness, health, and death—but also by problematizing, and eventually improving, the health discipline closest to the social sciences, namely, public health.

This book also emerges from a concern for the relationship between international health cooperation and national health systems during the second half of the twentieth century, a relatively new topic for both historians of medicine and public health scholars. For most of that period, Latin American public health, and many of the public health systems of developing regions, were intertwined with the international health activities promoted by the United States. Today, however, international health cooperation is beginning to be assessed, questioned, and reconsidered. During the past few years, some agencies and scholars have proposed that the new concept of "global health" should replace international health. Other institutions resist the change and believe that "global health" is an "old wine in a new bottle." The aim of this book is not to take sides in this ongoing debate but to examine a recent major intervention of international health, to demonstrate that the story of international health in the second half of the twentieth century is a rich and fascinating area of research for historians of medicine, and to identify the lessons of this story for the contemporary discussion of international public health cooperation.

Because some of the questions that have inspired my research have been raised by my students, I want to express gratitude to them and to my home institution, the School of Public Health of the Universidad Peruana Cayetano Heredia in Lima. Shortly after its creation in the early 1990s, this school made an unusual decision for one of its kind: to make "the history of public health" a required course for students pursuing a master's degree in public health. I am also grateful to Jorge Lossio, José Carlos de la Puente, Julio Nuñez, and Carol Pasco, my research assistants in Lima, who, unlike those preparing for work in public health, developed a vocational interest in the history of medicine or in social history.

I have been fortunate to discuss all or part of my research with friends and colleagues in the Americas: Marta de Almeida, Jaime Benchimol, Anne-Emanuelle Birn, Theodore M. Brown, Elizabeth Fee, Gilberto Hochman, Ronald L. Numbers, Diana Obregón, Steven Palmer, Emilio Quevedo, Darwin Stapleton, Alexandra Stern, Nisia Trinidade Lima, and Adam Warren. In Mexico, I was kindly helped and guided by Claudia Agostoni, Irma Betanzos, Ana Maria Carrillo, Paul Hersch, José Moya, and Ana Cecilia Rodríguez de Romo.

I have been fortunate to have had the opportunity to travel to several cities to do research for this book, thanks to support from a number of grants. The first institution that supported my travels and investigation for 2001 and 2002 was the Council for the International Exchange for Scholars, which organized the international New Century Scholars Program titled "Challenges of Health in a Borderless World." I want to give special thanks to three individuals who organized the program, Micaela Iovine, Ilona Kickbusch, and Patti McGill. Because of the program, I was able to use the library and archives of the World Health Organization in Geneva, where I always found the help of Ineke Deserno, Bernardino Fantini, Carol Modis, Marie Villemin, and Eugenio Villar. The New Century Scholars Program included a semester at Columbia University as a visiting researcher. During this semester, I was affiliated with the Center for the Study of Society and Medicine at the Columbia College of Physicians and Surgeons and with the Department of Sociomedical Sciences of the Mailman School of Public Health. At Columbia, I received great feedback from Ronald Bayer, Gerald M. Oppenheimer, Richard Parker, David Rosner, David Rothman, and Nancy Leys Stepan. Over the years, I have been fortunate to enjoy Nancy Leys Stepan's support and comments. In 2003, I received the John J. Pisano Travel Grant administered by the History Office of the National Institutes of Health. I am grateful to Pedro Brito and Victoria Harden, who made possible a very productive period of investigation at the National Library of Medicine in Washington.

The first time I presented the preliminary results of this work was at the Institute for the History of Medicine of Johns Hopkins University in 2002. In the spring of that year, a Johns Hopkins professor, Harry M. Marks, asked me to discuss malaria eradication in Mexico with an audience of graduate students and professors. Two additional presentations allowed me to refine and polish this work: in November 2003, as the Speaker of the Manuel Ancizar Chair at the Universidad Nacional de Colombia; and in February 2004, as the Chauncey and Mary Leake Lecturer in Medical History at the University of Wisconsin–Madison. I made significant progress with the first version of the manuscript for this book during the spring of 2004, when I was a resident fellow at the Woodrow Wilson International Center for Scholars. Several people at the Woodrow Wilson Center were extremely helpful during that period, among them Andrew Selee and Joseph S. Tulchin of the Latin American Program. I am also very grateful to Francisco Reyes, a remarkable research assistant who helped me during my stay at the Woodrow Wilson Center.

I responded to the insightful comments of the reviewers in Palo Alto, California, during the spring quarter of 2006, thanks to the invitation to be the Edward Laroque Tinker Visiting Professor at the Center for Latin American Studies of Stanford University. I am very grateful to Herbert S. Klein, director of the center, not only for inviting me to apply for this position but also for his sustained encouragement and advice for many years. At Stanford I was assisted by Erica Lorraine Williams, Megan Gorman, and Omar Ochoa. I also offer many thanks to James Dunkerley and the other editors of the *Journal of Latin American Studies,* who have allowed me to include excerpts from my article, "Appropriation and Resistance: Responses to Malaria Eradication in Mexico," which appeared in volume 37 in 2005. My special gratitude goes to Joseph Brinley and Yamile Kahn, respectively the director and editor of the Woodrow Wilson Center Press, who assisted me during the whole editorial process, and to my copyeditor, Alfred F. Imhoff. Finally, this work was only possible because of the patience and love of my family. To them, and all the above, *muchisimas gracias.*

A Note on Sources

This study is based on relevant archival and library materials from Mexico, Europe, and the United States. I have consulted newspapers and publications from Mexico's Biblioteca Nacional and Archivo General de la Nación, along with the papers of the antimalaria unit in the superb Archivo Histórico de la Secretaría de Salud, all located in Mexico City. In this collection, I found scores of boxes from the unit in charge of malaria eradication that no one had used before. In Oaxaca, Mexico, I also made good use of the regional Archivo General del Estado de Oaxaca, the municipal library, and the library of the Fundación Cultural Bustamante Vasconcelos.

The Secretaría de Salubridad y Asistencia was created in 1943. In 1983, its name was changed to Secretaría de Salud. An archive (Archivo Histórico de la Secretaría de Salud) open to researchers was founded in 1986. Part of its holdings are described in *Guía de la Sección SubSecretaría de Salubridad y Asistencia, Fondo Secretaría de Salubridad y Asistencia, Oficialía Mayor, Centro de Documentación Institucional Departamento de Archivo Histórico,* by Secretaría de Salud (Mexico City: Secretaría de Salud, 1994); and *Guía del Fondo de Salubridad Pública,* by Secretaría de Salud Centro de Documentación y Archivo Histórico (Mexico City: Secretaría de Salud Centro de Documentación y Archivo Histórico, 1991). For more information, see http://www.bireme.br/crics5/E/grupos/grupo1/Barnard.pdf and http://www.salud.gob.mx/unidades/cdi/presentcdi.html. I especially relied on 139 boxes (in Spanish, *cajas*) of the collection (*sección*) titled Comisión Nacional para la Erradicación del Paludismo of the record group (*fondo*) titled Secretaría de Salubridad y Asistencia, which comprises 1,421 boxes. A guide to this collection is kept at the Archivo Histórico de la Secretaría de Salud. From the same record group Secretaría de Salubridad y Asistencia,

I used the collections titled Secretaría Particular, Subsecretaría de Salubridad y Asistencia, Subsecretaría de Salubridad y Asistencia, Subsecretaría and Asistencia, and Subsecretaría de Salubridad (which have no series). In the notes, I also use the term in Spanish for folder, *expedientes.*

In the United States, I made extensive use of the congressional, presidential, Department of State, and bilateral agencies' papers and rare publications held at the National Archives in Washington and suburban Maryland. Archival and published materials from the National Library of Medicine in Bethesda (e.g., the Fred L. Soper, Eugene Campbell, and Louis L. Williams Jr. papers and diaries), and materials from the Rockefeller Archive Center in New York City (e.g., the Paul F. Russell Diaries) were essential to my work. The books, pamphlets, and rare publications held at the Library of Congress in Washington, the Library of the New York Academy of Medicine, the Library of Stanford University, the Library of the University of California at Berkeley, and the New York Public Library have also been extremely useful. Finally, I made extensive use of the remarkable collections of reports and publications held at the libraries and the archives of the World Health Organization in Geneva and of the United Nations Children's Fund (UNICEF) in New York City.

Cold War, Deadly Fevers

1

Introduction: The Burden of an Infection

Malaria has been called the "the king of diseases" and the "world's worst health problem" because it has been, and still is, one of the major infectious diseases on the globe.[1] Every year, more than 300 million people seek medical treatment for malaria, and 1 million die from this insect-borne, typically rural, disease.[2] Efforts to control malaria in the developing world have an intricate and fascinating history that has not been fully explored. Moreover, the lessons of this history—the advantages and limitations of what has been done—have received little attention and thus so far have mostly been lost. This book seeks to examine the interplay of medical, political, and cultural factors in the development of a major effort to eliminate malaria during the 1950s in one of the biggest Latin American countries, Mexico. Malaria eradication became an absolute between 1955 and the late 1960s, and it elicited contradictory processes of local appropriation and resistance.[3]

Malaria's basic symptoms, etiology, and transmission were established at the turn of the twentieth century by Italian, British, and French scientists.[4] Malaria is usually characterized by intermittent fevers, teeth-chattering chills, the shakes, headaches, a feeling of unbearable cold, uncontrollable shivering, profuse sweating, and occasionally brain damage. These symptoms may last from a few weeks to a few years. In addition, where malaria is common, people often acquire resistance after contracting the disease several times, often making its symptoms less severe in adults and acute in children from these endemic areas. Newcomers to malarious areas also suffer more intense episodes of the disease.

Of the more than four hundred species of the *Anopheles* mosquito, approximately seventy are vectors of malaria. The two most important species in Mexico during the 1950s were *A. pseudopunctipennis* and *A. albimanus*.[5]

Malaria is caused by a parasite protozoa of the genus *Plasmodium*. Natural infection occurs when the female *Anopheles* injects the *Plasmodium* while probing for human blood to produce its eggs. Humans are commonly infected by four species of this parasite: *P. vivax, P. falciparum, P. ovale,* and *P. malarie. P. vivax,* also known as "benign" or "tertian," was the most common of these four species in Mexico and Latin America during the twentieth century. The terms "benign" and "tertian" indicate that the fever that comes every three days is rarely fatal. Though people who contract this type of malaria usually do not die immediately, they are debilitated and experience relapses of drastic fevers. Cases involving *P. falciparum,* or "malignant" malaria, were common in Latin America, especially Brazil, during the late twentieth century.[6] The term "malignant" conveys the commonly fatal outcome of this type of the disease, which usually occurs within a few days or weeks.

Malaria transmission is different from yellow fever, another mosquito-borne infection important in Latin American medical history. The urban version of yellow fever is transmitted by the female *Aedes aegypti* mosquito. The preferred breeding places for this mosquito are domestic and artificial water containers and clear reservoirs where it deposits its eggs. This species is rarely found far away from habitations and has difficulty flying long distances.[7] In contrast to the *Aedes aegypti,* the female *Anopheles* prefers swamps and ponds as breeding sites, avoids light, feeds and is active at night, and usually does not live next to human residences. In sum, it is a stronger insect. An important feature of the *Anopheles* is its ability to fly longer distances than other blood-sucking insects. Another significant difference is that once yellow fever is contracted, it can, unlike malaria, confer lifetime immunity.

The Origins and Development of Malaria Control Efforts

In 1900, shortly after the Spanish-American War was fought partly in Cuba, a commission of the U.S. Army in Havana used the ideas of Carlos Finlay, a Cuban physician, to demonstrate that yellow fever was transmitted from a sick person to a healthy one by the *Aedes aegypti* mosquito. In 1901, the American colonel William Gorgas ended the fever by ridding Havana of *Aedes.* He later applied his method in Panama, which enabled the construction of the canal from 1904 to 1914. These achievements convinced private philanthropic organizations such as the Rockefeller Foundation that campaigns conducted in a military style would get similar results elsewhere. During the 1920s, the foundation launched anti–yellow fever campaigns in a number of Latin American cities, including those in Mexico and Peru. Yellow fever control operations and the new medical specialty of tropical medicine became an important instrument in the international expansion of European and American influence.

Although formerly found throughout much of the world, including temperate zones in Western Europe and the United States, starting in the late nineteenth century, malaria became restricted to tropical and subtropical regions, particularly in poor countries with little rural sanitation such as Mexico. During the first half of the twentieth century, two different malaria control efforts had contradictory effects on international efforts to fight malaria.

The first malaria control effort stemmed from two crucial decisions made by the U.S. government as it sought to eliminate the disease from the American South. First, the Agricultural Act of 1933 forced rural shack dwellers to move to bigger towns and to other healthier parts of the country where health services were available. This decision not only diminished the possibilities of contact between humans and mosquitoes but also made possible medical help in case a person acquired the disease. Second, during the 1940s, the New Deal's Tennessee Valley Authority (TVA) implemented a vast array of measures, such as environmental sanitation. These included building dams and draining swamps, providing quinine to people suffering from recurrent fevers, screening windows and doors in rural areas, promoting health education, and undertaking other control efforts. As a result, malaria became a rare occurrence in the southern United States.[8]

The second and very different malaria control effort occurred in Ceará, a state in northern Brazil, which was invaded by the dangerous *Anopheles gambiae* from Africa during the 1930s. By using potent larvicides in stagnant water and following a strict military-style discipline, Fred L. Soper, an officer of the Rockefeller Foundation, controlled the malaria epidemic and destroyed all remnants of this species.[9]

The experiences of Soper and the TVA suggested to medical experts that malaria was controllable, although it was not clear if the more flexible, integrated methods tried in the United States were more effective than the focused methods Soper used in Brazil. This question would not be settled until a few years later, partly because malaria was no longer significant in the United States and Western Europe by the mid–twentieth century. Rather, it had become associated with remote countries and hot climates. The disease would only become important again with World War II, when American soldiers fought in malarious areas and fell prey to intermittent fevers more frequently than to enemy bullets. New techniques related to military medicine appeared, such as using the insecticide DDT and the synthetic drug Chloroquine, which were crucial for the Allies in Italy, Northern Africa, Greece, and the Pacific and later became the technical cornerstones of the 1950s eradication operations.[10] The experiences of the military would be later used to argue that Soper's antimalaria techniques were more effective and cheaper than the TVA's malaria control program.

The technical name of the white, waxy powder known as DDT is dichloro-diphenyl-trichloroethane.[11] Although it was originally synthesized in 1854, its insecticidal properties were only discovered in 1939 by the Swiss researcher Paul Muller while he was working in Switzerland for a German subsidiary of the German Bayer Company. DDT was first used in 1944 to control epidemic typhus, a disease transmitted by the human body louse, which had killed millions at the end of World War I. At the time, there was a great fear that World War II would create similar conditions for the spread of typhus. At first soldiers, and later civilians and survivors of concentration camps, were literally dusted with the new insecticide.

However, DDT also soon began to be used to eliminate the *Anopheles* mosquito. During and immediately after World War II, the staffs of the Office of Malaria Control in War Areas of the U.S. Army and the United Nations Relief and Rehabilitation Administration (which was created by the Allies, with headquarters in Washington) began to glorify DDT and became convinced that epidemic disease control was possible without significant public health improvements.[12] In the wake of the war, a series of DDT-based malaria projects were successfully carried out in several smaller countries and islands such as Corsica and Greece, as well as in disease-ridden regions of such larger nations and territories as Italy, Venezuela, and British Guiana.

The story of Chloroquine was also related to World War II. Quinine, the traditional remedy for malaria, became scarce for Allied forces in 1942 after the Japanese occupied its primary world supplier, the Dutch East Indies. A U.S. Army Malaria Drug Development Program was rapidly established, and by 1942 it was testing and producing powerful new synthetic antimalaria drugs such as Chloroquine, Atabrine, Primaquine, Proquanil, and Pyrimethamine. As in the case of DDT, there was a link to previous German medical discoveries. The suppressive and therapeutic powers of the most effective of these drugs, Chloroquine, were first discovered in 1939 by German Bayer chemists, who called it Resochin. In 1941, thanks to a commercial agreement between Bayer and a French company, the drug's development was moved to Tunisia for clinical studies. When the Allied forces overran Tunisia in 1943, French scientists working there passed their clinical information and the remainder of their stock to the U.S. Army. Shortly thereafter, Chloroquine began to be used to protect American soldiers. In 1946, the U.S. Army made the drug available for civilian populations, and it began to be produced by the American company Winthrop Steams.[13] These developments were parallel to research on other antimalaria drugs. In 1938, Winthrop Steams gave the U.S. Army samples of Atabrine, a drug that had also been synthesized earlier by the Germans. By 1942, Atabrine was being issued to troops in the southwest Pacific. However, Chloroquine encountered less resistance and became the drug of choice because it did not discolor the skin (other drugs turned the skin yellow) and was more effective than Atebrine.

The main spin-off of the American military's experience with malaria was that in the 1950s, this disease became the quintessential theme for new health agencies working in developing countries, just as yellow fever had been for the military and the Rockefeller Foundation during the early twentieth century. In 1955, the World Health Organization, the United Nations Children's Fund (UNICEF), and U.S. bilateral assistance agencies launched a campaign to eliminate malaria from developing nations.[14] As a result, the military campaigns and technologically focused initiatives that had been carried out against malaria became the basis for new worldwide efforts to fight the disease.

A discussion of malaria eradication needs to be framed by the politics and rhetoric of the first two decades of the Cold War between the United States and the Soviet bloc, from the late 1940s to mid-1960s.[15] This period was marked by U.S. government efforts to prevent the spread of communism in developing countries. At the same time, the United States was not only playing a leading role in the United Nations and its specialized agencies such as the World Health Organization but was also starting to develop its own network to provide bilateral, country-to-country aid. Both these types of interventions by the United States were considered essential for "national security." Multilateral aid and American bilateral technical aid were reinforced after the death of the Soviet dictator Joseph Stalin in 1953.

An important characteristic of U.S. Cold War foreign policy during the 1950s was that, with few exceptions, it was basically a rhetoric that avoided direct military confrontation and emphasized competition with the Soviet Union that included a race in science and technology. During the 1950s, the

U.S. Department of State considered foreign technical aid essential to preventing communism in developing countries. A group of American social
scientists, supported by universities, foundations, and the government,
polished an antipopulist modernization model that supported bilateral programs in "underdeveloped" countries to educate technical elites and transfer modern technology to overcome poverty and disease.[16] In 1956, an
officer of the Department of State praised modernization and international
health programs in poor countries not only for their medical outcomes but
also because they "decrease[d] the possibilities of infiltration of those ideologies to which needy populations are often susceptible."[17]

Starting in 1950, private, multilateral, bilateral, government, and university institutions in the United States worked to consolidate international
health as a field of thinking and practice that would leave behind the limitations of the sanitary codes and quarantines of the turn of the twentieth
century, and the limited interventions concentrated on port cities and areas
related to export economies.[18] Also in contrast to those earlier limitations,
newly created international health agencies such as the World Health Organization included in their goals reaching remote regions in developing
countries, such as rural areas that experienced malaria, as a way to "modernize" backward health systems and societies. As a result, international
health cooperation—the mixture of activities of new multilateral and U.S.
bilateral agencies—and malaria eradication became instrumental for American Cold War objectives, just as tropical medicine and yellow fever control had been portrayed as tools for the expansion of empires at the turn of
the twentieth century. Malaria eradication continued as a priority of U.S.
foreign policy after eradication programs were enhanced by the 1959 Cuban
revolution and by an initially major "friendlier" development project, the
Alliance for Progress. Although malaria eradication dwindled in the aftermath of the Cold War—particularly during the late 1960s and after the inception of the "détente" foreign policy of U.S. president Richard Nixon—
it left an important legacy for international health and foreign aid.

The idea of promoting international health programs as a Cold War strategy was clearly expressed by James Stevens, who served as chief of preventive medicine for the U.S. Army during World War II and later as dean
of Harvard University's School of Public Health. Beginning in 1950, Stevens
organized a series of "Industry and Tropical Health" meetings for the leaders
of the medical departments of the biggest U.S. corporations. During his welcome address to the first meeting, he explained:

Powerful Communist forces are at work . . . taking advantage of sick and impoverished people, exploiting their discontent . . . to undermine their political beliefs. Health is one of the safeguards against this propaganda. Health is not charity, it is not missionary work, it is not merely good business—it is sheer self-preservation for the United States and for the way of life which we regard as decent. Through health we can expand industrial production, strengthen our military forces, and maintain the high morale of all our people. Through it we can prove, to ourselves and to the world, the wholesomeness and rightness of Democracy. Through health we can defeat the evil threat of communism.[19]

Organizing Principles for This Volume

Recent studies of the diplomatic, economic, and political aspects of the Cold War have demonstrated how important ideology was to the period and have suggested that it was an all-encompassing culture in both developed and developing countries.[20] This book contributes to this literature by examining a little-studied aspect of the Cold War, the technical and political dimensions of malaria eradication. The book thus helps to create a more comprehensive, multidimensional history of the Cold War by moving beyond the superpowers' diplomatic struggles and analyzing new, complex dimensions of national security concerns and their combination with altruistic motivations toward "underdeveloped" countries. The book also contributes to studies of the cultural and social impact of the Cold War outside the United States and the Soviet Union that attempt to trace a relationship between high-level politics and everyday life.[21] Furthermore, it amplifies histories of science that have examined the Cold War's role in the organization of research in the physical sciences related to atomic power, the influence of military patronage, and concerns for national security in post–World War II America.[22]

International health programs, though an apparent symbol of neutrality and rationality, were actually framed by political ends, especially in the rhetorical and the symbolic uses of code terms that validated an ideology of anticommunism. These programs also created political consciousness and loyalties, and they defined a political agenda to win "hearts and minds."[23] Cold War crusaders eagerly promoted the belief that solving important rural health problems in poor countries would consolidate commercial agriculture and prevent the spread of communism to these areas. Scholars such as Trout have analyzed how the United States' propaganda used symbolic terms such as "free world" to advance its superiority in the international arena.[24] This propaganda attempted to validate the position of the United States as the "humanitarian" leader of a so-called democratic-capitalistic world confronted by the Soviet Union, which was presented as dictatorial, exploitative, and evil. Barnet has shown how both sides of the Cold War resorted to metaphors of nature and disease to build their political consensus and discredit the opposing system. For example, U.S. government officials characterized communism as a "virus," whereas Soviet officers characterized capitalist culture as "in decay," "rotten," or a "cancer."[25] Using these terms made these systems appear more menacing to the public. "Campaign," a term used in malaria eradication, had a relationship with the military's medical experiences during World War II and with international yellow fever work done in the early twentieth century that frequently aimed to completely eliminate the disease.

"Containment" was a term used during the Cold War that had a special significance for international health cooperation in the 1950s. Although malaria eradication was sometimes referred to as a "global," uniform program, it eventually became a localized "containment" strategy fraught with ambivalence and contradiction. Shortly after its launch, the campaign' organizers decided that it would not actually "eradicate" the disease worldwide, as a literal reading of the word might convey. Instead, it was portrayed as a "demonstration" campaign for some countries and even for some regions of malarious countries; for example, Africa and large tracts of the Brazilian Amazon River Basin were explicitly excluded. In short, the campaign became a defensive strategy that would not result in interventions in a significant part of the world. It resembled the resigned approach of U.S. foreign policy, implied by a similar use of "containment," which accepted the fact that part of the world was under Soviet totalitarianism. The ultimate goal of malaria eradication was to "contain" malaria—not to eliminate it.

Malaria eradication contributed to a public health pattern described in this book as a *culture of survival,* in which health interventions were planned not as definitive solutions but as temporary responses, with the awareness that they would not completely solve the main disease issues of poor nations. The ultimate preoccupation of these interventions was to enhance the role of new medical technology and experts over community participation and to keep the most dangerous disease outbreaks in check. And these interventions were reinforced by the fact that poor people in rural Mexico did not at the time conceive of sanitation as a right that could be demanded from the state by its citizens.

The problematic legacy of this culture of survival was that many poor people in developing countries sincerely believed that public health efforts were simply responses to emergencies, embodied in the provision of vaccines, drugs, and hospitals and the arrival of foreign experts. In sum, prevention—the cornerstone of truly effective public health efforts—was delayed and replaced by mending patches. Another negative impact of this limited understanding of public health work was the production of short-term results that in turn created the basis for other temporary solutions. As a result, a vicious circle emerged between temporary solutions and epidemic outbreaks. This cycle, reinforcing a better-known cycle between poverty and disease, postponed health emergencies, which remained recurrent disasters waiting to happen.

During the 1950s, the Latin American region was apparently a remote arena for Cold War politics. However, the U.S. government actively sought to secure unquestionable loyalty and maintain internal order in this southern half of the Western Hemisphere, which was considered within its sphere of influence. It is true that during the 1950s, in its search for bulwarks against communism, the United States backed some military regimes under the assumption that they would guarantee private investment and political stability and firmly oppose communist penetration. However, such support for authoritarianism was also part of the antipopulist understanding of modernization, which assumed that all change would come from above, led by a small group of technical experts. In addition, the 1950s was also the beginning of bilateral programs that began to encourage orderly societal change through a modernization model of development that promoted foreign investment, industrialization, and commercial agriculture. Frequently, U.S. policymakers expressed a belief that Latin America's dictatorial regimes could accomplish these changes without social upheavals.

In the post–World War II period, Mexico was willing to follow this modernization model of development, which enabled it to overcome a long history of conflict with its northern neighbor, to soften the radical edges of its 1910 social revolution, and to validate its postwar position as a loyal U.S. ally. This third goal was important not only because of the economic and political gains Mexican regimes could obtain but also because they could use this support to impose their position on provincial authorities and extend their official "nationalistic" discourse throughout the nation. After the war, Mexican administrations embraced probusiness industrial and commercial agricultural policies close to the market-oriented economy promoted by U.S. modernizing advisers. Modernization meant the transformation of the "traditional" sectors of society and the elimination of such barriers as the major rural disease, malaria. Health officials working for these Mexican administrations strove to spread scientific medicine to rural areas, an attempt that could be traced to the 1930s but found sufficient resources and political commitment in the 1950s.

Post–World War II Mexican administrations made remarkable efforts to promote an official, standardized version of nationalism as a form of political validation and assimilation for the country's diverse ethnic groups. Schell has studied the interweaving of educational and hygiene policies in early-twentieth-century Mexico, and the effort to "nationalize" children, an attempt that the Catholic Church and the state both regarded as essential for the country's development.[26] Vaughan has pointed out how, in the 1930s, Mexican education also became a tool for political legitimacy, the Mexicanization of the nation, and the perpetuation of pro-natalist policies. Similar developments occurred in public health in Mexico during the 1950s. Previous attempts have been studied by Kapelusz-Poppi, who shows that there was a concern for creating modern medical services in the countryside in the 1930s.[27]

Educational and medical precedents would become important for Mexico's malaria eradication effort because this health intervention was seen as a way for the federal health and political authorities to assert their power over the corresponding state and provincial authorities. Simply put, the malaria eradication campaign was part of a process of state building and political centralization. Malaria eradication was also portrayed as a tool that would increase the Mexican population. The influence of Catholicism and nationalism resulted in a strong tradition in Mexico and other Latin American countries to consider their territories underpopulated. Preventive and curative medicine, as well as public health work, were portrayed as means to increase the number of rural inhabitants and to produce healthy, hard-working, nationally committed citizens.

A recent body of scholarship on the development and reception of international health efforts outside the centers of European and U.S. medicine during the early twentieth century has underlined how the arrival of Western medicine in colonial and postcolonial countries often elicited local processes of adaptation, recreation, and even rejection, and meant setting new health priorities.[28] The priorities of Western medicine included protecting economic operations as well as controlling or "assimilating" indigenous populations into Western culture. The link between the Cold War and malaria eradication has been discussed in brilliant essays by Packard, Litsios, and their colleagues. However, to this day, scholars have yet to undertake a comprehensive and detailed study of the eradication campaign in a developing country.[29]

Latin American diseases have been the subject of the attention of a new generation of social and medical historians, who have demonstrated how foreign or official health authorities located in the capital cities dictated which diseases were important and worthy of research and which control methods would be used.[30] These historical studies have included an examination of the Rockefeller Foundation's role in organizing public health systems and medical reform during the early twentieth century.[31] Some researchers have also emphasized the receiving part of the story—the negotiation or resistance from unofficial health practitioners or provincial communities and the construction of heterogeneous medical systems adapted to local needs.[32] Peard, Stepan, and others have convincingly argued that in the face of American and European fatalism about health care in tropical countries, Brazilian and other Latin American physicians in the nineteenth and early twentieth centuries rejected notions of the inherent inferiority of native people and local medical researchers. Furthermore, they believed that social conditions would improve only if large issues such as education and public health systems were addressed.[33] Palmer and Sowell have revealed the complexity of Costa Rican and Colombian local medical trends by analyzing the coexistence, complementarity, and even rivalry that marked the relationship between popular and professional medicine.[34] And drawing on sound anthropological perspectives, Farmer, Briggs, and Parker have demonstrated the usefulness of understanding indigenous discourses and popular reactions to recent official public health interventions against AIDS and cholera in Haiti, Brazil, and Venezuela.[35]

Plan of the Book

There are two gaps in the recent literature devoted to examining Latin American medical history. First, few studies have analyzed developments during the second half of the twentieth century. Second, few have attempted to provide an integrated perspective combining the metropolitan, national, and local dimensions of a health intervention. This book intends to partly fill in these gaps by studying the interaction of the contradictory processes of launching an international health campaign, its appropriation by Mexican authorities, and the local response (and sometimes resistance) it generated.

In other words, this volume considers three important dimensions of an international health campaign in a developing country: the complex web of metropolitan and national motivations for its support, its design and the technology it used, and the local responses it elicited. The study is organized as a triptych with three main chapters. Chapter 2 examines the emergence of the field of international health work and the humanitarian, economic, and political motivations of the multilateral and bilateral agencies that implemented the malaria eradication campaign. The three main assumptions, or requirements, for the success of eradication were that it was biologically feasible; that it yielded benefits in excess of the cost of other forms of interventions, such as malaria control; and that government political commitment was possible. The chapter also examines the reasons for the decline in the global commitment to eradication that were evident in the late 1960s, including the concern that DDT was contaminating the environment and was a death-deferring tool that contributed to overpopulation.

Chapter 3 begins in 1956, when thousands of Mexican health workers used hand pumps to spray a film of DDT on the walls of homes to kill mosquitoes and combat malaria before or after the mosquitoes had dined on human blood. The chapter focuses on the Mexican government's validation of this malaria eradication campaign and its appropriation by local medical personnel during a period marked by de facto one-party dominance, political stability, and economic growth. During this post–World War II period, Mexico's authoritarian regimes and probusiness political leaders saw the eradication campaign as part of their effort to develop capital-intensive agriculture, and it served as a basis for extending public health services to rural areas. For this purpose, Mexican administrations actively used mass media in health education. An important dimension of the campaign was the incorporation of Westernized or Americanized Mexican political and medical leaders, who adapted malaria eradication to the national context while enhancing their own positions as experts and as leaders of the country. The hegemonic trend among local health workers was the appropriation of the international campaign. Moreover, many of these workers went beyond what official agencies expected and combined their work with broader health activities and themes of popular nationalism. What was remarkable about this appropriation was how local medical personnel strove to use the antimalaria campaign as a springboard for further rural sanitation.

Chapter 4 deals with local responses to the malaria eradication campaign. Medical anthropologists and local physicians criticized the campaign. Though they often used inconsistent arguments, they revealed their lack of an intercultural perspective and, consequently, an important cultural mismatch. For example, according to the campaign's original design, blood samples obtained from a finger prick were necessary to confirm the presence of malaria. However, some Indians rejected these examinations because they believed that blood was related to individual strength, fertility, and protection from "magical" harm. Their resistance also highlighted the challenges that rural people faced with the penetration of international health initiatives, the commercializing of agriculture, and the emergence of an increasingly interventionist state. Public health doctors perceived malaria eradication as an entry point for Western medicine and aimed to overcome this resistance, which they believed was a result of "ignorance" and "remnants" of traditional medical practices.

Chapter 4 also examines the few cases of indigenous revolt against malaria eradication, which were especially intense in southern Mexico. Although the archival records give no definitive indication of the extent of these criticisms, they appear to be marginal to the hegemonic official anti-malaria campaign and to the pattern of local appropriation. However, these criticisms suggest that the lack of an intercultural perspective limited malaria eradication in rural areas.

Chapter 5 briefly discusses malaria developments from 1970 to the present. It stresses the legacy of short-term health interventions as reinforcing short-term expectations for public health. And it describes recent malaria outbreaks and assesses the efforts in Mexico and abroad to deal with the disease. Among them are the Roll Back Malaria program and the Global Fund to Fight AIDS, Tuberculosis, and Malaria, which overemphasize new technologies—such as the development of new drugs and vaccines and the distribution of bed nets impregnated with pyrethrum—and do not sufficiently emphasize the community-based prevention and management of malaria.

The title of this book reflects the coexistence between a dramatic disease and the ambiguities and contradictions of the Cold War period, when politicians exacerbated political tensions, stopping short of an actual full-scale military conflict. Simultaneously, common people in poor countries such as Mexico suffered real and tragic diseases such as malaria, which was marked by potentially "deadly" fevers, for which hopes of a definitive solution were raised but not met.

At a time when malaria, along with AIDS and tuberculosis, is once again a concern for international health agencies and there is a tendency to overemphasize the impact of using bed nets, new drugs, and a future malaria vaccine, this volume underscores the need to be suspicious of new "magic bullets" that might appear as the single way to eliminate malaria. Furthermore, it emphasizes the need to understand the complex dynamics among politics, ecology, international health agencies, and local forces, and to seek a balance between technical interventions and socioeconomic developments. Both past and present malaria eradication efforts demonstrate that the most important investment is not only in new medical technologies but also in building local and sustainable human capacities that can respond to specific and diverse challenges.[36]

This book does not dismiss the advantages of an eradicationist perspective for specific diseases in developing countries or the positive role of new medical technologies. Rather, its aim is to examine a historical case in order to convey a long-term, flexible, and integrated public health perspective for these nations, a perspective that entails overcoming the culture of survival.

2

Global Designs

Malaria eradication achieved a hegemonic position among international agencies and U.S. foreign policy from the mid-1950s to the early 1960s. Apparently, the driving force in malaria eradication was new biomedical knowledge framed around urgency. Its assumptions were, first, that the female *Anopheles* mosquito that transmits the disease could be killed because it rested on the DDT-sprayed walls of its victim's house after sucking her blood meal (it was assumed that it was too heavy to go beyond).[1] To be effective, insecticide spraying had to be applied thoroughly in two intense annual cycles because DDT would maintain its "residual" power on the walls for six months. Comprehensive spraying was as essential because uneven and mild spraying encouraged some mosquitoes to develop resistance, in which they began to tolerate doses of insecticide that would be lethal to the majority of members of their species. From 1951 on, there were reports on the resistance to insecticides within a portion of the population of some species of *Anopheles* as a result of natural selection pressure.[2]

A second assumption that sustained eradication was that the parasite *Plasmodium* could be defeated with new synthetic drugs, particularly Chloroquine (only after 1956 was resistance of *Plasmodium* to Chloroquine suspected for the first time, though this scientific fact was not confirmed until the 1960s).[3] Achieving, and maintaining for three years, a combination of no infected humans (with parasite reservoirs) and no infected mosquitoes (carrying *Plasmodium*) was malaria eradication's basic hope. According to a malariologist, the trick involved "striking both links of the chain."[4]

The decision to launch malaria eradication involved not only what appeared to be undisputable biological facts. Despite experts' efforts to portray eradication as nature's competition—as "one of the most exciting races ever run" between science and the mosquito—there was a fundamental interaction between the political context, the institutional actors, and the economic implications of the decision to eradicate malaria.[5] Eradication merged biological challenges and political opportunities. This accommodation of diverse institutional interests produced a symbiosis between the U.S. Cold War ideology and international health agencies that led politicians and health officers to share code words and euphemisms, such as "enslaving," "liberating," "war," "crusade," "golden opportunity," "enlightened self-interest," and "perfection."

This symbiosis created the basis for recurrent master metaphors, for example, between "malaria" and "communism" ("enslaving" conditions for developing countries) and "malaria eradication" and "modernization."[6] This metaphor validated the assumption that developing nations followed the path of industrialized nation as "liberating" processes for these countries. One important function of these euphemisms was to reinforce the legitimacy of political and medical authorities and elicit the conformity of common people regarding decisions made from above. Important precedents of the interweaving of medicine and politics were the military health campaigns developed in Cuba during the Spanish-American War and the medical work that contributed to the construction of the Panama Canal and World War II. These events witnessed the establishment of military terms such as "campaign" for any health intervention, "attack" for the beginning of health operations, and "enemies" for diseases, microbes, and vectors. These terms were later used during malaria eradication.

This symbiosis between international health cooperation and politics strengthens the idea commonly held by several Cold War historians, mentioned in the introduction, that during the 1950s, the superpowers portrayed their differences as a "moral" dilemma separating "good" from "evil." I contend that in the case of U.S. Cold War foreign policy, the ideology of anticommunism was also applied to matters of health and disease.[7] American policies encompassed many layers of society—including those considered neutral, such as international health cooperation—and attempted to narrow political divisions within developed and developing countries. In both types of nations, there were those who were "loyal" to the ideals of freedom, such as the U.S. Republicans and the Mexican government, and those who were said to be communist or soft on communism, such as the Democrats in the United States or the "fellow travelers" of communism in Mexico.

Political rhetoric influenced the language and practice of Latin American health officers, indicating that technical knowledge was not separated from propaganda in malaria eradication. Another important mixture of medicine and politics was the denomination of DDT as "the atomic bomb of the insect world."[8] This mirroring of politics and malaria eradication was instrumental in sustaining the public anxieties typical of the Cold War. "Military" euphemisms were found even for problematic scientific facts. For example, mosquitoes that avoided walls sprayed with DDT were "evasive," malaria-persistent regions were called "problem areas," and public acceptance of health interventions was a result of the effective educational work of "sensitization," or, in Spanish, *canalización,* which meant to make people comply with malaria eradication measures.

The ties between international medicine and politics validated a claim often made by military leaders: that it was necessary to promptly seize a unique opportunity so that prior achievements would not be wasted. For those who supported this idea, malaria eradication could not wait. Although it was a radical departure from the past, it also combined the best of prior efforts against the disease. These efforts were generally known as malaria control. During the first half of the twentieth century, malaria control sought to reduce the incidence of the disease by destroying breeding places such as draining marshes and clearing swamps, and by using petroleum oils and a copper-based powder (called Paris green) that floated in stagnant water and poisoned surface-feeding mosquito larvae. Additional methods used by malaria control were the protection of humans from *Anopheles* bites by screening windows and doors, and treating the sick with quinine.[9]

As I have shown in the introduction, a major malaria work experience that moved medical thinking toward eradication occurred during World War II. The U.S. Army, convinced that there was no time for broad public health programs, developed "magic bullet" interventions such as DDT and Chloroquine. Strict military enforcement of DDT use and new drugs significantly reduced malaria among soldiers. By 1953, federal support for DDT and other malaria control activities in the continental United States was temporarily discontinued because the disease had been eliminated from the country. However, the medical-military experience was already inspiring eradication efforts in other parts of the world.

Foreign Aid and the Cold War

An examination of the Cold War context, and the prominence of health agencies created or renovated shortly after World War II, enables one to understand the emergence of malaria eradication. International science and medicine are important and understudied dimensions of the early Cold War period, and they are related not only to the scientific race between the United States and the Soviet Union but also to postwar developments, such as the consolidation of U.S. bilateral cooperation in medicine, science, and culture; modernization proposals for developing countries; and the emergence of a web of multilateral agencies.

The U.S. Department of State was a key institutional actor in these developments. Before World War II, there was no real U.S. agency making foreign policy, especially in the field of sustained bilateral aid on public health, education, and social development. Official missions in Latin America during the interwar period (1919–39) were usually attached to the military, or were sporadic advisory missions for economic, communications, health, or educational projects. In addition, work in international health cooperation was fragmented and barely connected to American political interests. During the interwar period, a private philanthropic agency, the Rockefeller Foundation, was virtually alone in the field of international health programs in developing nations. This organization operated under the assumption that Western science and medicine were universal aspirations for all cultures and societies. The Foundation engaged in efforts to control or eliminate hookworm, yellow fever, and malaria from a number of countries around the world. These were debilitating human diseases for which there was a "magic bullet," or new medical technological solution. One of the most important campaigns of the foundation, mentioned in the introduction, took place during the 1930s in Brazil, where in a matter of months the experienced Rockefeller officer Fred L. Soper eliminated the dangerous *Anopheles gambiae* mosquito that had invaded the country from Africa.

The Rockefeller Foundation's relationship with American foreign interest was subtle. Although it tried to appear unconnected with the work of U.S. foreign policy, its ultimate goal was the well-being of the capitalist system as a whole. However, several events of the post–World War II period had an impact on both the foundation and U.S. foreign policy: China's rejection of capitalism after the 1949 revolution, the political independence of former European colonies in Asia and Africa, the confrontation of Argentinean president Juan Peron with the United States (Rockefeller had established an important field office in Buenos Aires in 1941), and the so-called Iron Curtain. After 1951, the Rockefeller Foundation decided to close down most of its international health work. Instead, it concentrated on new endeavors, such as agricultural development in a few countries. The United States and a number of new agencies stepped into the field of international health cooperation and began to administer significant resources.

The Cold War between the Soviet Union and the United States pervaded all aspects of society and culture, making health and developmental work in developing countries an arena for political dispute. The growing disintegration of the colonial European framework of domination provided opportunities for the United States and the Soviet Union to enlarge their spheres of influence on other continents, where countries were important for the superpowers because of their large populations and their vast resources of raw materials.

An important Cold War personality of the malaria eradication period (the mid-1950s) was John Foster Dulles, the controversial, assertive, and sometimes arrogant U.S. secretary of state from 1953 to 1959 (during the two terms of President Dwight Eisenhower).[10] Dulles, the grandson of a former secretary of state, came from Sullivan & Cromwell, the prestigious Wall Street law firm that represented several corporations including the United Fruit Company, which had a monopoly on Central American banana's production and maintained important investments in the Caribbean and Colombia. Under Dulles's direction, the State Department became the main operating as well as policy-determining agency of U.S. foreign relations. Dulles was determined to consolidate the United States' international power and to undermine the standing of the Soviet Union. Despite the fact that, in the 1952 electoral campaign, both he and Eisenhower denounced the "futile" policy of containment against communism, once in power, they followed and expanded Truman's foreign policy of containment (originally designed by George Kennan, the leading American foreign policy expert on Soviet affairs). Besides the well-known chapters of the Cold War of the early 1950s (the War in Korea, the tensions in Berlin, and the invasion of Hungary) and Dulles's exploitation of anticommunist anxieties (even considering the possibility of a nuclear war), Dulles made a point of containing the Soviet Union's exportation of its ideology to the so-called third world.[11]

Under Dulles, the State Department experienced organizational changes. It energized its regional operations, including an American Republic Affairs Office and an assistant secretary for inter-American affairs; consolidated its Bureau of International Organization Affairs, which was created in 1949 to support the United Nations and its specialized agencies, such as the World Health Organization; created a departmental science adviser position in 1951; and regularly published the Department of State Bulletin as a monthly periodical.[12] During the 1950s, the assistant secretaries heading the Bureau of Inter-American Affairs and Bureau of International Organization Affairs were vocal supporters of foreign aid, and their speeches and articles appeared frequently in the *Bulletin*.[13]

The active participation of the Department of State in the UN system was something new in American foreign policy. During the interwar period, the U.S. Congress and American foreign policy were marked by noninterventionism. Congress refused to join the League of Nations, which had been founded after the Paris Peace Conference of 1919. Yet shortly thereafter, U.S. federal organizations, such as the United States Public Health Service, did participate to a limited extent with agencies linked to the League, such as the League of Nations Hygiene Organization based in Geneva. In contrast, after World War II, the UN and the World Health Organization (WHO) emerged with decisive U.S. support. The UN was founded in San Francisco, and U.S. presidents and diplomats played an active role in its establishment.[14] In 1956, the United States contributed over $23 million to the UN and its ten specialized agencies. This sum accounted for 31 percent of these organizations' total assessments.[15]

There were several reasons for this support. First, the United States sought to take part in international assistance to increase its image of humanitarianism and heighten its global economic and political hegemony. According to the U.S. representative to the UN, "to carry out our own foreign policies under the aegis of the United Nations, helps America directly, as we then get credit for practicing altruism instead of power politics."[16] Francis O. Wilcox, the Department of State's assistant secretary of international organization affairs, explained the insufficiency of existing world trade to secure American economic well-being. It was necessary to create new markets, increase the purchasing power of people in areas where per capita income was low, and raise their standards of living, so that they would be able to participate in the world economy.[17] A corollary opinion was provided by the State Department's director of the Office of International Trade, when he remarked that the United States cannot be prosperous and secure in an impoverished world; it cannot "sell unless others buy." A unit of the department applied the same idea to international health work: "Good health contributes to economic progress."[18]

A second reason that explains the United States' active participation in UN programs was that it sought to share the cost of American bilateral activities. The UN's pool of labor power and training resources was greater than what the United States could provide. As a result, U.S government officials hoped that some of the technical experts working in these agencies could carry on the projects supported and promoted by the United States. Third and finally, because many developing countries were protective of their newly won sovereignty, they preferred to receive aid from multilateral agencies rather than from one of the Cold War superpowers.[19]

The support that the United States provided to the UN agencies also reinforced the modernization scheme designed in the 1950s by establishing priorities, reinforcing the role of elite experts, and following an orderly planning process—instead of violent social changes produced by revolutions—in less developed countries. In 1956, U.S. bilateral agencies discussed the criteria for choosing priority health programs because the gap between needs and funds was significant. These included programs that were technically feasible, that had a greater impact on a larger proportion of people, that had a real possibility of strengthening the economy, and that would "improve citizen morale" and "contribute to our political objectives," including ensuring that American personnel be "highly welcomed."[20]

During the early 1950s, the UN and WHO were perceived by the Soviet Union as linked to the United States. Moreover, between 1949 and the 1956, the Soviet Union and several Eastern European communist countries withdrew from WHO, accusing it of not doing its job and suggesting that it was an instrument of U.S. imperialism.[21] The USSR also boycotted the UN Security Council and did not join other UN agencies. The USSR's additional motivation for these decisions was the resentment it felt because it had paid a high price during World War II in human and material destruction but had received little from the UN in general, and U.S. bilateral assistance in particular, especially after it became clear that the Marshall Plan for the reconstruction of Europe was aimed at Western European democracies. Ideology also played a role, as is shown by this excerpt from a speech by the delegate of Poland to the 1949 World Health Assembly:

WHO, like many other international organizations, has become the battleground of two opposing points of view. Two rival camps face each other. The camp of peace, standing for the interest of humanity, which demands that the attainment of medical science should serve the whole human race, is represented by the USSR and the Popular Democracies, while the capitalist camp represents the interest of a minority who consider science as a source of income and as a weapon of war. The activities and behavior of the majority of members of the Executive Board, as well as the administration, prove that WHO inclines towards the capitalist and imperialist camp.[22]

When the USSR and other communist countries returned to WHO, a Department of State officer declared to Congress that it was "even more important than ever that the United States should continue the support" of WHO.[23] An officer of the Department of State explained the accommodation of Soviet leaders in the following terms: "[They] realized that the economic and social services performed, largely under U.S. leadership, by the United Nations and the specialized agencies, threatened the communist plans in the world. They were impressed and frightened by the impact made upon the underdeveloped countries by free-world aid."[24] As this quotation suggests, modernization and international health programs were seen not only as a means to solve problems of poverty and disease but also as a way to halt communism that could capitalize on long-forgotten social issues.[25] In his 1952 State of the Union message, President Eisenhower stressed the promotion of "world health," namely, aid to WHO and U.S. bilateral health programs, as "essential in the fight on reds."[26]

The State Department *Bulletin*'s articles during the second half of the 1950s emphasized foreign aid as essential for economic hegemony, national security, and self-protection. The department weighed the dimension and nature of technical and economic aid for developing countries as tools to repel Soviet influence. Latin America was important to the United States because of its size (over two and one half times the United States); its increasing population, with an annual growth rate of 2.5 percent, or 190 million in the mid-1950s; and the significant U.S. commerce and investments in the region.[27] The bonds between the United States and Latin America were also influenced by fear of a world conflict, as U.S. security was linked to hemispheric security. For officers of the State Department, the Western Hemisphere was more than just a world sphere of influence; it was the "inner citadel" of the United States.[28] In the words of an American expert: "A Latin America friendly to the United States can be a source of great strength. . . . If unfriendly, it could adversely affect our national welfare."[29]

This concern for regional security also stemmed from the increasing number of Americans living in Latin America after the World War II. According to a 1959 study, more than 1.5 million American citizens lived outside the United States. Most were running embassies, administering foreign aid, and maintaining military garrisons. However, a significant number were engaged in private business, as well as in research, teaching, and missionary activities.[30]

Since 1947 a mutual defense pact, the Inter-American Treaty of Reciprocal Assistance, also known as the Rio Treaty, had created closer military and political links between the United States and Latin America. It was part of a series of international treaties (e.g., NATO for Western Europe, and SEATO for Southeast Asia) that sought to confirm alliances during the Cold War. In the 1950s, the agreement for the Americas was interpreted as the possibility to use force to "protect" the nations from communist aggression. A corollary development was the recreation in 1948 of the traditional Pan-American Union, which had originally been organized as a commercial office in the late nineteenth century and staffed by diplomats living in Washington. After World War II, the union, having acquired more relevance and funds, changed its name to the Organization of American States (OAS) and begun to recruit more Latin Americans with diverse fields of expertise to work in its staff. The treaty, OAS, and other inter-American agencies received strong support from the United States. By 1956, the American contribution to the OAS was $2.3 million (66 percent of its total assessments).[31]

By the mid-1950s, the number of political and military agreements in the Americas increased. The Department of State became convinced that military aid by itself was not enough—a small but active Latin American program of technical cooperation was required to deal with poverty, malnutrition, ignorance, and sickness. These were portrayed as social weaknesses that created the basis for political insecurity. Some years later, Dulles would explain his foreign aid "philosophy" for the region as an "admixture of altruism and enlightened self-interest."[32] Similar terms were used a few years later by a member of the U.S. Congress on the Committee on Foreign Relations, who declared that international technical cooperation in health services would help "our . . . self interests" because it would help new nations to resist "the totalitarian aggression . . . [of] the Cold War—aggression which thrives on conditions of want and privation in disadvantaged nations."[33]

Common economic interests were another reason for renewing ties between the United States and Latin America. In 1955, about half of Latin American foreign trade was conducted with the United States, as compared to only one-third of Latin American trade before World War II. In that same year, 37 percent of the total U.S. private investments made abroad took place in Latin America.[34] In addition, Latin America was, after Western Europe, the second largest market for U.S. exports, receiving 27 percent of the total. Latin America also provided 34 percent of total imports, including important primary goods such as oil, sugar, minerals, and coffee. If only the seventy so-called strategic materials for stockpiling—a list established during World War II—were counted, Latin American imports represented 30 percent of total U.S. imports. Moreover, tourism, with the emergence of new summer resorts such as Acapulco, was becoming a crucial link between the United States and Latin America. In 1955 alone, American tourists spent an estimated $330 million in Latin America, of which more than 75 percent was in Mexico.[35]

Deepening the relationship with Latin America was also important for political reasons. In the first place, a substantial number of Latin American votes could be cast in meetings of UN agencies—in the early 1950s, over half the votes that generally seconded U.S. proposals were from Latin American governments.[36] Second, there was fear that Soviet propaganda might attract Latin American intellectuals and politicians with appealing opportunities for fellowships, aid, and trade or appeal to opportunistic local politicians ready to "fish in troubled waters and find unwary customers."[37] U.S. economic and technical aid in Latin America would help to demonstrate that orderly social progress, without a revolution, was possible. This meant a gradual elimination of evil social forces, such as extreme poverty, acute inequalities, and strident nationalism, which could be manipulated by communists to feed what U.S. officers thought of as "false panaceas."

By the mid-1950s, tensions between the Soviet Union and the United States were high. The Soviets already possessed atomic bombs and were developing a nuclear arsenal—facts that shattered American overconfidence in having a monopoly on these destructive weapons. In addition, U.S. soldiers had died in a Cold War–motivated conflict fought in Korea (1950–53) that stopped short of a third world war. U.S. foreign policy responded to the perceived threat of nuclear annihilation with comprehensive programs. In addition to a military build-up, bilateral technical and nonmilitary aid programs began to be emphasized. These were portrayed as pivotal resources to maintain loyal allies not only in the Western Hemisphere but also in other parts of the world.

Nonmilitary aid became important in the campaign that ended with Eisenhower's first electoral triumph in late 1952. The president had promised to reduce the government's deficit by trimming the budgets of military and public projects and by balancing the federal budget. U.S. government officials tried to economize on military foreign aid by stressing the peaceful applications of nuclear science and enhancing the role of the United States as the world's humanitarian benefactor diffusing new technologies such as radioactive isotopes, nuclear medicine, miracle drugs, and DDT. Eisenhower and Dulles practiced a "rhetorical" diplomacy that implied belligerent speeches against communism but little practical support for "liberation" movements in countries regarded as "satellites" of the Soviet Union.[38] U.S. foreign policy began to back away from the reckless provocations against the Soviet Union that were typical of the beginnings of the Cold War, and it reframed how the ultimate goal of rolling back communism might be achieved. For U.S. government officials, it was not just an issue of military power, with the obvious exception of Vietnam, but also the promotion of technical bilateral aid. Future U.S. administrations would increasingly attempt to compete with the Soviet Union in economic, political, and scientific terms without resorting to an open conflict that neither side could win. It was truly hoped that the strength of American ideology and technology would undermine any efforts to develop communist ideologies in these nations.

The trend toward a greater role for nonmilitary aid was strengthened by an important Cold War event: the death of Joseph Stalin in March 1953. During the following three years, although it was unclear who the real leader of the Soviet Union was, there was a fear in U.S. government circles that the incipient de-Stalinization would appeal to politicians and intellectuals from developing countries. An interest for these countries was reflected in the broadcast made by Nikolai A. Bulgarin, one of the ephemeral heads of the Soviet Union between the death of Stalin and the rise of Nikita Khrushchev in 1956. Bulgarin encouraged Latin Americans to expand their diplomatic, economic, and cultural relations with the USSR. This was the first time a top Soviet official made a special call to Latin America. The U.S. authorities noted the relationship between an increase in Soviet shortwave propaganda broadcasting in Latin American and other developing areas of the globe and a new and "menacing" Soviet expansionism.[39] American fears increased when Khrushchev rose to power because he intensified de-Stalinization, postulated the principle of peaceful coexistence, praised national liberation movements in developing countries, offered to help new "third world" nations end their dependency on former colonial powers, envisioned diverse paths toward communism, and prophesied the emergence of socialism all over the world.[40]

Considering that communist parties were small, or illegal, in most Latin American countries, the Department of State warned of camouflaged "front demagogic organizations" that hoisted broad and noncontroversial causes such as peace, economic independence, and labor rights, and publicized the scientific achievements of the Soviet Union.[41] The Department strongly believed that the leaders of these organizations maintained secret links with the Kremlin. According to State Department, Latin American front organizations provided Soviet fellowships and grants to indoctrinate intellectuals, politicians, and labor leaders. An "enslaving" conspiracy was denounced by the *Department of State Bulletin.*[42]

The 1954 events in Guatemala, in which President Jacobo Arbenz confiscated most of the United Fruit Company's lands and legalized the Communist Party, convinced the Department of State that the communist menace did indeed exist in the Americas, and that a "red beachhead" might appear there and elsewhere. An Inter-American Conference held in Caracas, shortly after a coup orchestrated by the U.S. Central Intelligence Agency deposed Arbenz, established a suitable principle for the Cold War: The control of an American nation by "international" communism was a threat to all states and would enable a collective "response."[43] After the meeting, the U.S. Congress Committee on Foreign Affairs received a report from the secretary of state declaring that "other steps" should be taken because "living standards in most Latin America are low and there are large and vocal elements who seek to place the blame on the U.S."[44] This statement strengthened the trend of supporting nonmilitary aid.

Some years later, another political event became a concern for the Department of State: the stormy eighteen-day goodwill tour of Vice President Richard Nixon to the capitals of South America. In May 1958, Nixon began the tour with an unruly reception in Montevideo, and he ended it with mobs in Lima and Caracas attacking him as a symbol of U.S. imperialism. The Eisenhower administration characterized this failure as the result of communist infiltration. The events in Guatemala and Nixon's negative reception were read inside the State Department as an indirect call to take care of Latin American social ills—unstable economies; reliance on one exportable cash crop in the world market; and sick, poverty-stricken peasants. It was feared that in this dismaying context poor Latin Americans would be tempted by faux communist propaganda. In response, President Eisenhower launched "Operation Pan-America," which was suggested by Brazilian President Jucelino Kubitschek to promote both democracy and economic growth. In addition, in 1960 Eisenhower visited Brazil, Argentina, Chile, and Uruguay to build up friendship and stress "collective security" against communism. Although this "Operation" was not significantly funded, it was the beginning of concern among the makers of U.S. foreign policy for integral development models in the Western Hemisphere that could alleviate misery and rural poverty in the region.[45]

This concern was renewed after the Cuban revolution of 1959 and prompted an intense development program known as the Alliance for Progress. Launched by President John F. Kennedy in 1961, this program pledged $20 billion in regional assistance for the next ten years.[46] This was the biggest U.S. regional foreign aid program to date, after the Marshall Plan for the economic revival of Western Europe. To counter the allure of revolutionary Cuba, the Alliance coordinated bilateral programs aimed at promoting democratic regimes, limited land reforms, better housing, and extended educational and medical services in shantytowns and rural areas.[47] According to the deputy assistant secretary for inter-American affairs, the Alliance provided a real alternative for development and forced Latin Americans to make an urgent and inescapable choice "not just between the Communist bloc and the United States but between communist domination and independence."[48] In 1962, a former assistant secretary of state for inter-American affairs explained the relationship between the Alliance, social progress, and communism: "With the achievement of better education, improved housing, higher health standards and enhanced dignity, . . . the masses will then have a stake in freedom and will not fall prey to Communist deception."[49]

A study by Leeds argues that the Alliance for Progress was not so different from Eisenhower's policy towards Latin America—both shared a fear of communist expansion in the hemisphere and made used of technical aid as an integral part of foreign policy.[50] By the early 1960s, the makers of U.S. foreign policy shared the belief that preventing communist penetration in the Western Hemisphere and other developing regions of the world required not only military force but also the promotion of social reform. For a State Department officer, the United States' fortune was inextricably bound up with the "fate of the billion and a half people living in the lesser developed areas of the world. . . . Our survival no longer depends upon guns and tanks and bombs alone."[51] Another officer combined a missionary zeal with the American nonmilitary aid provided to the Western Hemisphere in a clear challenge: "whether Latin America shall grow and flourish in freedom or as a province of overseas communist empires. This depends in part on us."[52]

During the Kennedy and Johnson administrations, there was continuity with Dulles's policies, thanks to Dean Rusk, the new secretary of state. Having been assistant secretary of state for United Nations affairs during the

Truman presidency, in 1952 he became president of the Rockefeller Foundation, where he was in charge of a number of programs in developing countries. Also, thanks to President Kennedy, modernization as an ideology of U.S. foreign policy received a boost with the appointment of Walt W. Rostow, a professor at the Massachusetts Institute of Technology, to the coveted post of deputy national security adviser.[53] Rostow, who possessed a solid reputation in economic studies and international affairs—he was the author of *The Stages of Economic Growth: A Non-Communist Manifesto* (1960)—served first as the head of the State Department's Policy Planning Council and later as national security adviser, during the early to middle 1960s. He shared the goals of the Alliance for Progress of giving impetus to social progress, and he was convinced that a massive transference and diffusion of U.S. technology would prepare the conditions for an economic and political "take-off" of Latin American nations. Modernization was, for Rostow, a positive, achievable alternative to communism that would be led by authoritarian managerial elites who could convince backward people of the advantages of Western culture—or who could inject or impose the spirit of this culture. Rostow would also resort to medical metaphors to validate his claims. In an article for the *Department of State Bulletin,* he characterized communism as "a serious disease."[54]

Rostow believed that the main tension within an "underdeveloped" country was between its "modern" pole—usually urban, commercial, and industrial—and its "traditional" pole—usually rural, stagnant, and formed by closed units that were self-sufficient, relatively isolated from the rest of the country, and inhabited by non-Spanish-speaking people who lived on a subsistence level.[55] Rostow's idea that the stimulus for modernization would come from the modern pole was consistent with antimalaria campaigns that were launched from capital centers by Latin American medical elites toward the rural areas of their countries.

American economic and political validations for increased foreign aid in the region were combined with a search for cultural hegemony. During the 1950s, U.S. agencies became aware that there was minimal European bilateral aid and that the traditional European cultural influence on Latin America had diminished. This represented a radical change, for during the first half of the twentieth century, Latin American science, medicine, and culture were strongly influenced by European, particularly French, educational models and ideas. New American programs, such as the Fulbright, affiliated with the Department of State's International Educational Exchange Service (IEES), increased the exchange of humanities and sciences graduate students and scholars in the Americas. Private philanthropic organizations such as the Rockefeller Foundation also joined the effort. For example, between 1952 and 1955, more than $208,000 was awarded to the Mexico City–based Mexican-American Cultural Institute, one of a series of binational cultural centers that emerged in Latin American capitals after the mid-1940s.[56] These institutes taught English, trained English teachers, organized art exhibitions, and became a meeting place for pro-American local intellectuals. By the early 1950s, U.S. universities were the favorite choice for Latin American university students pursuing training abroad (in 1958, over 75 percent of all Latin Americans who studied abroad went to the United States).[57] As a result of Nixon's trip to Latin America, a White House Cabinet meeting requested a substantial increase in the exchange of all Latin American and U.S. professors from IEES, the Mexican-American Cultural Institute received an additional congressional appropriation of $2 million earmarked for Latin America.[58]

These activities intensified the Americanization of Latin American culture, medicine, and science, a process that can be traced to the first Rockefeller Foundation programs of the 1920s, and that dramatically increased in the wake of World War II. Americanization was linked to modernization and the abandonment of Latin American stereotypes. In the words of a State Department officer, the region no longer wasted its time with "*sambas* and *mañanas.*" On the contrary, it was an "area of dynamic progress . . . whose government and peoples look to the U.S. for leadership and support, whose ideals and aspirations are more and more akin to our own."[59]

A related development that consolidated American cultural predominance in medicine was a greater dependency on drugs and medical supplies produced in the United States. U.S. pharmaceutical purchases in Latin America increased 522 percent from 1942 to 1953—from $18 million to $119 million. A high officer in the Department of State noticed this trend, and he explained the growing presence as partly the result of the training of Latin Americans in the United States and a marked decline of European influence.[60] These medical developments validated U.S. foreign aid in Congress as an instrument for fostering economic expansion, creating new clients overseas and building new markets in which U.S. enterprises would dominate.

American cultural hegemony in the region also included the 1953 creation of the U.S. Information Agency (USIA), a formally independent organization within the U.S. government executive branch that consolidated different propaganda programs and diffused information about the United

States with crusading zeal.[61] After the mid-1950s, an increasing amount of attention was spent on "targeting" countries in Africa, Asia, and Latin America with pro-American propaganda to avoid any communist "deviance" of uncommitted, confused, or doubtful individuals. This propaganda and educational exchanges, as well as the threat of force and covert operations, were all seen as important tools of psychological warfare that was justified by the anticommunist "noble" end. Policy guidance for USIA propaganda came from the Department of State, and its official aim was to promote "friendly" ties with other nations. This agency translated and distributed hundreds of films, books, and other publications, including anticommunist cartoons, films, and comic strips especially designed for Latin America. One of USIA's best-known activities was "Voice of America," a large broadcasting network launched in 1954 that interviewed Latin American university students studying in the United States.[62] USIA also publicized joint health programs and other cooperative activities in the region that were championed by U.S. bilateral assistance.

IEES and USIA energized an important cultural change in the region. Though Latin American elites considered French the foreign language with the highest reputation throughout the early twentieth century, in the 1950s English was quickly becoming the most popular foreign language among Latin America science and medical elites.[63] Americanization found advocates among several local intellectuals, who were instrumental in overcoming resistance from academic institutions. Eventually, Americanization was welcomed, and during the 1950s, there was an intense local competition to take advantage of U.S. fellowships and grants.

How did Cold War motivations influence health agencies? In the first place, a relationship was established between health and national security. A U.S. officer conceptualized disease as a global phenomenon when he said, "Germs go from one country to another without passports or visas."[64] The American ambassador in Chile insisted on U.S. incentives for participating in health programs abroad to improve "the well-being of people [and] to avoid epidemics of external origin." In more colloquial terms, he explained that "to keep our yard clean we sometimes have to clean up our neighbor's."[65] For another State Department officer, aid aimed at international health created a sound basis for "a lasting peace" (another code term of the Cold War).[66] International health and WHO programs were usually portrayed in U.S. official publications as a means to reduce the tensions and the vicious circle of poor health and poverty that could explode into war.

An important reorganization measure taken within the Department of

State was the formation of the International Cooperation Agency (ICA) in June 1955. This agency was the main nonmilitary bilateral agency until 1961, when it was replaced by the U.S. Agency for International Development (USAID).[67] The ICA was a semiautonomous organization with its own budget and personnel offices that consolidated a series of foreign economic and technical assistance programs. These included the Technical Cooperation Administration; an ephemeral Foreign Operations Administration that functioned between 1953 and 1955; and the Institute of Inter-American Affairs, created by Nelson Rockefeller in 1942 as a unit of the Department of State and the first U.S. bilateral program. These agencies institutionalized bilateral, or country-to country, approaches to technical cooperation, including agricultural, transportation, health, and housing programs.[68] The ICA was responsible for all U.S. foreign assistance, except military projects, including the American contributions to the UN and other international organizations. ICA activities abroad were funded through Mutual Security legislation, which was originally authorized in the June 1950 Act of International Development. This Act had a larger scope, for it included all military, economic, and technical assistance programs that were portrayed as valid "instruments" of U.S. foreign policy.[69] About $27 million was used to start assistance programs related to this Act.[70]

The Act of International Development was based on the fourth point in President Harry Truman's 1949 inaugural address, which called for increasing the international exchange of "know-how," and facilitating the flow of investment capital to developing countries. The Act defined international development as a mixture of military aid, economic support, and technical projects. In 1955, these projects amounted to $3.5 billion. The act allowed the U.S. government to arrange contracts with individuals, corporations, and foreign governments to pursue technical programs. In 1955, Dulles made public his decision to maintain and increase programs in military and technical assistance overseas.[71] He was responsible for the policy guidance given to the ICA's director, who reported to the secretary of state on all operating programs. The ICA had country desks that paralleled the regional bureaus of the State Department.

John B. Hollister, a corporate lawyer from Cincinnati, was the ICA's first director, from July 1955 to September 1959. Hollister had previously been the law partner of Robert A. Taft, a Republican senator and leading isolationist during the 1940s and early 1950s. Hollister's appointment was perceived as President Eisenhower's bid for the support of right-wing Republicans. Like Dulles, Hollister believed that as long as the Soviet Union

existed, American technical aid programs overseas were essential. Hollister organized a "global" plan to strengthen the United States' ties with the
rest of the world, and he established ICA offices in a number of Latin American capitals.[72] The ICA also organized a public health unit (initially named
the Public Health Division and later called the Office of Public Health)
within the office of the ICA's deputy director for technical services.

In 1956, the ICA's personnel included 325 Americans serving in public
health programs overseas. Another indicator of its relevance is the fact that
in same year, 553 of the ICA's American experts, or 28 percent of its employees in all fields who worked abroad, were stationed in Latin America.[73]
A few years later, 37 percent of all ICA staff were placed in Latin America.
Among the ICA technical staff—which included mostly educators, and
agricultural, mining, and civil engineers—American health officers represented 12 percent of all expert personnel. These officers worked on the
control of specific diseases such as malaria and yaws, ran environmental
sanitation projects such as building water systems and rodent control, constructed and operated health facilities, and trained local health personnel.
Between 1954 and 1960, the ICA trained 2,452 physicians, nurses, sanitary
engineers, and other health professionals from all over the world, most of
whom attended courses at U.S. universities.[74]

Following the lead of the Rockefeller Foundation's programs, the ICA's
public health activities assumed that developing countries were at a stage
comparable to the nineteenth-century United States, and, consequently, that
the solution to their health and disease difficulties should follow the path
indicated by U.S. American bilateral assistance. The State Department exalted the contributions of multilateral health agencies and let them take the
credit for international health programs, usually over its own bilateral agency,
the ICA. This was done despite the fact that the multilateral health agencies
received fewer U.S. funds than bilateral programs and had a smaller budget
than the ICA. By 1956, all U.S. bilateral programs in over forty countries
totaled $33 million, an amount higher than the $21 million provided by the
U.S. government to international multilateral organizations such as WHO,
the Pan-American Sanitary Bureau (PASB), and the United Nations Children's Fund (UNICEF).

One important difference between the Rockefeller Foundation and the
ICA was that while the former searched for a low profile to avoid political
controversies in the U.S. and overseas, the ICA was more concerned and
willing to participate in public debates, especially in Congress. A pamphlet
directed to American audiences played down the significant amount of fi-

nancial resources given to bilateral aid by stating that it only represented 1.3 percent of all federal and state health expenses spent at home.[75] It was important for government officials to underscore this proportion, especially when discussing foreign aid with Congress, which usually tried to reduce the number and size of U.S. foreign grants and loans. In 1956 the director of the International Health Division of the U.S. Public Health Service explained to members of Congress that if the sum of all the funds used in technical projects (including health, but excluding military activities) were prorated among American citizens, it "would amount to a pack of cigarettes per person."[76]

International Health Cooperation

Leaders of international health agencies adapted and used Cold War policies and motivations. At the same time, they interacted with U.S. bilateral programs. The names of these key players in malaria eradication were Fred L. Soper, director of the Pan-American Sanitary Bureau (after 1959, the PASB was called the Pan-American Health Organization); Marcolino Candau, director general of WHO; Maurice Pate, executive director of UNICEF; and Eugene P. Campbell, chief of the International Cooperation Administration's Office of Public Health. They sought validation and credibility for their institutions, which were all created or renovated during the 1940s. All the leaders had sound backgrounds in international work, knew their jobs inside-out, and intertwined humanitarian, economic, and political arguments to persuade nonmedical audiences.

These leaders portrayed malaria eradication as an unavoidable battle in history. From their perspective, it was a moral obligation, a crusade against the single most important disease in the world. In addition, wiping out malaria would make a lasting contribution to the world economy and help in the fight against communism. The new commitment to malaria eradication was supported by American professional organizations and by the widely respected Rockefeller Foundation, which was the leader in international health during the interwar period. In 1951 the U.S. National Malaria Society organized a symposium titled "Nation-Wide Malaria Eradication Projects in the Americas." The participants in this meeting were confident that malaria would be eliminated if trained personnel, proper equipment, and political will existed.[77] These conclusions were followed by international meetings, such as the fifth and the sixth International Congresses on Malaria

and Tropical Medicine, which fully ascribed to the idea of malaria eradication.[78] According to a Rockefeller Foundation report, the need for food,
land, and security partly produced by malaria could "drive some communities toward communism," and therefore malaria eradication would help
the fight against it.[79] A similar, but more elegant, statement full of Cold War
metaphors was written by an important Rockefeller officer in 1955: "Malaria
is a factor that, among others, helps to predispose a community to infection
with political germs that can delay and destroy freedom."[80]

The first international meeting with government representatives that
fully endorsed malaria eradication was the Fourteenth Conference of the
PASB, held in Santiago from October 7 to 22, 1954. The conference was
attended by Soper, Candau, the Mexican minister of health (who would later
direct the first malaria eradication campaign in Latin America), and Rockefeller Foundation delegates.[81] Soper, who was director of the PASB from
1947 to 1959, played a critical role in making the PASB the leading agency
in malaria eradication. Soper, who had graduated from Chicago's Rush
Medical College and the Johns Hopkins University School of Public Health,
had worked for Rockefeller, mainly in Brazil, for over twelve years.[82] During World War II, he served as an Army adviser in Egypt and Italy. Like
many Rockefeller medical officers, he found new institutions for his career
after the foundation decided to shift from international health programs to
agricultural development. He was elected the PASB's director thanks to the
support of the United States and a number of Latin American governments.
As director of the PASB, Soper increased the budget, created field offices,
and signed agreements with the OAS and WHO. By 1956, the PASB received
a sizable annual contribution of over $3 million from the U.S. government.
After the OAS, the PASB was the inter-American agency receiving the most
funds from the United States.[83]

Soper and the Argentinean Carlos Alvarado, another PASB officer who
was known for having led a remarkable malaria control campaign in northern Argentina, elaborated a report that explained the rationale for malaria
eradication to the delegates attending the Santiago meeting.[84] According to
the report, malaria was one of the region's main diseases, affecting about
143 million people in Latin America—36 percent of its total population.
The all-or-nothing proposal was possible thanks to DDT indoor spraying
and new antimalaria drugs. Moreover, according to the report, eradication
was an intervention with "no secrets," namely, with no insurmountable technical problems. Any country in the region with the proper equipment, good
administration, and sufficient political commitment could eliminate malaria

in a few years.[85] The operation was presented as technically feasible, with clear advantages over malaria control in results and finances and in ease of obtaining a political commitment from governments.

The report portrayed eradication as urgent because the success gained in prior malaria control programs had generated complacency and relaxation. Moreover, it contributed to a potential crisis because the intermittent and uneven application of insecticides increased mosquito resistance. In attendance at the meeting in Chile was the Italian Emilio Pampana, the first director of WHO's malaria unit, who fully supported the antimalaria report. Pampana had lived and worked for seven years in El Choco, a tropical rural location in Colombia, where he had firsthand experience with malaria, held a degree from the London School of Tropical Medicine, had worked on the successful campaign against malaria in Rome shortly before World War II, and was a former officer of the League of Nations Health Organization.[86] The report was also validated at the conference by a working group of distinguished Latin American malariologists, who prepared a draft resolution calling for all governments in the region to embrace malaria eradication and to create within the PASB a special and flexible fund capable of collecting voluntary contributions.

A few representatives at the Chile meeting raised some doubts about the malaria eradication decision. Among them was the Chilean Amador Neghme, who was responsible for the elimination of malaria in the northern section of his country, and who believed that a previous detailed investigation on mosquito resistance to insecticides was a prerequisite for launching malaria eradication. The representatives of Nicaragua and El Salvador questioned the decision, not only because of the lack of research on the mosquito's resistance, but also because of the absence of a vaccine (something that would take years to develop). For them, malaria eradication was unfeasible.[87] They correctly explained that although the original idea of eradication had appeared in 1950 when DDT resistance was unknown, the definitive decision was made after the first reports of resistance appeared and its implications had not yet been fully assessed. It was true that a 1950 PASB Conference approved malaria eradication before reports of mosquito resistance appeared. However, in that year there were no PASB funds to enforce the decision, and the campaigns took place in only a few countries.

In responding to some of the criticisms, Soper and Alvarado advocated an optimistic interpretation of what mosquito resistance to DDT meant for antimalaria work. They believed that only a few small pockets of resistance existed, and that precisely this factor made eradication urgent: Only a comprehensive and relatively short-term intervention would eliminate malaria before resistance spread all over the region.[88] For Soper, a clear mandate from the Conference, the creation of a new malaria eradication office in the PASB, and the approval of sufficient financial resources were absolutely necessary to carry out the campaign.[89] He felt that approving the resolution was not an option, but an obligation for every representative. If one country did not embrace eradication, it would endanger its neighbors and the whole investment, and thus his generation was responsible for "freeing future people from the bondage of malaria"—or not. This imperative tone would persist and filter down to health workers in the following years. According to a high officer of the PASB around 1957, "control" was a word that the agency's personnel were forbidden to use. Instead, they used "eradication" because the staff was convinced that malaria eradication was clearly "in sight."[90] The connotation of loyalty and obedience resonated not only with the military metaphors of medical operations of the early twentieth century but also with the commanding style of Cold War politics.

As a result of the 1954 conference, a Special Office of Malaria Eradication in the PASB and a fund of $100,000 were created. Initially, the office did not establish clear guidelines, a definitive deadline, or an estimated cost for the whole intervention. These decisive issues would be addressed in the following years by other agencies. After the Santiago meeting, Soper championed malaria eradication. In an effort to raise funds, he discussed the new PASB malaria project with Nelson Rockefeller, Rockefeller Foundation President Dean Rusk, and World Bank President Eugene Black. Although they decided not to openly oppose malaria eradication, they were unconvinced of its feasibility.[91] Soper would find, however, enthusiastic support from UNICEF and U.S. bilateral assistance.

UNICEF, the second multilateral agency to join the eradication crusade, was a new actor in the international health field. It was created in 1946 as the United Nations International Emergency Children's Fund to carry out relief work in post–World War II Europe. Although the words "emergency" and "international" were later dropped, it maintained the acronym "UNICEF" and was also known as the UN Children's Fund. During its first years, it had to renew its UN mandate frequently because it was created as a temporary organization. Only in 1953 did it become a permanent specialized agency, thanks to a decision of the UN General Assembly.

During the second half of the 1950s, UNICEF's niche became secure. A UNICEF Executive Board, formed principally by representatives of the

Economic and Social Council of the UN, met twice a year to select proposals deserving support. What began as a small office located in the UN headquarters became in a few years a full-fledged organization with headquarters in New York City, an experienced international staff, and Latin American field offices in Bogotá, Guatemala City, Lima, and Mexico City. Latin America's UNICEF regional director was the Frenchman Robert Davee, a magnetic personality and a sound planner.[92] UNICEF's financial resources and flexibility were significant. Although the secretary general of the UN appointed its executive director, the position allowed a great degree of autonomy in day-to-day operations. It was the only UN agency that did not establish its budget according to a quota proportional to its population by each nation-member of the UN but based its income on unlimited governmental and public voluntary donations. UNICEF began with a remarkable gift of $15 million.[93]

An indication of UNICEF's relevance is that in the early 1960s, governments donations reached $22.7 million a year, and public donations from churches, women's groups, and individuals provided about $2.7 million. In addition, UNICEF recruited some of the first lobbyists for humanitarian foreign aid in Congress, among whom were Eleanor Roosevelt and Virginia M. Gray. Partially thanks to their help, the U.S. government was UNICEF's largest contributor. In 1955, the United States funded over 57 percent of UNICEF's budget, followed by Germany and France.[94] Another indication of the United States' backing was its 1956 contribution, $14.5 million, an amount almost three times what it gave to WHO and the PASB combined.[95]

The prominent financial position achieved by UNICEF was also the result of the prestige of its first leaders. During its initial years, its chairman was the renowned Polish medical doctor Ludwig Rajchman, who was director of the League of Nations Health Organization before World War II. Its second-in-command was the American Maurice Pate, a charismatic executive director who occupied this position from 1946 to 1964. After Rajchman's retirement in the late 1940s, Pate was for all practical purposes the head of the agency.[96] Pate was a Princeton graduate who worked on relief operations in Europe shortly after World War I, worked in private business in the 1930s, and joined the American Red Cross during World War II to assist prisoners of war. These experiences prepared him to combine humanitarianism and free enterprise. By the mid-1950s, he was known as a skilled fundraiser and Republican gentleman with a self-effacing personality. He changed UNICEF's original emphasis from relief during emergencies to medium- and long-term projects in health, nutrition, maternal care, and child care. In addition, he contributed to a shift in UNICEF's activities from Europe to the less-developed world.

From 1947 to 1950, 76 percent of UNICEF funds were spent in Europe. This proportion diminished in the years 1951–52 to 13.3 percent, and to only 4 percent in 1953. In contrast, Latin America, which represented only 3 percent in the first period, rose to 15.5 percent between 1951 and 1952. By 1953, 18 percent of UNICEF funds were spent in Latin America.[97] This transformation had a symbolic component, as poor countries were portrayed as children in need of guidance. Food and emergency assistance were not sufficient for the population, and permanent health programs, including the control of malaria, tuberculosis, leprosy, and other diseases, also became important dimensions of the agency's work. In 1955 UNICEF was assisting 268 programs in more than eighty countries around the world.[98] A year later, UNICEF estimated that it reached 45 million mothers and children all over the world. Thanks to Pate, UNICEF consolidated the public image of benevolent work with children of underdeveloped countries.

To dismiss the initial concern that UNICEF might be treading on WHO territory, a WHO-UNICEF Joint Committee on Health Policy was created in the 1940s to define the scope of both agencies. Rather than operate field projects of its own, UNICEF endorsed programs run by governments, WHO, and the PASB. Consequently, UNICEF became a "supply" organization providing financial resources for buying equipment and materials for health interventions usually designed and directed by WHO officers. The first UNICEF-PASB campaign was the eradication of yaws from Haiti in the early 1950s. It began with a three-party agreement, signed by the PASB, UNICEF, and the Haitian government, that became a model adapted to malaria eradication in Latin America.[99]

According to this model, UNICEF was in charge of providing vehicles, medicines (penicillin), and other equipment, and the PASB was in charge of the direction of the campaign through expert personnel working in the field. The host government was responsible for providing buildings and local health workers, promising to continue work after the end of the international agencies' campaign, and facilitating the intervention through tax exemptions. This type of agreement was based on the Rockefeller Foundation concepts of an explicit request of help from host governments and of "matching funds," in which local authorities were required to demonstrate their willingness and ability to complete the project by doubling the donation coming from abroad, although they usually waived a strict enforcement of this requirement. The model agreement of the PASB and UNICEF was also instrumental in appeasing members of the U.S. Congress who were concerned that a foreign government would not appreciate American largesse or would not maintain the burden of a program initiated by foreign aid. Not only were these arrangements portrayed as an ideal blend of humanitarianism and pragmatic administration, but they also reinforced the prestige of UNICEF and the PASB as "technical" institutions that could deal with foreign politicians while remaining essentially neutral, noncontroversial, and trustworthy.

UNICEF had worked in malaria control in developing countries almost from its inception. The fact that pregnant women and children were particularly vulnerable to malaria placed the disease firmly within UNICEF's scope of action. A significant number of miscarriages, maternal and infant deaths, and low birth weights were well known to be associated with the disease in developing countries. Between 1949 and 1953, UNICEF used an average of over $1 million a year in malaria control activities around the world.[100] In March 1955, a meeting of UNICEF's Executive Board considered the PASB's request to shift from control to eradication. Soper, a special guest at the meeting, made a vivid plea for the latter:

> Malaria populations tend to live on a bare subsistence basis, contributing nothing to the common good. Even where the incidence of infection is relatively low, there is a surprising inhibition of both mental and physical effort. Malaria is a serious burden on the economy of every malarious country. It has been well said that, where malaria fails to kill, it enslaves. It is an economic disease. No infected area may hope to meet the economic competition of non-malarious regions. . . . As a primary basis of economic development, malaria must be suppressed.[101]

With encouragement from Pate—and from Davee, UNICEF's regional director—the UNICEF Executive Board decided to join the campaign, and it provided the funds needed for insecticides and equipment.[102] Simultaneously, the Eighth Session of the WHO-UNICEF Joint Committee on Health Policy, attended by Pate, Alvarado, and Pampana, endorsed the decision.[103] From 1955 to 1958, UNICEF allocated over $22.7 million for malaria projects worldwide. UNICEF's donations for malaria activities comprised its single largest project. In 1956 alone, almost 50 percent of UNICEF's program budget was absorbed by malaria work.[104] Most of these funds went to Latin American countries. UNICEF's commitment to WHO's decision was portrayed as a demonstration that national health organizations should shift as soon as possible from malaria control to eradication, and that doing so would make more funds available for health work. According to one expert, UNICEF was willing to "multiply by four or five times the amount of supplies now furnished to antimalaria activities of governments, but only if the program is one of eradication."[105]

UNICEF's Executive Board insisted on a clear division of labor for malaria eradication. Its primary responsibility was to provide and ship insecticides, spraying guns, laboratory equipment, vehicles, drugs and other materials that were not locally available. UNICEF was reluctant to pay salaries to local health workers because it was not an operating agency. The PASB facilitated professional advice and sent foreign experts as advisers to work in the field. Governments were supposed to provide buildings, hire and pay local health workers, and appoint the local medical leaders who would direct the campaign. In addition, host governments were required to demonstrate strong political commitment, launch aggressive antimalaria propaganda, enact appropriate legislation such as tariff exemptions for the campaign's imported materials, and guarantee the right of health officers to enter all premises in search of mosquitoes and malaria cases.

At the Eighth World Health Assembly held in Mexico City in May 1955, two months after UNICEF's Executive Board sanctioned malaria eradication, WHO approved the new policy.[106] It was the first WHO Assembly to meet in the Western Hemisphere. The Assembly, attended by representatives of ministries of health in eighty countries, was the supreme decision-making body of WHO.[107] The location of the conference in Mexico was unusual because WHO meetings usually took place in Geneva. The meeting was housed in the National University's splendid Library building, decorated with frescoes that had been dedicated by the Mexican authorities just three years before. The Program Commission and the main Plenary Session took part in extensive discussions about the eradication of malaria. Only one other topic merited the attention received by malaria eradication: the use of atomic energy in medicine. As a concern of the Cold War, this issue was related to the notion of peaceful uses of nuclear energy.

WHO's decisive orientation toward eradication was made possible due to the election of Marcolino Candau as director general of WHO two years before the Mexico meeting. After graduating from Rio de Janeiro's School of Medicine and the Johns Hopkins University, this Brazilian native worked with the Rockefeller Foundation in Brazil at the time when Soper directed the Brazilian field office. Candau was under Soper's supervision during the fight against the *Anopheles gambie* in the Brazilian Northeast—an important precedent for eradication programs. He would remember calling Soper *"comandante"* during those years. Candau later served in a special public health service in Brazil funded by U.S. bilateral assistance.[108] In 1950 he initiated an international career and became head of WHO's Division of Organization of Health Services in Geneva, and after two years, he moved to Washington upon Soper's request to become the assistant director of the PASB. In 1953, Candau was elected WHO's second director general, replacing the Canadian Brock Chisholm. Candau was reelected three more times, directing WHO between 1953 and 1973. During this period, his support for malaria eradication was unwavering.

The appointment of Candau implied a friendly relationship between WHO and the PASB, during a period when WHO was setting up its six regional offices around the globe. PASB became the regional arm of WHO in the Western Hemisphere.[109] Candau's election was also well received by the U.S. Department of State, which saw the Brazilian as advocating methods similar to the philanthropic and public health traditions of the United States. From 1954 to 1959, the U.S. government supported WHO, covering 55 percent of its budget—in 1956 alone, the U.S. contribution was $3.4 million.[110]

An indication of the growing importance that disease-oriented projects acquired with Candau was that in 1959, of the nearly 800 projects developed by WHO around the globe, 200 were control or eradication "vertical" campaigns against communicable diseases, and of these 59 focused on malaria eradication.[111] WHO increased its prominence under Candau's leadership. By the mid-1950s, the agency included eighty-eight countries—several of which were not members of the UN—its budget was $13.5 million, and it had about 900 employees. In contrast, in 1948—when the first World Health Assembly took place—only twenty-six nations were officially members of WHO and its budget was $5 million.[112]

At the Mexico meeting, Candau exalted malaria eradication as one of WHO's primary activities in the near future. His opening speech underscored malaria as a killer that afflicted approximately 200 million people a year worldwide, killing 2 million. He also addressed some of the growing concerns of experts. As Soper had explained to delegates at the PASB meeting, Candau believed that insecticide resistance, and the recently discovered issue of some species of mosquitoes in Panama that "learned" to avoid DDT surfaces, made an energetic malaria eradication campaign imperative. A new argument presented by Candau to validate the urgency of the decision was that the initial commitment of politicians and governments who were willing to support malaria eradication might wane if a decision was not made rapidly. For Candau, malaria work was at a "crossroads": one direction was an uneven application of insecticides and flimsy political commitments that would result in an unlimited explosion of malaria. He advocated following an alternative path that would completely give up on malaria control and concentrate on energetic and thorough eradication.[113] As there was no longer a dilemma between cautious control and a risky eradication operation, the choice was now—for Candau—between malaria eradication or an uncontrollable epidemic outbreak.[114]

According to Candau, the window of opportunity created by the confluence of biological and political factors should not be lost. The "urgency" of the situation was another instance where the resonance with military and Cold War metaphors was clear. Candau underscored another by-product of eradication—that it would "cement" WHO's role as the "directing and co-ordinating authority" of international health, the "trusted instrument in the service of all countries."[115] In other words, malaria eradication would secure WHO's leading position among the multilateral and bilateral health agencies created after World War II.

Candau's proposal was enthusiastically supported by experienced and legendary antimalaria health workers such as Paul F. Russell, a Rockefeller Foundation officer who excelled in the Mexico Assembly by providing coherence and consistency to the proposal. His medical career began at Rockefeller's malaria training station in Leesburg, Georgia. Later he was in charge of malaria studies in the Philippines and was director of the foundation's antimalaria work in India from 1934 to 1942. During World War II and in its aftermath, he was the architect of U.S. Army malaria control operations. He served as medical adviser to General Douglas MacArthur in the South Pacific, who feared losing more men to malaria than to enemy bullets. In 1944 Russell personally directed DDT spraying in Castel Volturno, Italy, in the first attempt to control malaria in an entire civilian community. By the early 1950s, he was North America's foremost malariologist. He is credited with the forceful slogan: "No country is so poor as to afford *not* to control malaria."[116] Although the Rockefeller Foundation did not then have a program in international health, he acted as a consultant on malaria eradication for other agencies. His prestige was connected to his publications, such as *Man's Mastery of Malaria,* a book that insisted on eradication.[117] Russell also had disciples and followers from around the world, such as the Mexican Luís Vargas, who not only translated his book but also applied Russell's methods for identifying *Anopheles* in his home country.

Russell's arguments in the Health Assembly of Mexico inspired practical idealism about malaria eradication and downplayed fears of resistance to DDT. He argued that although the complete worldwide eradication of malaria might have appeared as a utopian dream "ten years ago," after "several field trips" around the world, he was convinced that it was completely achievable. For Russell, resistance was a minor danger. Only about four or five of the approximately fifty *Anopheline* species identified at that time as major carriers developed resistance to DDT. He complemented the argument with a warning that used a military term: Unless something was done immediately, more species would join the resistance "front."[118]

Russell's arguments found advocates among several of the Latin American representatives attending the WHO Assembly—thirteen of the twenty-eight countries that submitted the draft resolution for malaria eradication were from Latin America.[119] The Cuban representative urged a positive decision, because "if the trend continued, health authorities would find themselves completely defenseless."[120] Haiti's representative answered skeptics' requests for more investigation by claiming that the matter required no further study. He asked a pivotal question: Who would "simply sit down and watch the house burning because he was not sure of the efficacy of the water available?" This question held those who were unsupportive of an immediate campaign accountable for the devastation that malaria would cause throughout the world.[121] Furthermore, these comments revealed that clear, firm, unquestionable decisions, such as those made by generals and Cold War politicians, found a comfortable audience among some health representatives.

On the critical side of malaria eradication were representatives from the United Kingdom, France, and Belgium. Germany and Norway were the only two Western European countries that signed the draft resolution. The European critics complained that they had had little time to study thoroughly a proposal in which "efficiency was surely more essential than haste." The date of Candau's proposal reveals the rush: It was dated May 3, 1954, just seven days before the Mexico meeting's inauguration, which meant that most representatives only read the proposal upon their arrival in Mexico. Furthermore, the "draft resolution" was dated May 18, which suggests that it was elaborated in Mexico and not previously circulated with other resolutions. The British representative found it difficult to identify the finances needed to apply the program at its full intensity for the required number of years.[122]

Similarly, the Belgian representative argued that Candau provided few details on the precise financial resources that were needed. The proposal included only a rough estimate of malaria eradication's total cost: $427.56 million for the period 1954–64.[123] The Belgian representative predicted that health officers would lose the confidence of their governments if they requested supplementary appropriations for malaria eradication after a few years.[124] Another interesting criticism came from an African country. Revealing the different degrees of progress in developing nations, the Liberian representative argued that eradication was only possible in "advanced" developing countries, "such as Venezuela," but was unachievable in Africa because of stark realties such as bad communication with remote rural towns.[125]

Russell's response to these objections is significant because it was followed by other advocates of malaria eradication. According to Russell, eradication was unavoidable, and it was imperative to go forward at a rapid pace. Moreover, Russell stressed that only a few experts really understood the complexity of eradication, suggesting that not any health worker could give informed advice on this issue. He arrogantly argued that regardless of what WHO delegates at the assembly decided, eradication was unpreventable and was already well under way in several countries. Eradication was snowballing, and Russell hoped that WHO would not "be left behind." Some years later, another malariologist described the malaria eradication determinism that emerged from the assembly: "Those who did not share the prevailing euphoria and expressed some caution were treated as retrograde obstructionists or enemies of progress."[126]

The U.S. representative addressed the criticism against eradication by attempting to find a smoother position. His intervention at the assembly offered an alternative path, relieved the financial burden on the United States, and justified the exclusion of Africa from the whole enterprise, a possibility that had been previously discussed by experts in a meeting that took place in Kampala in 1950.[127] The American calmly clarified that WHO's proposal did not call for eradication everywhere; the southern part of Africa was excluded because it would be "premature" to enforce a major health operation in countries that lacked public health systems. The Costa Rican representative similarly contended that whereas eradication was not appropriate for every developing country, it was a legitimate enterprise for Latin American nations. In agreement, Russell claimed that African countries could begin with pilot projects, and later they could follow the rest of the world. Eradication could be planned in consecutive stages, eventually covering a whole country.[128] The compromise appeared in the resolution's wording: Malaria eradication "might not be feasible on every continent."[129] Eventually, almost all of Africa was excluded on the grounds that eradication would be unattainable in such a vast area with a mobile and rural population and little health infrastructure.[130]

This double decision—to call for global malaria eradication but to limit the work to some regions of the world—was consistent with the double political discourse of the period. President Eisenhower and Secretary of State Dulles used belligerent rhetoric in public speeches against the Soviet Union, but they used a moderate discourse in discussions in closed American circles of power.[131] Their real aim was to contain communism to particular regions of the world. Malaria eradication also became a containment strategy that resembled the actual practices of U.S. foreign policy. As a result, what might appear as a fantastic operation covering the whole globe was really understood by health experts and politicians as a limited, and defensive intervention.

The officers of the PASB, UNICEF, and WHO also believed that it was best to proceed with a full eradication program only in specific regions as an example to be imitated later by other nations.[132] They even contemplated the possibility that eradication could be achieved in certain sections of a country, while malarious areas could persist in other regions. To sustain these ideas, examples of successful "limited" eradication campaigns of the 1940s and 1950s were held up as models. These included the work of the Italian George Giglioli in British Guiana as head of a mosquito control service for the Sugar Producers Association.[133] Other remarkable examples were Alvarado's work in northern Argentina and Brazil's heterodox technique that provided Cloroquinated salt for domestic use, such as cooking. The medicated salt was used to reach remote rural communities where malaria control could not be implemented by other means. This method was implemented by Mario Pinotti, the powerful director of the Brazilian National Malaria Service.[134] The most spectacular example was led in the mid-1930s by the Venezuelan Arnoldo Gabaldón, a medical doctor who studied at the Johns Hopkins University. As chief of the Malaria Division of the Ministry of Health and Social Welfare, Gabaldón created a Malaria School in Maracay that attracted students from all over the region.[135] When DDT became available for civilian use in Latin American countries in 1945, Gabaldón was the first to use it on a nationwide scale, spraying more than 507,000 houses over an area of approximately 600,000 square kilometers. Shortly thereafter, he became a champion of DDT. Thanks to his reputation, Gabaldón was elected chairman of the Malaria Expert Committee of WHO and was a member of this committee from 1948 to 1970. The fact that by the early 1960s he was appointed as Venezuela's minister of health and was a strong candidate in the election for the position of PASB director were other indicators of his prominence.

Assuming that eradication would be implemented regionally, a WHO resolution was unanimously approved by the Health Assembly gathered in Mexico, which meant that eradication would first be tried first primarily in the Americas and later in the Western Pacific and Southeast Asia. Following the decision made by the PASB that created a special office headed by Alvarado, the assembly created a WHO Division of Malaria Eradication and a fund for the purposes of seeking voluntary contributions from governments and private donors.[136] A detailed program of eradication would only appear later.

In 1956 Russell, Gabaldón, and Alvarado, while attending a meeting of WHO's advisory Expert Committee on Malaria in Athens, produced a blueprint for malaria eradication to be followed everywhere. It was titled the *Sixth Report* to underline its continuity with the committee's earlier reports.[137] A table in the report praised eradication because it set a definitive end point and was cheaper than control in the long run. The table also explained the distinction between control and eradication and used the term "perfection" as the gold standard. A great deal of "perfection" was certainly necessary for a pervasive, countrywide operation to stand on its own. This table, which is reproduced here as table 2.1, gave consistency and clarity to health workers.

In establishing a model for a standard operation, the main premise of the *Sixth Report* was that eradication could be accomplished with energetic campaigns lasting roughly five to eight years, and self-sufficient special units operating outside the regular budgets and routine work of health ministries. These malaria eradication services needed efficient management, clear lines of command like an army, full economic support, and political backing. Its staff would be hired on a full-time basis, departing from the tradition of part-time jobs typical of ministries of health of developing countries.[138]

According to the report, the eradication plan consisted of four phases: preparation, attack, control, and consolidation. Preparation, which usually lasted about a year, concentrated on exploratory surveys, recruitment and training of staff, and a pilot project. The attack phase was a massive national indoor spraying of all rural houses in the malarial area with insecticides, mainly DDT. It was hoped that spraying DDT two times a year would kill

Table 2.1. Comparison of Malaria Control and Malaria Eradication Programs

Aspect	Control Program	Eradication Program
Objective	The reduction of malaria	The definitive suppression of malaria transmission
Area of operations	May depend on degree of endemicity, on accessibility	Wherever transmission takes place
Minimum acceptable standards	Good: reduction of transmission to a level at which it ceases to be a major public health program	Perfect: Transmission must be interrupted in the entire area
Duration of operation	Without limit	Program concluded when malaria transmission has been ended for three years
Economic aspects	Expenditure constantly recurring	Expenditure will represent capital investment and not a permanently recurring cost
Integration with other insect-control programs	Often convenient and feasible in program	Not always feasible
Case finding	Of secondary importance	Of primary importance
Parasitological verification of suspected cases	Relatively unimportant	Of primary importance

Source: Expert Committee on Malaria, World Health Organization, *Sixth Report* (Geneva: World Health Organization, 1957), 9.

the female mosquito that rested in her victim's sleeping quarters after sucking blood. During the third phase, any remaining cases of malaria were identified and treated with drugs. It was assumed that the reduced number of mosquitoes would diminish the risk of transmission, and that the parasite would naturally die in the human host in about two and a half to three years. If there were no new malaria cases and no more *Anopheles,* it would result in no new individuals infected, thus breaking the transmission cycle. The criterion of the achievement of eradication was the absence of any new malaria cases for three years. The consolidation phase lasted as long as malaria existed in a neighboring country. At this phase, national health services absorbed the eradication service. A desired by-product of the campaign was to teach health workers how to run an efficient vertical campaign and provide a nucleus to move public health interventions to other diseases.[139]

The *Sixth Report* praised new diagnostic techniques that later became controversial. A new method of diagnosis—finding malaria parasites within the red blood cells in stained smears—was apparently simple and low technology. In addition, it was portrayed as more efficient than older techniques. Identifying *Plasmodium* parasites was considered better than the traditional "inaccurate" estimations of malaria previously undertaken in control operations against the disease, such as counting people with recurrent fevers or the percentage of people with an enlarged spleen.[140] These traditional techniques were discarded because, although palpation of the spleen in children was easy given that the immune response was building up, it was more difficult in adults because they had usually experienced prior attacks of malaria. They were also discarded because feverish individuals could have illnesses that mimicked malaria, and because little-noticed transmission still occurred in places where the disease seemed to be at a vanishing point. Thus, according to the *Sixth Report,* there was only one way to identify the real incidence of malaria: to visit all localities and rely exclusively on the blood examinations obtained through blood-stained smears of all fever cases.

There was a parallel between the new system of identifying malaria cases and a Cold War fear. The new laboratory techniques implied that symptomless carriers could harbor invisible germs that could spread malaria in a healthy population. Likewise, in Red-Scare America of the 1950s, communism could exist in a few apparently normal people who could "contaminate" other citizens and an entire society. It was of the utmost importance that infected individuals—carriers of malaria parasites or communists in disguise—were isolated and treated so that they would not become dangerous, and even fatal, to the rest of society.

The new diagnostic techniques of malaria eradication were difficult to enforce due to the fact that the laboratory facilities and technical competence needed to be able to take a clear blood sample were not always in place in developing countries. Great care had to be placed on doing blood smears; it was essential for health workers to learn how to perform the difficult "thick blood film" technique. The sanitarian had to prick the person's finger deeply with a sharp stab so that the blood would well up. After the first drop of blood was wiped off with a piece of cotton, the finger was squeezed gently until another drop of blood was forced onto the surface of the finger. A clean slide was lowered to the finger's fresh blood and then covered immediately. This was in itself a difficult operation because there were a number of technical details to consider: slides tainted by grease, dust, or sweat; and the repetitive use of slides that could get scratched or corroded.

Another essential technique for malaria eradication operations was the use of drugs, especially Chloroquine, which inhibited the formation of parasites in the blood.[141] This and other new synthetic antimalaria drugs were regarded as more effective than quinine, which had been used in malaria control. Chloroquine's rapid attenuation of clinical symptoms, its minimal side effects, and its lower degree of toxicity in comparison with pre–World War II drugs such as Atabrine contributed to its popularity and explained why it was entrusted to nonmedical personnel. Chloroquine retained its popularity after the early 1950s appearance of pyrimethamine and primaquine, two synthesized antimalarials that required a monthly or weekly administration and carried the risk of failing to kill the parasite if used indiscriminately. The latter was a serious consideration because health authorities feared that local health workers might distribute the drug indiscriminately if pressured by popular demand for medicines.[142]

Because of the WHO Expert Committee's comprehensive design, malaria eradication campaigns were ready by the end of 1956. One year after the Mexico meeting, a WHO press release announced the annual health day's theme: "War to insects, carriers of disease," using military terms as "*lucha sin cuartel*" and "crusade." The release included an excerpt from Marson Bates's book *The Natural History of Mosquitoes,* in which he stated, "The control of diseases transmitted by insects has removed the only and true obstacle created by the environment to stop the progress of the tropics."[143] Not only does this quotation—which encapsulates the hopes of European tropical medicine at the turn of the twentieth century—suggest the political overtones that malaria eradication was acquiring, but it also serves as a good introduction to the reencounter between international health and U.S. foreign policy. To finance malaria eradication, another player had to be brought to the fore: U.S. foreign aid. The U.S. government's participation in the campaign was facilitated by the convergence of three international agencies, the PASB, UNICEF, and WHO; the matching funds formula; and the elaboration of an expert definition and plan for eradication as opposed to control. The United States' incorporation into the global operation came with an estimation of expenses, clear deadlines, and a more complex economic justification that appealed to politicians and nonmedical audiences.

The Encounter of International Health and Politics

In 1956 and 1957, the U.S. federal government made a definitive commitment to malaria eradication. At the beginning of that year, the ICA requested and received a proposal on new foreign aid programs from an International

Development Advisory Board that had been created in 1950 to advise the president on foreign aid. The board, which included Paul F. Russell, strongly recommended doubling the funds available for malaria eradication and promoting the transformation of malaria control programs into eradication ones.[144] The board's proposal followed Soper's rationale and even repeated a term that he frequently used—"time is of the essence"—to underscore the importance of a rapid and energetic campaign to avoid increased mosquito resistance to DDT. Despite the fact that the board's recommendation was approved by the State Department and the ICA, and efforts were made to implement it in the fall of 1956, the plan was dropped because Congress was not in session and the ICA did not want to announce a program without official approval from Congress. Another important reason for the abandonment of the plan was the fact that Eisenhower was running for re-election that same year.

A final factor that influenced the ICA to temporarily drop the plan was the meeting in May 1957 of a special committee of the Senate to examine U.S. foreign aid. At this meeting, questions were raised about the ultimate goals and effectiveness of foreign aid and about whether aid was motivated by altruism or was simply a strategic tool to secure friends abroad. And an ICA representative spoke in support of the bilateral assistance given to poor countries in the preceding few years as the greatest in history, praising it as an act that benefited commercial interests and was a sound mechanism to remove immediate social dangers of flourishing communist subversion or to "keep nations with uncertain loyalties in a state of neutrality between the communist and the free worlds."[145]

The year 1956 was devoted to a number of intergovernmental meetings that polished the arguments on malaria eradication to be used in Congress in 1957. The American political decision to fully endorse eradication was orchestrated by Eugene P. Campbell, the head of the ICA. He was a medical graduate of the Johns Hopkins University with a wealth of experience in Latin America. He joined the Institute of Inter-American Affairs during World War II to serve as the American director of a special bilateral health service in Guatemala. In 1945, he was appointed field director of all United States–sponsored health services in South America, and a few years later he was put in charge of medical bilateral programs in Brazil. He served as acting chief, deputy chief, and chief of the ICA's Office of Public Health, located in Washington.[146] He relied on U.S. federal and state health agencies that played a decisive role in polishing the techniques of eradication. For example, by the mid-1950s, the Centers for Disease Control and Prevention

(CDC) established the specifications for an effective water-dispersible insecticide powder that was later used in all malaria eradication campaigns
(In addition, a CDC facility in Savannah was used to train Mexican malariologists.) He also followed the transformation of the traditional sprayers
from a home-garden type apparatus to a rugged piece of application equipment that was easy to use, and the development of alternative insecticides
such as Malathion.[147] One of the few articles Campbell published explained
that bilateral health and Western medicalization would contribute to a civ-
ilization process that would do away with primitivism: "Just as many of the
newly developing nations have bypassed the horse-and-buggy days to leap
into the air age, so it has been in the field of health—from primitive cures
and witchcraft to the primary functions of medicine: prevention and cure of
disease."[148] During the mid-1950s, the ICA organized a series of meetings
that resulted in its decision that malaria was the number one preventable
disease in developing countries, and that the ICA should concentrate on the
eradication campaign in Latin America.[149]

Campbell's activities were complemented by the work of Henry van Zile
Hyde, the main U.S. representative to the WHO Executive Board between
1948 and 1952 and a strong advocate of malaria eradication. Hyde also
made a distinguished career in bilateral health projects, had been director
of the Health Division of the Institute of Inter-American Affairs and director of Health and Sanitation of the Technical Cooperation Administration
(the organization that preceded the ICA), and had been the head of the International Health Division of the U.S. Public Health Service since 1950.[150]
The responsibilities of van Zile Hyde's division included professional advice to the ICA and the training of international medical students in the
United States.

In 1956, a series of meetings among U.S. agencies and the PASB discussed how to secure "U.S. financing" for the eradication program in the
Americas and "incidentally in the world." An account of one of these
meetings reveals the anxiety of its participants to appear in Congress as a
united front to overcome the hesitation of politicians. The tension among
different agencies was apparently a concern of U.S. members of Congress.
One of Campbell's diary entries relates that a "minor" obstacle to malaria
eradication that came from the "technical side" was to get rid of the perception that "certain PASB" officers might try to "get the United States
out" of malaria work by exacerbating nationalism in the host countries.
Campbell also suggested that part of the tension within agencies was due
to the unsolved question of who controlled the malaria eradication proj-

ect. Initially, Campbell expressed his concerns as an ambivalence. He was not certain of the ICA's precise role in the whole enterprise: "Should we give some yearly grant to the PASB and expect them to do the job? Should we reserve some funds for bilateral activities? Should we find some matching formula with OAS [the Organization of American States] or [the PASB]?" These questions were raised candidly in a meeting with Soper, who had definitive answers.

For Soper, the matter was clear: With the exception of Cuba, which was considered an "unstable" political situation, Latin America was ready for malaria eradication. He was convinced that the bulk of foreign aid to the region "must come from the U.S. Treasury" as part of "the President's support of inter-American agencies," but the program should be implemented by multilateral agencies. He requested—almost demanded—a large ICA malaria fund for Latin America that would be available to countries once eradication programs were negotiated with the PASB. Defending the supremacy of his agency, he insisted that a better job would be done only if the PASB dealt with governments alone and controlled the funds provided by the U.S. federal government. He was also adamant that malaria eradication "will only be successful" if accomplished in the Western Hemisphere first by the PASB and then "pushed to other parts of the world" by the ICA.[151]

Soper's comments demonstrated his strong opinion on the merit of multilateral agencies such as the PASB over bilateral agencies. He believed that international agencies such as the PASB were not simple followers of individual governments, nor should they limit their activities to the elaboration of codes and quarantine regulations. On the contrary, Soper conceived of these agencies as leaders in national, regional, and global programs, willing to work in the field attacking "communicable diseases in their endemic haunts."[152] In a mid-1950s diary entry, he lamented the fact that bilateral organizations were "inevitably nationalistic political enterprises . . . and as such have limited acceptability and utility."[153] On the contrary, he believed that multilateral organizations had greater leverage and enjoyed a better reception abroad. He sincerely believed, as did other leaders of multilateral agencies, that his agency was partially autonomous from the strict enforcement of Cold War foreign policies.

Confident that he could handle Soper's reluctance to coordinate with his bilateral agency, Campbell knew that other PASB officers were more flexible.[154] In a meeting organized by the ICA, the Argentinean Alvarado appeased ICA officers by emphasizing that "it would be very difficult, if not impossible, to obtain malaria eradiation in the Western Hemisphere without the aid of the ICA."[155] In the same meeting, the WHO malaria adviser for Southeast Asia made two important remarks; first, he dismissed the "erroneous impression" that WHO dominated the program, and second, he claimed that the ICA's role in eradication should not be minimized. Campbell corroborated the ICA agreement with these comments, and he expressed a wish that all agencies would receive full public recognition for eradicating malaria.[156]

Eventually, after a few meetings where complementary functions and planning were clearly established, the tension between bilateral and multilateral organizations was diffused and brought under control. The collaboration that malaria eradication prompted had no precedent. Usually health agencies had different approaches to diseases, concentrated on a specific issue, or had limited activities related to the control of epidemic outbreaks.[157] The new interagency coordination was portrayed as a much more efficient tool to overcome the traditional fragmentation of international health efforts.[158]

Interagency coordination was instrumental to polish the arguments validating malaria eradication for nonmedical audiences. The arguments used usually revolved around the economic benefits of the health program. In a meeting organized by the International Health Division of the U.S. Public Health Service, Russell underscored the economic feasibility and advantages of malaria eradication. He pointed out that politicians, governments, and donors would presumably become enthusiastic about eradication because DDT-spraying operations were cheaper than traditional antimalaria control methods. Thus, the possibility of achieving rapid success at a low cost made the health intervention appealing. Russell emphasized, again, that there was a unique window of opportunity for eradication that should not be lost, stressing that that biological and political circumstances favorable to malaria eradication should be grasped while they lasted. He also agreed with other experts that although worldwide eradication was still "far off," Latin America was ready. In his words, "there can be eradication from the Americas."[159]

In another meeting devoted to polishing the arguments for malaria eradication to be used with government nonmedical institutions and donors, a speaker argued that malaria eradication should be introduced as a "capital investment" in human resources rather than as a "give-away program."[160] For its advocates, malaria eradication should be portrayed as an impulse for the economic modernization of developing countries: Healthier and more vigorous people were better for the local and world economies than were those sick. Russell appreciated the well-defined single objective implied in malaria eradication: It was a positive characteristic that yielded predictable and measurable results for those responsible for economic policies and who usually dominated government bureaucracies. According to Russell, the concentration on one goal was in opposition to the inefficient governmental practices at home and abroad of attempting to attain several goals simultaneously, such as the control of a number of diseases.[161] The real test for all these arguments came in 1957, when the ICA discussed malaria eradication in Congress.

In a journal entry for September 1956, Campbell meditated on different aspects related to the next move of malaria eradication:

> As is often the case, not until a project actually gets to the final steps in planning do the real feelings and interests get smoked out. . . . In the year-long struggle [1956] to get an effective malaria eradication project off the ground, we have encountered all the road blocks that any good project could encounter. It now appears that we have overcome them all.[162]

This quotation was written a few months before the beginning of the "budgetary battle" in the U.S. Congress, also known as the "malaria eradication hearings." An event that marked these hearings was a State Department donation made earlier that year using funds that did not need to be approved by Congress.[163] In a ceremony attended by Soper, the secretary general of the OAS, Jose A. Mora, and Milton S. Eisenhower, the president's brother and his adviser on Latin America, the ICA gave the PASB a check for $1.5 million. The speakers underscored that malaria was the most urgent health issue in the Americas and demanded first priority.[164]

Later in 1957, the ICA and the State Department were ready to convince the House and Senate of the urgency of malaria eradication, a task that would require skill because the Democrats narrowly controlled of the Senate.[165] In addition, major decisions had previously been discussed in specialized committees that had been increasing their importance after World War II, such as the Senate Foreign Relations Committee, the House Foreign Relations Committee, and the Senate Appropriations Committee. Before the war, these committees relied upon executive agencies to obtain information and make decisions. However, after the war, most congressional committees created small staffs, developed their own sources of information, supervised ongoing governmental operations, insisted on consultation between the executive and legislative branches, sought bipartisan consensus, and formed independent opinions. In addition, the fact that the experienced Texan Democrat Lyndon B. Johnson was the majority leader of Congress during the second half of the 1950s made political negotiation necessary. It is also important to mention that the Red-baiting tactics of Joseph McCarthy against the State Department—claiming that it harbored communists—were condemned by the Senate before the discussion of malaria eradication began. As a result, there was an opportunity for more foreign aid programs and for a renewed leadership of the State Department. According to a representative: "Democrats didn't like Mr. Dulles and his policies, but we did not have any big hassles."[166]

To testify in Congress, Campbell made use of impressive charts and maps of the world showing the dramatic widespread distribution of malaria and the economic estimation of malaria spraying. He also obtained letters of support from the U.S. Public Health Service and the U.S. Department of Defense, and he recruited Russell and Louis L. Williams Jr., among other experts, to testify.[167] The participation of Williams was important because he was a patriarch of public health and a prestigious veteran of malaria control in the southern United States. He believed his embracing of eradication to be the most worthy transformation of his career—a conversion that convinced many of the trustworthiness of the cause. Williams's participation in the congressional hearings was also instrumental in emphasizing malaria eradication's "historical dimension," or the idea that there was some continuity between past and modern efforts to fight the disease.[168] During the hearings, Williams would underline that the "all-or-nothing" proposal was inspired by the best lessons of the past and could be done.

The hearings discussed three main themes: the role of foreign aid, the social implications of eradication, and the economic dimension of malaria eradication. A few spirited members of Congress—Democrats and Republicans alike—questioned the proposal on the principle that they were against any increase in foreign aid. They considered it wrong to use taxpayers' money to assist other nations, to buy the allegiance of underdeveloped countries, or to prevent the Soviets from purchasing it. Although there had been a debate in Congress earlier that year, many Americans and their representatives still believed that the fate of developing countries should not be a concern of the federal government. Skepticism about the motives of foreign aid included criticism of the large spending on military aid abroad, the risk of creating dependent nations, and the fear that bilateral programs might be unwelcome overseas.[169] These ideas also inspired proposals to provide foreign aid to Latin American countries only in the form of loan disbursements with stringent obligations to repay, leaving no room for grants, which were largely outright gifts for which no payment was expected. Campbell was confident that grants and malaria eradication would win the day. He knew that although the House might slice the administration's foreign aid program, the Senate was willing to endorse the proposal. In his diary, he wrote: "It appears that malaria is a good case for the ICA to justify grants and a bad one for the . . . loan boys to justify their position."[170]

During the hearings, Campbell, Russell, and Williams underlined the global dimensions of malaria. Campbell made a clear, poignant illustration of the estimated 2 million people killed by malaria: "It is equivalent to destroying a city the size of San Francisco every day." The three leaders also criticized the irrationality of retreating to isolationism from a medical perspective that was reminiscent of Dulles's policies in the State Department. Disease had no frontiers, and the United States could not be secure or prosperous in a sick world. Consequently, it was necessary that America assume medical world responsibilities during the Cold War. The fear seemed especially real for the Southwestern part of the United States, where four states had frontiers with Mexico—California, Arizona, New Mexico, and Texas—and received a sizable flow of migration that could become an entry point of the disease.

Moreover, the campaign was portrayed in the hearings as a means to win "tremendous numbers of friends for the U.S. at all levels."[171] Campbell, Russell, and Williams also warned that not moving immediately on the five-year campaign "may cause irreparable damage." The deadline established in the original design made it important to launch the campaign as soon as possible and to provide it with the necessary financial resources, partly because the proposals for an increase of foreign aid in Congress were always granted on a short-term basis (at least during the Truman and Eisenhower administrations). The promise of eliminating malaria—resorting to terms such as emergency, recovery, and self-help—was important for overcoming isolationist objections that opposed permanent foreign aid programs. In prior discussions on foreign aid, there had been efforts to establish a terminal date for U.S. grants. From 1954 on, a compromise was established that stipulated that there would be no terminal date for ongoing programs but that Congress would appropriate the needed funds for foreign aid each year.[172]

Campbell resorted to terms familiar to international health experts but new to members of Congress: It was a "unique" moment in the history of man's attack on one of the "oldest and most powerful disease enemies."[173]

A convenient way to frame the proposal was to underscore that eradication would be implemented gradually, as approved by WHO in Mexico. This meant the creation of malaria-free areas, or "islands of eradication." The goal was that these areas would expand until their borders overlapped and a full protection from the disease would be achieved.[174] The metaphor was consistent with the "demonstration" system that Rockefeller Foundation public health programs had organized in the U.S. South and abroad. In addition, Campbell underscored the need for an official request to develop the campaign from local governments, the cost-sharing concept, the idea that foreign aid was a spark rather than unilateral intervention, and the promise that host countries would take over malaria eradication efforts in the future. The U.S. technical programs were expected to have a definitive end point, something that pleased many legislators. As a result, the limited scope of the real implementation of "global" malaria eradication was presented as an advantage. Setting an example that would be imitated was portrayed as a cautious method, an example of American philanthropic traditions, and the best method to extend foreign aid.[175]

A second issue discussed in the hearings was the social consequences of malaria eradication in poor countries where there was no control over the rapid increase of their population. Some members of Congress were concerned that malaria eradication might contribute to a world population explosion, a theme that was beginning to achieve notoriety in the United States. The argument revived Malthusian worries on the gap between uncontrolled population growth and limited natural and food resources. DDT, as well as antibiotics and sulfa drugs, were considered death-deferring tools in poor countries where birthrates were high. From this perspective, the elimination of malaria contributed to the economic burden of these countries. An example usually cited was Ceylon, where a DDT campaign launched in the mid-1940s contributed to diminishing death rates by 40 percent in a few years, despite the fact that poverty indicators remained unchanged and even worsened. Latin America was also a concern because, in comparison with other developing regions of the globe, its population grew at a faster rate. Between 1920 and the mid-1950s, the Latin American population more than doubled, totaling approximately 190 million inhabitants.[176]

Campbell responded to this criticism by arguing that overpopulation was a relative term because it depended not only on the existence of a healthy population able to sustain itself but also on areas free of disease that could be added to agricultural exploitation.[177] For him, any "excess" population produced by the antimalaria program would move to areas liberated from

malaria. Campbell was convinced that the best way to respond to the out-
stripping of agricultural outputs by population growth was to create more
disease-free agricultural workers and more disease-free land for cultivation.
His argument complemented the idea of experts at the time, who hoped that
technology would always be capable of producing food, medicines, and
goods. Simply put, good health was a sound population policy. A State Department officer also insisted in dismissing any link between overpopulation
and WHO by arguing that healthier individuals would be able to produce
more.[178]

In any case, there was no profound debate on the relationship between
malaria eradication and overpopulation until the mid-1960s. A discussion
of population growth and foreign aid was postponed because President
Eisenhower believed that population control was not the business of the federal government. Even in 1960, the State Department's assistant secretary
for international organization affairs argued that in the case of a rapid
growth of the world's population, the solution was simple: "World production must increase faster than people."[179] During the 1950s, most UN
agencies avoided the theme of overpopulation, partly because of the risk
that birth control programs would be rejected in pro-natalist Catholic countries such as Mexico.[180] Consequently, the concern for overpopulation was
dismissed in the malaria eradication hearings.

The third topic discussed in Congress was the cost of malaria eradication. According to its supporters, the campaign might be regarded as expensive, but it was less expensive than the economic losses produced by
malaria. An example cited was that before 1946, malaria in the United
States cost the U.S. economy about $500 million a year, but after ten years
without malaria, the country had saved $5 billion. Just as Soper had done
for UNICEF's Executive Board, Campbell, Russell, and Williams portrayed
malaria in the hearings as an economic disease, in which eradication efforts
would save significant funds in both developed and developing nations.[181]

Moreover, Campbell, Russell, and Williams all sincerely believed that
malaria was the world's "most expensive disease" because of the permanent drain produced by medical care, drugs, and hospitalization, because
of the loss of labor power that resulted from premature death, and due to
the decline of the working time needed to produce in agriculture.[182] A study
estimated that each infected adult suffered from at least one annual attack
of malaria that incapacitated him for six days. This study computed the
total number of malaria cases and the percentage of the economically active
population in several countries. In 1955 in Mexico, for instance, the loss of

working time due to malaria was the high figure of 4 million person-days. Finally, malaria presented a serious economic issue because it wasted great tracts of potentially fertile land that were abandoned or undercultivated.[183] The definition of malaria as an economic disease was enriched by WHO, which portrayed malaria as an impediment to the full development of the economic and social potentials of "underdeveloped" areas of the world. For this multilateral agency, malaria was "one of the most important factors in the vicious circle of disease, poverty, and ignorance."[184]

The benefits of malaria eradication were portrayed in economic terms. The campaign would save the life of rural workers, increase agricultural productivity, reduce medical budgets, revert depreciation of rural estates, and energize development in poor countries.[185] The campaign was also depicted as an obligatory requirement for all developmental programs; no other bilateral or multilateral social program would be effective unless malaria was eliminated.[186] Eradication would also benefit the economies of industrialized nations because the agricultural imports of developing malarious countries carried an additional cost created by labor inefficiency and high absentee rates. Moreover, campaigns would get rid of a "hidden malaria tax," estimated at 5 percent of the price paid by importing countries.[187] According to a 1956 study, U.S. importers lost $300 million with the so-called hidden malaria tax.[188]

More sophisticated economic arguments for malaria eradication appeared when the cost of the operation was actually estimated, something that was not done when the proposal was first launched by the PASB or WHO. The ICA's proposal to Congress estimated $519 million for a worldwide campaign with a duration of five to ten years. The U.S. share of this amount would be about 20 percent, or $100 million, and the rest would be paid by benefiting nations, WHO, UNICEF, and the PASB. A *New York Times* article saw this as a great matching scheme in which the United States would contribute approximately one-fifth the total amount, international organizations another one-fifth, and the host countries the remaining three-fifths.[189] These calculations excluded Africa, Borneo, New Guinea, and a number of other "highly malarious areas" of the world, where rapid success was perceived as more difficult.[190]

Estimates for Latin America also appeared. From an initial vague sum of $100 million, the total cost of eradicating malaria in the Americas over a five-year period was established at $144.4 million.[191] The total international contribution to this sum was an anticipated $40 million, of which the PASB would contribute approximately $20.2 million and other agencies and host governments would provide the rest. It was also expected that part of the funds coming from Latin American really came from bilateral assistance.

Taking into consideration these calculations, Campbell's office cut the initial request to Congress to a "solid bedrock" figure of $23.3 million, of which $16.3 million would be used directly as bilateral assistance to convert control programs to eradication ones, and to support malaria eradication programs. This was a sum that Campbell believed marked the beginning of a sustained backing for eradication programs. It is important to note that to receive a special assistance fund and secure the support of the program, the proposal was presented separately from the Mutual Security bill submitted by the Eisenhower administration to Congress. The decision was also instrumental in raising the status of the ICA health unit. It was no coincidence that when the proposal was submitted, the ICA's health office became the Office of Public Health with a similar ranking to other offices at the State Department.

The definition of malaria eradication's cost came with a deadline. According to the PASB, malaria would disappear from the Americas in 1966. A *New York Times* article said the same would occur in the rest of the world one year later.[192] The forecast reinforced beliefs in the power of science and technology over nature and disease. In 1958 an optimistic Candau declared that most communicable diseases would be wiped out within "a foreseeable future," like malaria, which was "definitely on the way out"; later yaws, syphilis, smallpox, tuberculosis, leprosy, and eventually cancer and heart disease would "yield to science."[193]

There was one final and important economic reason to support malaria eradication for Congress. In one of his 1957 interventions in Congress, Campbell explained that "less developed countries do not manufacture insecticides, house spraying equipment nor automotive machinery, and are not able to supply the dollars to procure these manufactured products, which one finds, mainly produced in this country."[194] Campbell was responding to members of Congress who questioned foreign aid programs because they might put American industries out of business. As these remarks suggest, buying American insecticides and pharmaceutical goods was a factor in sanctioning malaria eradication.[195] For Campbell, buying insecticides, drugs, and equipment in the United States was necessary because of the ability "of our own manufacturers to meet peak requests." In addition, he pointed out that this was not a new trend by assuring that in the mid-1950s, 96 percent of all ICA purchases were made in the United States.[196] In 1959, a decision by Congress cemented the trend by establishing a preferential position for

American bidders over foreign producers on government contracts linked to bilateral assistance.[197] As a result, foreign aid became an indirect subsidy to American business.

Drugs, hand compression, sprayer equipment, and insecticides were the most significant expenditures for malaria eradication.[198] By the mid-1950s, the antimalaria drug Chloroquine became widely used and would retain a position as a leading pharmaceutical until 1990, when it became the third most widely used drug in the world.[199] Another indication of its importance to bilateral programs was the fact that nearly 90 million Chloroquine tablets were purchased by the ICA to be distributed overseas in the 1960 fiscal year. Two years later, this figure increased to 137 million tablets.[200] The increased commercial importance of Chloroquine was related to the international expansion of U.S. pharmaceutical industries after World War II by corporations such as Pfizer, Lilly, Merck, Squibb, Winthrop, and Parke-Davis. These companies created the emergence of a dependent market overseas that included not only Chloroquine but also new "wonder" antibacterials such as penicillin, which was effective against a series of infections; streptomycin, which was the first antibiotic remedy against tuberculosis; and plasma, which transformed surgery. These products were extolled to health professionals, hospitals, international health agencies, and consumers for improving individual health, medical practice, and public health. They were also regarded as decisive factors in changing the disease patterns of society from one in which infectious diseases predominated to one where chronic ailments were more significant.[201]

Insecticides and drugs, significant investments and key weapons for any malaria-eradication operation, were produced and shipped from the United States to different parts of the world. Although DDT was first discovered in Europe, its production was mainly done by American petroleum and chemical businesses engaged in the elaboration and sale of pesticides for agriculture since the 1940s. After World War II, the oil and chemical branches of these companies devoted to insecticide and pesticide production dramatically increased their activities in research, patenting, production, advertising, and large-scale sales, resulting in coherent, vertically integrated operations.[202] An indication of this growth was the creation of Shell Chemical in 1950, a division of Shell Oil Corporation, the patent-owner and exclusive seller of the two powerful insecticides, Aldrin and Dieldrin. There were great hopes for the residual powers of Dieldrin, which had longer lasting effects than DDT, despite the fact that it cost about twice as much as DDT. A few companies did not come from the oil business but rather specialized in the production of pesticides. One such company was Montrose Chemical Corporation of California, which had been producing DDT since 1947 and would continue until 1982. As the largest producer of DDT in the late 1950s, Montrose participated in the bid for insecticides for the international health programs sponsored by the ICA.

In addition, Monsanto, Hercules, DuPont, and Merck usually kept a convenient low profile but soared in sales in the growing and profitable business of pesticides for commercial agriculture.[203] Likewise, Hudson Manufacturers from Chicago, a company that had been producing compressed-air equipment for insecticide spraying since World War II, became the main supplier of hand compression sprayers and other spraying equipment for insecticides and pesticides. By the mid-1960s, some of the companies had established subsidiaries and affiliates in a number of countries, including Mexico City.[204] These companies adapted this equipment from what was used by the Army in World War II and elaborated simple and solid pumps that produced a uniform dosage on sprayed surfaces and a controllable nozzle that could be used with minimal technical knowledge.[205] Because pumps would be handled mostly by health workers with little training, this was considered essential for malaria eradication operations in Latin America.

By the mid-1950s, Shell was delighted to report remarkable sales of Dieldrin, thanks to demands from the "World Health Programs of the United Nations agencies and public health authorities." It also predicted that "Dieldrin would continue to experience increasing demand as a result of its successful fight against malaria."[206] In 1955 alone, 128 million pounds of DDT were manufactured by several companies in the United States, mostly for use abroad.[207] By the end of 1957, the ICA had purchased 22.5 million pounds of DDT, or more than half the 40 million pounds that was to be exported by U.S. manufacturers that year. In addition, during the fiscal year 1957–58, the ICA exported 1.5 million pounds of Dieldrin.[208] The trend was confirmed later: During the first six months of 1958, the ICA bought more than 33 million pounds of DDT and shipped it overseas.[209] The trend of U.S. bilateral agencies buying insecticides continued in the following years. For example, USAID purchased and shipped more than 74 million pounds of DDT in 1961, which amounted to nearly one-third of all the insecticide manufactured in the United States that year.[210] A letter from the deputy chief of the Malaria Eradication Branch of USAID, the agency that replaced the ICA, indicates the continuation of the trend: "The largest proportion of AID malaria eradication funds expended during the recent years has been for DDT, accounting for more than half the dollar costs of this program to AID."[211]

The coherent economic, political, and humanitarian arguments presented by Campbell, Russell, and Williams to the U.S. Congress received a boost in the middle of 1957, when a bill authorized the president to spend up to $23.3 million in malaria eradication during the next fiscal year. This sum was expected to be part of the $107.2 million invested by all nations and international agencies committed to the health campaign.[212] The result was a victory for the ICA and for the emerging international health web formed by the State Department, UN agencies, and U.S. bilateral institutions that had eagerly advocated malaria eradication. In the following years, the ICA secured similar or slightly higher contributions for malaria eradication from Congress. For example, for fiscal years 1958 and 1959, more than $27.2 million and $26.2 million, respectively, was appropriated for malaria eradication. In 1959, the amount represented 43 percent of all health activities supported by the U.S. government overseas, including its aid to multilateral agencies.[213] It was also expected that $32 million would be provided by the United States in 1960.

When the political, technical, and economic aspects of the decision were clear, the humanitarian dimension of malaria eradication became more visible and acquired a political connotation (figure 2.1). President Eisenhower urged an all-out attack on malaria in his 1958 State of the Union message because it was the "world's foremost health problem" and it was "practicable to end" the "scourge in large areas of the world."[214]

Propaganda for the program intertwined humanitarianism with stereotypes of poor rural people in developing countries. Among these stereotypes was the idea that malaria was a manifestation of a natural inclination to poverty, laziness, resignation, and fatalism of peasants—ideas that proved instrumental to the construction of a racialized version of the disease, in which indigenous people were disease carriers and their culture was an obstacle to progress. The perception had precedents in provincial Mexico. In the 1920s, a medical doctor explained the combined effect of the physical and moral harm that malaria produced among peasants: "The inhabitants become apathetic and indolent . . . lie down or sleep. Their appearance notes fatigue, indifference."[215] A pamphlet and poster produced by the PASB for the campaign used an image of a peasant sitting on the front porch of a crumbling hut with a skinny dog, with a caption emphasizing the relationship between poverty, malaria, and apathy.[216] This perception persisted, as suggested by a 1967 Mexican publication in which the population suffering

Figure 2.1. *The face of malaria: A Mexican woman shakes with the all-too-familiar fever (1968).*

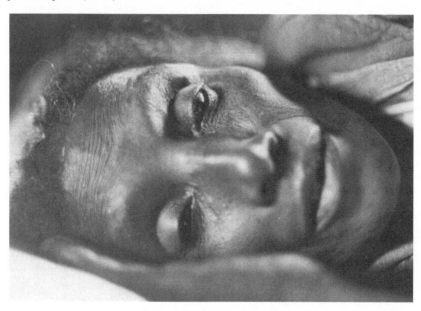

Source: Photograph by Peter Larsen. Courtesy of the World Health Organization Archives.

from malaria was described as tied to "chains of misery . . . a human being whose initiatives are not advanced and who is discouraged because his efforts are useless gives to certain fatalism."[217]

A corollary idea was that U.S. foreign aid and medical science would remove tradition and create a desire for better living standards. The belief that malaria was a drag in backward countries was expressed in the intervention of a member of the House of Representatives in the malaria hearings who underscored that development meant "less malaria and more vigor."[218] According to a *New York Times* article, the greatest havoc of the disease was the destruction of the "will" of individuals. It also cited the opinion of experts to blame the anemia produced by malaria as the source of lethargy: "Malariologists point out that it's common to regard people in tropical countries as indolent. One doctor stated, 'They are not lazier than people in temperate climates. . . . They merely have malaria.'"[219]

Cold War anxieties inspired a recurrent metaphor cited at the beginning of this chapter. Not only did malaria kill some people, but it also "enslaved" its sufferers, causing the disability, immobility, and impairment of the majority of the rural population of developing countries. "Enslavement" was also frequently used to describe people living under communist regimes.[220] The notion of malaria as an external force restricting freedom was consistent with U.S. foreign policy during the early Cold War.

Several journalists in American newspapers commented on the coincidence of the decision to embark on malaria eradication and the launching of the Soviet satellite *Sputnik* into orbit in October 1957. *Sputnik* alarmed the American public because it questioned the scientific capacity of the West and created a fear that Soviet superiority in rocketry could lead to an intercontinental attack with nuclear missiles. The impact of the event in the U.S. public imagination was portrayed as a conspiracy by an article titled "Communism in the Americas" in the *Department of State Bulletin,* which described how "Soviet propaganda boasts following the *Sputnik* launchings conveyed veiled military threats against the free world."[221] A newspaper article in the *New York Times* compared the Sputnik with malaria eradication. It depicted malaria eradication as part of "a far more important battle" with a broader political connotation in developing countries, which facilitated the control of "the inner space in the minds and hearts of mankind throughout the world."[222]

The impact of Congress's decision on malaria eradication was crucial. During 1957, the PASB received an additional donation of $2 million, and WHO received its first donation of $5 million. For Secretary of State Dulles, who presented the check in a special ceremony to Soper and Candau on behalf of the PASB and WHO, respectively, these donations were made to fight "the greatest single source of death and sickness in the world" and "to harness together . . . the total capabilities of freedom-loving people to achieve lasting peace with justice and lift from the backs of mankind the burdens of poverty, hunger and disease." This sentence was part of a speech that demonstrated a command in blending political and medical terms according to the Cold War context.[223]

This rhetoric would be followed abroad by Latin American dictatorial regimes that wanted to demonstrate their loyalty to all actions launched by the U.S. government. Seeking additional validation for his unpopular rule of the Dominican Republic and its discrediting abroad, the dictator Rafael Trujillo donated $500,000 to the fund created by the PASB for malaria eradication. The Dominican ambassador in Washington gave a first check for $100,000 with a blunt speech toying with Cold War terminology: "In our country malaria will be something of the past. . . . In the moral order we occupy the first place among nations that firmly fight against any infiltration of the mortal virus of international communism."[224] The first check was supposed to be followed by four more similar installments, but Trujillo did not live up to his promises and never donated the remaining checks. So as not to be left behind, the unpopular Venezuelan military regime of Marco Perez Jimenez added $299,600 to the PASB Fund. Thanks to these and other contributions, the PASB Fund, which began in 1954 with $100,000, had $4.3 million by the end of 1957. The amount was taken as sufficient to cover the expenses for the first two years of antimalaria work.[225]

However, despite profound economic and political backing, by 1959 Candau was concerned about the small sums received by WHO. He complained in a letter to a Mexican health authority that the $9.5 million in WHO's malaria fund was insufficient and came mainly from one source— the United States.[226] The situation suggests a cold reception of malaria eradication by European governments. Despite their doubts, they never confronted directly the decision. The situation was not much better two years later, when the United States provided $11 million of the $11.6 million WHO funds.[227] As a result, WHO eagerly sought voluntary contributions for its antimalaria fund, and it had to support malaria eradication by taking financial resources from other activities, resulting in a deficit for the tasks that were initially planned.[228] Another result of this development was that Latin America, though initially presented as the entry point of a global program, became, along with India and a few other developing nations, the only real areas where malaria eradication was fully enforced.

In part as a response to the concern that malaria eradication might not receive full funding and might not sustain its international scope, the ICA formed a panel of twelve experts in late 1959. Headed by Soper, who by then had retired from the Pan-American Health Organization, the panel included Russell and Williams, who had to assess the progress of worldwide malaria eradication and determine the United States' future participation in the program. In August 1960, the panel produced an optimistic, reassuring, and lengthy report underscoring the historical dimension of the campaign: "the greatest single international cooperative activity ever undertaken in the field of health," that would go down in "history as one of the greatest works of man." Moreover, the campaign was portrayed as "the most significant program sponsored by the U.S. foreign aid policy."[229] The report recommended several technical adjustments—including a more intense search for donors; improved surveillance of malaria cases; the use of a new insecticide, Malathion, in places where DDT and Dieldrin found mosquito resistance; building better administrative capabilities of national programs; and greater coordination among international agencies and national ministries of health.

The costs of eradication were also addressed by the report, which estimated that the financial sources used for global programs from 1958 to 1960 totaled over $299 million, of which U.S. bilateral assistance had given 23 percent and UNICEF had given 9 percent. The United States had given significant economic resources to the world campaign in comparison with other countries—more than the one-fifth of the total cost initially expected. These calculations were followed by complaints that the campaigns appeared to be an American enterprise, and a greater participation of other industrialized nations was strongly recommended. This was exemplified in the statement that "[it] cannot be expected that this one-sided pattern will continue in its present ratio."[230] The report estimated that $1.3 billion would be needed for malaria eradication worldwide from 1960 until the end of the program. This figure represented a significant increase in comparison with the approximately $519 million estimated in 1957. About 12 percent of the new figure should be used in Latin America, as it was considered the most advanced region in malaria eradication.[231] The panel was confident in the ability of governments and agencies to obtain the funds.[232]

The report was widely diffused, because it became a fifty-page article in the prestigious *American Journal of Tropical Medicine and Hygiene* and was also translated into Spanish. For Campbell, it was a "milestone"—a sound instrument for his ongoing negotiations with Congress to secure funds, and a definitive demonstration "that taking into account all the problems, malaria can and is being eradicated."[233] Partly as a result of this document, more funds for malaria eradication were provided by the United States in the following years, and the campaign continued with vigor well into the early 1960s.[234]

Concluding Thoughts

From 1954 to 1959, a complex web of technical expertise, humanitarian motivations, economic interests, and political will was spun to support the largest international health program of the second half of the twentieth century. The emergence of a political, economic, and medical bloc made malaria eradication unavoidable for many countries. Even the Soviet Union became engaged in malaria eradication and followed the plans and methods established by the PASB and WHO.[235] By the late 1950s, plans were being implemented in more than seventy-five malarious countries with a combined population of more than 1 billion.[236]

Latin American programs, usually called *servicios* (or *comisiones*) *nacionales de erradicación de la malaria* (or *paludismo*), received a great deal of resources, and their members enjoyed high prestige.[237] Their strategies were similar and simple, with minor variations, and followed a standard pattern. Sometimes these units became "ministries" inside the ministries of health of their countries. What was formally a subunit of these ministries was run by experts who claimed that their methods and new technologies demanded complete autonomy. These experts knew what was good for the recipients and had no need to explain the benefits of the campaign to health workers involved in other programs.

The implication of these beliefs was that the inhabitants of underdeveloped countries were considered unable to make informed decisions and could not understand long-term goals of technical aid. The technology used by these experts was portrayed as unaffected by the diverse ecological, social, and cultural contexts of "backward" nations. Techniques were also part of a cultural diffusion effort that would create values of innovation and expertise among local professional elites that paralleled those of the sending nations. Following this rationale, international and local experts could do away with the need to consult beneficiaries affected by malaria eradication. This authoritarian understanding of international health as programs coming from above was consistent with the medical military tradition and an emergent Cold War tradition of secrecy in science. Orders, including health directives, were to be obeyed, not to be discussed.

A few years after its approval, WHO announced that malaria eradication in Latin America was in full swing. On March 14, 1957, a monument of a dead *Anopheles* mosquito was erected by the Lyons Club of Valencia Moron in Carabobo, Venezuela, to anticipate the celebration of malaria's end. Mexico, the most populous Spanish-speaking country of the region, became the first location where the large-scale program was launched. It was chosen to set an example for the developing world. A 1958 *Reader's Digest* article celebrated the Mexican campaign by resorting to a military metaphor: Malaria eradication had "generals [who are] physicians and doctors in science" and "soldiers . . . armed with guns that send out a spray of DDT. The enemy is mankind's most prevalent disease—malaria."[238] The campaign even acquired an esthetic flavor, unified people of the world, and achieved a consensus that overcame Cold War differences. According to the description of a writer:

A sprayman was working on the far wall of the López shack. He slowly waved the wand of his pump over the dusty surface of palm canes—a modern magician exorcising discomfort and disease and death. It was beautiful; beautiful not only in the slow, graceful movements of the sprayman as he moved the brass-tipped wand down and up, depositing two grams of DDT on each square meter of wall, but beautiful too as a symbol of something men the world over can agree upon. The young Mexican with the pump was a representative of all the scientists and technicians who are fighting to end the menace of mosquitoes that breed in the lime sinks of Georgia, the swamps of Panama, the treetrops of Trinidad, the gullies of the Sahara, the water jars of Engu-Ezike, the rice paddies of Formosa, the river potholes of Ecuador.[239]

The scientific-political battle was ready to begin.

3

National Decisions

In a nationwide radio broadcast on September 7, 1956, President Adolfo Ruíz Cortines announced the beginning of a national crusade for malaria eradication in Mexico.[1] His call was followed by a ceremony attended by Cabinet officers and health authorities. At the same time, state governors and provincial medical authorities held smaller similar events in the main squares of their towns and cities, indicating the national scope of the federal program. Important actors in the background of these rituals were the campaign's "soldiers"—the field sprayers of DDT. They were members of a new political and medical entity called the National Commission for the Eradication of Paludism (Comisión Nacional de Erradicación del Paludismo, CNEP), a special government corporation within the Secretariat of Health. The field sprayers appeared in the photographs of the launching ceremonies as a disciplined army wearing bright khaki uniforms and low black boots and carrying aluminum fumigating pumps. Using a familiar military metaphor of international health campaigns, one writer characterized the sprayers as members of "an army of liberation" ready to "drive out disease."[2] Local, national, and international newspapers celebrated malaria eradication as a milestone event.[3] A *New York Times* article described the day of the campaign's launch as "one of the really big days in Mexican history."[4]

The goals of this chapter are to describe the process by which the Mexican national authorities embraced the international campaign, the intersection of political and medical motivations in Mexico, and finally, the *Mexicanization* of the campaign, or its appropriation by local health workers.

Mexican Politics and Medicine

Malaria initially became a concern of Mexican politicians and medical leaders for humanitarian reasons. The disease was a tragic reality in rural and semirural areas where the majority of the people lived. Malarious areas in Mexico covered over 1.1 million square kilometers—approximately three-fourths of Mexico's territory—and spread from sea level to 2,000 meters of altitude. The disease was particularly intense in the Pacific Ocean and Gulf of Mexico southern slopes, the Yucatán Peninsula, and interior basins of the high plateau. In 1955 it was estimated that 2 million people a year suffered from malaria in Mexico. A death toll of 19,639 individuals made malaria the third largest cause of mortality in Mexico, following diarrheal diseases and respiratory infections. In some indigenous states, the disease was more acute. In Oaxaca, according to a report of the 1940s that described the situation of malaria as dreadful, the disease was the first cause of morbidity, surpassing diarrheal and respiratory diseases.[5] Moreover, malaria led to an increased vulnerability to other deadly and widespread killers in the country, such as tuberculosis.[6] According to medical doctors, all infectious diseases in Mexico became graver if preceded or accompanied by malaria. This was especially true among the rural inhabitants who experienced appalling health indicators, such as a low life expectancy and high infant and maternal mortality rates that doubled national rates.[7]

The economic impact of malaria was also a major issue that validated the campaign. Not only was the disease portrayed as an explanation for backward agriculture, but malaria eradication appeared as an essential tool to incorporate wide areas of the territory into the national development process. In the mid-1950s, agriculture was still the most important activity in terms of the number of people it employed—approximately 60 percent of the population—and it led Mexican exports. Livestock was another important rural economic activity. In addition to cotton and coffee, the two main profitable exports, the country also produced maize, fruits, beans, rice, sugarcane, cocoa, sisal, and wheat for national and international consumption. In addition, Mexico was a large producer of vegetable fibers used to make ropes and cords, and it produced about half the world's supply of fibers for harvester twine. Its total agricultural output for the period 1952–53 was valued at 4.6 million pesos, a slight increase relative to previous years.[8]

It was estimated that for the period 1949–53, the annual economic losses directly caused by the ravages of malaria's morbidity and mortality (including the loss of lives and working days; the decrease in work output; the depreciated value of land; and the loss of potentially rich land for agriculture, livestock, tourism, and petroleum exploitation) were more than $160 million.[9] This figure was later used to argue that one year of malaria in Mexico was more expensive than the whole eradication campaign.

The humanitarian, economic, and political validations for the campaign were seen as intertwined by both medical experts and the Mexican government. It was expected that with eradication, children and rural health workers would be saved and lands would be "liberated" from malaria, prompting commercial agriculture and livestock and mining industries. The campaign was also a means to incorporate indigenous rural inhabitants into a market economy. Moreover, it was portrayed as a demonstration that the government and the medical elite were fulfilling the mandate for better health of the 1910 Mexican Revolution.[10] According to the Constitution of 1917, the provision of public health services was a responsibility of the federal government. However, in the wake of the revolution, it was difficult to enforce this obligation because of political turmoil, civil war, and scarce resources. In addition, when the first solid public health networks began to appear in the mid-1920s, few human and financial resources existed to solve the sanitation problems in rural areas.

Official health policies were reinforced with the creation of a Secretariat of Health and Welfare (Secretaría de Salubridad y Asistencia) in 1943, which regulated all federal matters regarding sanitation, hospitals, and clinics. Created by President Avila Camacho, the secretariat signaled an important institutional reform common to several Latin American countries: founding cabinet-like positions devoted to providing basic health services to its citizens.[11] The secretariat resulted from merging the Board of Health, created in 1917, and the Welfare Secretariat, established in 1938. The Board of Health intervened in epidemic outbreaks, organized immunization campaigns (especially against smallpox), provided basic maternal and child health services, and supervised the construction of safe water systems in urban areas. The Welfare Secretariat coordinated "welfare societies" (*beneficencias* in Spanish) in charge of hospitals and cared for the poorest segments of the population. The organizational fusion was part of federal authorities' efforts to construct a centralized web of health institutions. The status of the secretariat was reinforced by the creation of new hospitals and specialized centers during the 1950s and 1960s.

The creation of a new and more powerful Secretariat of Health and Welfare was also the result of the demands of labor unions and peasant organizations that, after the 1940s, became important constituencies of the Institutional Revolutionary Party (Partido Revolucionario Institutional, PRI), the ruling political party that emerged after the 1910 Revolution. For example, the National Peasant's Confederation (Confederación Nacional Campesina), created in 1938 and supported by the government, included in its goals the extension of health and educational services.

The first health secretary was Gustavo Baz, an eminent physician and former president of the National University of Mexico. The second in command was Manuel Martínez Báez, a distinguished medical scientist from Morelia, Michoacan, who had been trained at the Medical School of Paris and the Institute of Tropical Medicine of Hamburg.[12] Martínez Báez, who had also studied malariology at specialized centers in Rome and Spain, was also close to American methods due to his Rockefeller Foundation fellowships and his role as a founding member of the World Health Organization (WHO). Not only had Martínez Báez supported malaria eradication since the early 1950s, but he had also published a textbook on medical parasitology that established his reputation as a malaria expert.[13] He conceived malaria as more than a simple infectious disease for his home country; it was "a social evil." This powerful comment evokes the political and economic connotations that were attached to malaria during the Cold War.[14]

During the malaria eradication campaign, several physicians with a wealth of experience in politics and administration were in charge of the Health Secretariat. The first was Ignacio Morones Prieto, appointed by President Ruíz Cortines, who held the position from December 1952 to November 1958. A native from Linares, Nuevo Leon, Morones Prieto obtained his medical degree from La Sorbonne in Paris when some Mexican physicians still admired French medicine. He returned home to become a professor at the School of Medicine at the University of San Luís Potosí in his home state, and he rose to the rank of president of the university. Later, he was appointed to high positions in the Health Secretariat in Mexico City, such as undersecretary of health during the years 1946–49. He finally made a decisive move into politics, becoming governor of Nuevo Leon from 1949 to 1952.[15] He would play an important role in the Pan-American Sanitary Bureau (PASB) and WHO meetings (e.g., Mexico's World Health Assembly, where he was elected president of the meeting and delivered the opening speech) that sanctioned malaria eradication in Latin America.[16]

In addition to the Health Secretariat, an important Mexican public health organization was the Social Security program (Instituto Mexicano de Seguridad Social), created in 1943 initially in the Federal District.[17] It slowly but steadily extended its activities to other provincial cities. Initially, it provided protection against accidents on the job, pregnancy, illnesses resulting from particular types of employment, and old age. It provided health services for workers with stable jobs, and it constructed and ran hospitals, sanatoriums, pharmacies, laboratories, and rest homes. The Social Security system was reinforced by Ruíz Cortines, who extended the role and network of medical establishments and health services that it regulated, and who also extended the Social Security program to rural workers in 1954.[18] However, during the mid-1950s, more than 70 percent of its beneficiaries lived in the biggest urban centers of the states of Mexico, Nuevo Leon, Jalisco, Puebla, and Tlaxcala.[19]

An enlarged scope for public health and malaria eradication fit the modernization framework initiated by the moderate probusiness Mexican governments of the post–World War II period. President Ruíz Cortines (1953–58) followed the policies of two former presidents, Manuel Avila Camacho and Miguel Alemán.[20] These postwar regimes sought industrial growth through import substitution, foreign investment, mild social reform from above, arbitration in any conflict between unions and industry, and improved diplomatic relations with the United States. An American official publication celebrated President Avila Camacho's inaugural address, in which he stressed that his aim was no longer "Revolution but Evolution."[21] The new social and economic policies contributed to an aura of modernization and to the adjective of "miracle" for the Mexican economy during the years 1945 to 1968. This development was consistent with the modernization model being promoted by U.S. foreign policy, which emphasized the creation of strong links between foreign investment and technology transfer, the promotion of secondary and higher scientific education, and the creation of a technical and managerial professional elite.[22]

Ruíz Cortines—a noncontroversial career civil servant—possessed a reputation as an honest and efficient administrator whose careful, detailed planning contributed to malaria eradication.[23] He joined the Mexican revolution as a civilian and gained experience in federal and state bureaucracies beginning in the mid-1940s. He was minister of the interior under the administration of Alemán. His reputation as a trustworthy and frugal administrator was instrumental for his presidency, due to the fact that accusations of corruption and cronyism had tainted the terms of his predecessors, and because government officers were perceived as inexperienced managers of the large, well-funded irrigation and electricity projects that were common in Mexico after World War II.[24] Shortly after his landslide election victory in 1953, Cortines filed a statement of his net worth, passed an anticorruption law, curbed lavish public spending, taxed luxury goods imports such as automobiles and jewelry, and nationalized a few properties of corrupt government officials.[25]

The decision to allow Acapulco to grow from a small town into a seaside tourist city that attracted a significant number of American visitors was a symbol of Mexican modernization during the 1940s and early 1950s. Also, women were granted the right to vote in elections for the first time, a milestone that was preceded by the recognition of their right to hold elective office. A third symbol of modernization was a bill sent to the Mexican Congress for the creation of a National Nuclear Energy Commission, a decision that was framed with a Cold War goal of the peaceful use of atomic energy. Another important post–World War II development was Mexico's active participation in multilateral agencies. The Mexican government contributed significant sums to the United Nations Children's Fund (UNICEF) and the PASB, and it expected to receive something in return for this support. In fact, the PASB and UNICEF had signed agreements of cooperation with the Mexican government before a malaria eradication agreement was finalized.[26] In negotiating these agreements, the Mexican regimes tried to maximize the benefits they could derive from international and bilateral programs.[27]

Mexican administrations believed that industrialization and substantial economic development required active government intervention in social areas such as public health.[28] The provision of medical assistance in underserved areas by the federal government was an opportunity to address Mexico's uneven development in public health services, such as its reduced number of provincial medical services and the persistence of preventable infectious disease in rural areas. By the early 1950s, the vast majority of Mexican physicians and medical establishments operated in the cities, and less than 15 percent of the rural population received medical attention.

Mimicking the tradition of self-help of American philanthropy established by the Rockefeller Foundation and revived by U.S. bilateral aid, President Ruíz Cortines declared that his government did not intend to maintain assistance to the indigenous communities in a "permanent state," but rather planned to provide the tools and guidance to achieve their integration into the economic and political life of the country as soon as possible.[29] Ruíz Cortines also regarded malaria eradication as a complement to official agricultural policies that, after World War II, concentrated on increasing the productivity of land by making technological improvements.

These policies deemphasized the creation of more *ejidos*—the community land expropriated from large private holdings that were designed in the original agrarian reform of the pre–World War II period as a tool for social justice. In fact, Ruíz Cortines expropriated and transformed fewer hectares of land into *ejidos* than any of his four predecessors.[30] Although he never abolished land reform because land distribution was clothed with revolutionary respectability, the government perceived the individually worked *ejidos,* which could not be mortgaged or sold, as unproductive, inefficient, and marginal to a market economy, and as a burden to the national economy. Moreover, backward systems of farming and the *ejidos* were portrayed as an obstacle to the use of modern machinery and a reason the country needed to import agricultural products. *Ejidal* credit was portrayed as complicated by the small size of the properties and the fact that the parcels were inalienable.[31] According to some contemporary scholars, there was an inherent contradiction between the *ejidos* and the commercial trend of Mexican agriculture promoted by the post–World War II presidential administrations.[32]

Indeed, in 1958, a Mexican Senate Commission that studied the agrarian reform described the situation as chaotic.[33] Post–World War II agricultural policies attempted to create additional arable land through irrigation works because most land suffered from a deficiency of rainfall or an oversupply of moisture, offered preferential credit for commercial crops, and encouraged large-scale agro-export enterprises. In 1954 Ruíz Cortines launched a program called "March to the Seas" with 250 million pesos aimed at moving and resettling millions of Mexicans from the central plateau to the less developed zones along the East and the West coasts.[34] In his first presidential address, he also pledged to supply ample foodstuffs at low prices to the Mexican people and declared war on food speculators. WHO agreed with these policies with the following statement: "The future of Mexico is on the roads to the sea, that is, in highly malarious territory."[35]

The Rockefeller Foundation's Green Revolution, an international project officially called the Mexican Agricultural Program, had been an important ally of Mexican agricultural policies since the 1940s. This project was aimed at research and increasing the production of basic food crops, particularly corn and wheat, through the use of improved seed varieties, fertilizers, and pesticides that operated in Mexico.[36] The foundation also engaged in campaigns against crop and animal diseases that used pesticides and developed rural health work on the side. A number of Mexicans became agricultural or medical experts acquainted with American methods and universities thanks to the training programs of the foundation.[37] A general count for the period 1917–60 gave the sum of 287 Mexican Rockefeller fellows in all fields, representing, after Brazil, the Latin American country that received most awards.[38]

During the 1940s, the Rockefeller Foundation also developed programs against malaria and increased the number of fellowships provided to young Mexican medical doctors who, upon the completion of their studies, returned to their home country to work in public health. In addition, since the early 1940s, the Foundation had paid the salary and laboratory expenses of the renowned physiologist Arturo Rosenblueth at the Instituto Nacional de Cardiología. He was an outstanding Mexican laboratory researcher who had worked at Harvard Medical School for fourteen years before moving to Mexico City.[39] Thanks to Rockefeller support for this and other academic centers, Americanized Mexican medical and scientific elites in agriculture and medicine were in place just before malaria eradication began. Their publications, access to funding, and talent would change the traditional European influence that had marked the development of Mexican medicine during the early twentieth century.

Despite political rivalries and linguistic differences, another example of the close relationship between Mexican and American medical doctors was the United States–Mexico Border Public Health Association, which was created in 1943 during a meeting held in Ciudad Juárez, Chihuahua, Mexico, and shortly thereafter in its twin city in the United States, El Paso, Texas, by medical representatives of the military, federal, state, and local health services of both countries.[40] The association was initially interested in health programs for the protection of U.S. medical personnel who visited Mexico. It's important to underscore that during the 1940s and 1950s, Ciudad Juarez and El Paso were by far, in terms of population, the biggest twin cities on the border between Mexico and the United States, with more than 100,000 inhabitants in the 1940s and 250,000 ten years later.[41] The medical interventions initially envisioned by the association included the treatment of tuberculosis and so-called venereal diseases. After the war, the association expanded its activities to other diseases that were of common interest to inhabitants of both sides of the frontier, such as smallpox, typhus, and malaria. During the following years, including the period of malaria eradication, meetings of this organization took place in the southern United States or in northern Mexico, and the president of the organization was chosen alternately from the United States and Mexico.[42]

Mexicans trained in the United States or institutions that received U.S. backing supported malaria eradication. Some dimensions of the campaign were not included in the initial rationale of eradication but were emphasized by Mexicans. For instance, the justification of the campaign as a means to populate the country was specifically emphasized locally and was aimed at convincing Mexican politicians with Catholic backgrounds who were advocates of high fertility and understood that a dimension of nationalism was to dismiss neo-Malthusian arguments on the dangers of overpopulation in developing countries. A strong government pro-natalist position could be traced to the 1947 General Law of Population, which restricted the sale of contraceptives and made abortion a crime.[43] Mexican public health experts and politicians as well as WHO officers thought malaria eradication would be a tool to alleviate demographic pressure in rural areas. The rationale for their argument was that the lack of space for people to settle in the highlands and the high plateau lands left only two options: a greater division of rural property, which would prevent the use of modern techniques in agriculture, or the creation of new lands thanks to malaria eradication. There was also a concern that after the civil war's violence during the wake of the 1910 Revolution, population growth was urgently needed to recoup population losses.

Mexican civilian politicians perceived malaria eradication as an opportunity to reinforce the subordination of military authorities to civilian governments, and the power of civilian federal authorities over provincial authorities, in which members of the Army were usually prominent. The government's demilitarization, initiated by Avila Camacho, the first postrevolutionary president who had no military background, implied the use of soldiers in public works, as it occurred in the antimalaria campaign. Eradication was designed to reinforce the strong centralized political and administrative Mexican federal system marked by the hegemonic rule of the PRI. The head of the PRI chose his successor and controlled the PRI's candidate lists to the most important offices, including state governors and highranking military appointments.[44]

Malaria eradication had another advantage for politicians. It was a way to reinforce the friendly relations between the Mexican and U.S. governments. Before 1940, wars, land disputes, and oil expropriations led to a tense relationship between the two countries.[45] In 1947, Mexico made a final payment for all outstanding claims related to the oil expropriation measures made by President Cardenas in the late 1930s. During World War II, relations between the two countries improved with the declaration of war on the Axis powers by President Avila Camacho in May 1942, the participation of Mexican aviators with the Allied forces in the South Pacific, a $40 million loan from the United States to complete the Inter-American

Highway, and the establishment of a Mexican-American Commission for Economic Cooperation.

Mexico's economic closeness to the United States continued during the 1950s, when President Ruíz Cortines enacted policies that encouraged U.S. investors and tourists by devaluing the peso and increasing commercial relations. By the mid-1950s, 50 percent of Mexican exports went to the United States, and 80 percent of Mexico's imports came from its northern neighbor. In addition, between 1950 and 1957, the American Export-Import Bank and the World Bank approved loans for $372 million for railroad construction, agricultural development, mining exploration, and electrification projects in Mexico. As a result, the credit standing and foreign investment in Mexico increased dramatically. In 1955, foreign investments totaled $112 million, of which 70 percent came from the United States. Two years later, U.S. investment in Mexico grew to $600 million. Chemical products and drugs, which mostly came from the United States, were the third item on the ranking of Mexican imports for 1955.[46] This meant a significant change from the pre–World War II situation, when German companies such as Bayer, with field offices in Mexico City and Monterrey, dominated the sale of chemicals and pharmaceuticals in Mexico.[47]

According to an article in the *New York Times,* the historical antagonism and "anti-U.S. feeling in Mexico" was easing after a long period of tough sledding and Mexican ministers "in the privacy of their offices expressed their warmest sentiments toward the northern neighbor."[48] The Mexican ambassador to the United States proudly declared in 1954 that relations between the two neighbors "have never been better."[49] President Ruíz Cortines and President Dwight Eisenhower maintained very cordial relations; they met two times, signed important agreements to control illegal fishing in the Gulf of Mexico, and cosponsored the Falcon Dam, a major hydroelectric and irrigation construction project on the lower Rio Bravo, near Laredo, Texas. The project was portrayed as not only important in itself but also as a symbol of how technology and modernity could conquer and utilize nature. A recurrent issue was the pirating by U.S. shrimp boats in Mexican waters. The agreements diminished or eliminated seizure of U.S. vessels by the Mexican Coast Guard, which was usually followed by a negotiation between the two governments. The two countries also tried to regulate an increasingly important problem: the flow of thousands of laborers entering the United States, pejoratively referred to as "wetbacks," who traveled back and forth across the border to work on farms in Texas and California.[50]

The cordial Mexican-U.S. relations continued after Cortines left power in 1958, as suggested by the participation of the U.S. secretary of state, John Foster Dulles, in the inauguration ceremony for the new president, Adolfo López Mateos (1958–64), a forty-eight-year-old lawyer and former minister of labor. Americans celebrated the fact that López Mateos's first cabinet was predominantly made up of experienced "technicians" with experience in administration under the outgoing administration of Ruíz Cortines, rather than political figures. Among the new secretaries were José Alvarez Amézquita and Jaime Torres Bondet, two people with distinguished careers in public office who were in charge of health and education, respectively.[51] Alvarez Amézquita was succeeded by the physician Miguel Bustamante, a graduate of the Johns Hopkins University School of Hygiene and Public Health who was the first Mexican with a Ph.D. in public health and later became president of the National Academy of Medicine.[52]

Although President López Mateos had a leftist inclination, he maintained anticommunist policies and signed more agreements with the United States to control and regulate migrant Mexican agricultural workers. He purged the teachers' union of its communist leaders, and he jailed some prominent members of the Communist Party, such as Demetrio Vallejos, the leader of the railroad workers, and David Siqueiros, the muralist.[53] Partly because of this policy, President López Mateos's honors included receiving an honorary degree from the University of California, once visiting Camp David, and meeting with Presidents Eisenhower, Kennedy, and Johnson six times. In 1963 these meetings resulted in a friendly arrangement on the long-disputed tract of land in El Paso, which had passed from Mexico to the United States after the Rio Grande changed its course. As a result, the Rio Grande became the definitive boundary between the two countries.[54]

The U.S. government was confident that the Mexican government would support the United States if Cold War tensions escalated. Dulles had no doubt that "in any crisis, Mexico would be on our side." In accordance, Ambassador Francis White observed in 1955 that "if the communists should force a showdown with us, Mexico would definitively be on our side."[55] Despite the fact that the small Mexican Communist Party was no threat to the political stability of the country, the Mexican and U.S. governments shared their uneasiness about the local and international menace of communism. Created in 1919, the Mexican Communist Party enjoyed the advantage of being legal, something rare in the region; it was one of four legal communist parties in Latin America. In his 1955 annual report to the nation, Cortines made a specific reference to Mexico's stand against communism. He also removed Narciso Bassols, an influential and well-known leftist and former ambassador to the Soviet Union, from his circle of advisers.[56] Bassols was credited with having played an important role in determining Mexico's abstention at the Inter-American Conference at Caracas, which took place in March 1954, and which validated the overthrow of Arbenz Guzman's regime in Guatemala.[57] In addition, although it was not officially endorsed by the government, in May 1954 a "Congress against Soviet intervention" took place in Mexico City.

Within its inner circle, the U.S. State Department warned vigilance because it believed that Mexican politicians were more "tolerant" of communists than Americans. An illustration of this leeway was the powerful influence of Víctor Lombardo Toledano, a lawyer, teacher, writer, union leader, political activist, head of a Confederation of Latin American Workers, and candidate of the Partido Popular in the elections of 1953. Toledano's political organization, created in the late 1940s, was defined by the State Department as a communist "front" organization, namely, a "fifth column." Toledano was also feared because he supported the Soviet position on international issues of the Cold War and personally admired Joseph Stalin. For Roy R. Rubottom, the U.S. assistant secretary of state for inter-American affairs at the State Department, Toledano was the "number one Communist labor leader" in the region.[58] Toledano was also a concern for PRI politicians, and he began to be stripped of most of his power in the Mexican labor movement during the late 1940s and early 1950s. There was also anxiety in the United States about the Soviet Embassy's influence in Mexico and about the proposals made by some politicians for the nationalization of basic industries owned by foreigners.[59] Anticommunist remarks were subtly used by Fred L. Soper to validate eradication in Mexico. In a 1954 meeting at the State Department, he emphasized that communists in Mexico were still very active and that "the flag of the Soviets" was "the only flag on the bier of Diego de Rivera."[60]

The preoccupation with a possible rapprochement between Mexico and the Soviet Union would continue after Ruíz Cortines left power. In 1959, Anastas I. Mikoyan, the premier of the USSR, visited Mexico for ten days to inaugurate a traveling Soviet industrial exhibition. His visit, which received a great deal of local media attention, included a tour of the steel mills of Monterrey and the government's petroleum industrial complex in southern Mexico. In a television interview, he emphasized that his country was not seeking world domination; on the contrary, it respected the "national sovereignty of each nation." He also discussed the possibilities of Soviet credits and industrial equipment with Mexican government officials.[61]

Occasionally, the Mexican administrations of the 1950s disagreed with U.S. foreign policy on the Cold War; an attitude that contributed to a self-cultivated image of autonomy, nonintervention, and sovereignty. Examples of Mexico's dissension were the cases of Guatemala in 1954 and Cuba in 1960. Mexican administrations initially resisted the immediate condemnation of Guatemala, although they later fell in line with U.S. policy. In the case of revolutionary Cuba, Mexico was against the trade embargo imposed by the U.S. government.[62] The Eisenhower administration tolerated Mexico's occasional defiance and waited patiently for it to reverse its stand. In general, as Niblo has argued, Mexican officials of the post–World War II period undermined their own autonomy from within by following the main U.S. Cold War foreign policy.[63]

The U.S. perception of the Mexican preference for an independent image in international affairs and its tolerance of mild communists had some effect on the style of bilateral cooperation. The State Department was aware that Mexican governments were subject to local pressures to adopt strong nationalistic attitudes and not rely too heavily on foreign aid. This also meant the existence of a proud local political tradition of Mexico solving social problems by itself. Intelligently, the U.S. government believed that this attitude should be respected as such; it appears in a health agreement signed in the early 1950s.[64] The U.S. ambassador in Mexico was urged by the State Department to emphasize "cooperation" and minimize the idea of a foreign-driven "operation" in bilateral programs. The reason for the emphasis was explained: "Communist and anti-American elements . . . seize every opportunity to convince Mexicans that the United States seeks to control and direct" segments of the Mexican national economy.[65]

Mexican Malaria Control

The Mexican health authorities and physicians had studied malaria and established an incipient medical network of public rural institutions before malaria eradication began. Foremost among the official institutions supporting antimalaria work was the already described Secretariat of Health and Welfare. During the late 1940s and early 1950s, two main features of this federal institution were strengthened: its power to enforce its policies in all twenty-nine states, one federal district, and two territories; and the organization of a series of "vertical" campaigns against prevalent infectious diseases such as tuberculosis, leprosy, and oncocercosis.[66] These campaigns received a boost in 1953, when a unit inside the secretariat (the Dirección General de Epidemiología y Campañas Sanitarias) was organized to coordinate these disease-driven efforts. Some states, such as Oaxaca, also organized regional meetings to support malaria control campaigns.[67]

Although the Mexican health care system of the early twentieth century usually focused on the urban population, some work was done in rural areas where malaria was a major concern. Moreover, the concept of eradication was not a complete novelty for the Health Secretariat before malaria eradication. For instance, an active campaign of vaccination in urban and rural areas achieved a victory in 1951 by eliminating smallpox from Mexico. Since 1947 the secretariat combined curative and preventive activities in rural areas by implementing a Board of Rural Hygiene and Social Medicine (Dirección de Higiene Rural y Medicina Social).[68] The board supported a national malaria control program to reduce mosquito-breeding areas in some regions. The tools of these programs were typical of malaria control: draining marshes and filling swamps to eliminate mosquito breeding, spraying larvicides on ponds to kill the mosquito's larvae, distributing antimalaria drugs such as quinine to treat the disease, and equipping houses with screens. Mexico even attempted to cultivate quinine in Chiapas during World War II, when the primary world source of quinine was cut off after the Japanese invasion of the Dutch East Indies.[69]

Before the onset of malaria eradication, the Mexican health authorities were already familiar with DDT, the insecticide that would become the weapon of choice against malaria. Shortly after DDT became available for civilian use, it was used for housefly control in dairy barns around Mexico City in 1944.[70] Between 1945 and 1951, more than 100,000 kilograms of DDT was sprayed against malaria mosquitoes in 358 towns and cities all over Mexico to protect 480,620 inhabitants.[71] DDT's early use in Mexico was partly due to the activities of the Oficina de Especilización Sanitaria, a Mexican health unit in the Health Secretariat organized by the Rockefeller Foundation with the assistance of the U.S. Department of Defense and the U.S. Bureau of Entomology and Plant Quarantine.

The Oficina de Especilización Sanitaria experimented with insecticides in malaria-infested areas, initially in the state of Morelos and later around Mexico City.[72] W. G. Downs, a member of the Rockefeller Foundation's Division of International Health and leader of the oficina, focused the work of the organization around two tasks: determining the best scientific methods to control malaria, and identifying cost-effective programs of malaria control. The preliminary results in Morelos were spectacular. After only one year of spraying, there was a drastic reduction in the number of *Anopheles* in houses and in nearby rice fields.[73] The oficina's trials with DDT in 1949 in Xochimilco, located near Mexico City, were also astounding.[74] After a short campaign in over five thousand houses, the malaria parasitic index was drastically reduced almost to zero.[75] A by-product of Downs's work was that until that date, some physicians questioned the existence of malaria in Mexico City. Downs demonstrated not only that it existed but also that it could be controlled.[76]

Since the late 1940s, DDT was used in several locations, including the northern camps of the national oil company (Petróleos Mexicanos, PEMEX), and a major government development project in the Cuenca del Papaloapan that included areas in the states of Veracruz, Oaxaca, and Puebla with a total population of 1.3 million.[77] These activities continued until the early 1950s, when all malaria control activities began to be coordinated by a National Department for the Control of Paludism, under a Board of Epidemiology and Sanitary Campaigns of the Health Secretariat.

Malaria control and public health activities were also part of the regulated migration from Mexico to the United States. Since 1949, the Mexican health authorities in Ciudad Juárez, the twin city to El Paso, had vaccinated Mexican *braceros* against smallpox and treated them against worms (*parásitos*) as a means of preventing them from being quarantined in isolation in U.S. territory. In addition, U.S. sanitary officers provided new malaria drugs, and when little was known of the toxic effects of the insecticide, DDT was sprayed on these workers (as in Europe, shortly after World War II) before they crossed to the United States. An interesting continuity with the recent worldwide conflict was that the DDT equipment installed in El Paso was a surplus of materials used by the U.S. military during World War II.[78]

These health care and antimalaria activities were discussed by medical associations, meetings, and publications, which debated the advantages and limitations of malaria control or eradication. For example, malaria was a frequent theme in Mexican medical theses and two national malaria congresses were held before the eradication campaign began.[79] Initially, malaria control workers distrusted DDT and were uncertain that the country was ready for a comprehensive eradication campaign. Galo Soberón was an important medical leader who disagreed with eradication. His strong background in malaria education was a result of study at the London Institute of Tropical Medicine and the School of Malariology in Rome after completing medical school in Mexico. Upon his return, he became a professor of parasitology at the National University, a researcher at a new Institute of Tropical Diseases, and an officer in the Health Secretariat. In 1936 he published a classic textbook on malariology.[80] In his capacity as chief of the Medical Section of the antimalaria work of the Health Secretariat in the early 1940s, he promoted a holistic attack on the disease by trying to improve the nutrition, living standards, and lifestyles of rural populations. Although he used DDT and the new antimalaria drugs, he was convinced that these should not be the only methods used against malaria.[81] He believed that urban malaria eradication was feasible, but the elimination of the disease in rural areas was impossible, both in technical and economic terms. In a 1951 publication, he considered "presumptuous" the term "eradication" and concluded that DDT had diverse effects in different areas of Mexico.[82]

Soberón also participated in the elaboration of a 1952 report of the National Commission of Malaria that disagreed with the radical solution of "extirpating from the roots" implied in the term "eradication" and recommended that the word should be used with great caution in public health work. According to the report, it was only possible to eliminate some species of mosquitoes, as Soper demonstrated in the campaign against the *Anopheles gambie* of Brazil. Pessimistic about complete malaria eradication, the authors of the report argued that it was more effective to concentrate on incidence reduction of the disease, or control, rather than eradication.[83]

However, Soberón found few followers. In the early 1950s, Mexican medical doctors gradually became convinced of the limitations of traditional malaria control and that the disease was *the* public health challenge for the country. Malaria control was portrayed as only capable of achieving temporary and specific success, suffering from discontinuity, occasional activities to destroy larvae, insufficient funding, and never being able to reach a national scope.[84] According to a report from Oxaca, malaria control and its results were palliative.[85] A testimony of Soberón's son reveals that in 1956 he disagreed quietly when the growing hegemony of malaria eradication became a dogma for Mexico's medical elite:

My father . . . was convinced that an isolated measure (DDT spraying) would not be effective and that it was necessary to reinforce an antilarva campaign as well as the identification and treatment of cases. However, the political pressure was overwhelming. . . . To rest his conscience he sent a letter to the National Academy of Science where he would state his skepticism. The letter should not be opened until his death.[86]

Two important medical events for the advocates of eradication were the 1953 Spanish publication of a textbook in Mexico by Paul F. Russell, the world's foremost malariologist.[87] A few years later, he also received the rare honor—for a foreigner—of being elected an honorary member of the Mexican National Academy of Medicine, an institution created in the mid–nineteenth century.[88] A second and more crucial event for the victory in Mexico of an eradicationist perspective on malaria was the Eighth World Health Assembly held in 1955 in Mexico City (described in chapter 1). According to an important Mexican health officer who attended the meeting, not only the well-being of "our motherland" relied on the results of malaria eradication in Mexico, but also the immediate future of the campaign in the rest of the world.[89]

By the mid-1950s, malaria eradication was fully endorsed by Mexican political and medical leaders. National and international agencies were confident that Mexico's fight against the disease would accomplish its intended purpose, be regarded by international agencies as a triumph, and set an example for the rest of the world.[90] The Catholic Church also joined malaria eradication. Mexico's archbishop blessed the campaign, announced that he prayed to the Virgin of Guadalupe—Mexico's most popular religious image venerated since the colonial period—for its success, and asked all Mexicans to collaborate with the health authorities.[91] Provincial authorities also joined the optimistic forecast that malaria would disappear.[92]

Organizing Malaria Eradication

In December 1955—a few months after the World Health Assembly was held in Mexico City and three months after UNICEF's board approved its first allocation for Mexico—an agreement for malaria eradication was signed in Mexico. With the characteristics of an international treaty, its chief signatories were Morones Prieto, the health secretary; the lawyer and ambassador Luís Padilla Nervo, the eminent Mexican minister of foreign affairs (who was Mexico's representative to the UN between 1945 and 1952); Maurice Pate of UNICEF; and Carlos Luís Gonzales, a PASB representative.[93] Its blueprint was the so-called Tripartite Plan signed by the PASB, the Mexican government, and UNICEF. The name was partially a misnomer, because an important portion of the funds would come indirectly from U.S. bilateral assistance through UNICEF and the PASB. The contribution of these agencies was conspicuous. The total cost of the campaign was estimated at $36 million, of which the Mexican government would provide $20 million; UNICEF, $10 million; and the PASB, about $1 million.[94] Eventually, UNICEF's contribution exceeded its initial expectation (about $15 million between 1956 and 1963).[95]

Initially, it was expected that the program would last only five years. The year 1956 would be used to test techniques and organize the administration details in a pilot project. Although the total sum of the operation in Mexico might appear impressive, at the time it became another opportunity for the advocates of eradication to establish a contrast with the economic losses produced by malaria. According to a PASB officer, the loss of salaries caused by premature malaria death in rural areas produced an unbearable drain: more than $156.7 million.[96]

The distribution and use of these funds responded to the local tradition of receiving foreign aid on a complementary basis and fit a design elaborated abroad. UNICEF took responsibility for providing equipment, vehicles, and material; the PASB facilitated technical guidance, granted fellowships to study overseas, and organized a Training Center for Malaria Eradication Field Officers in Mexico City; and the Ruíz Cortines administration provided labor and local leadership and enacted appropriate legislation. Consequently, and as part of its contribution, the PASB assigned six technical advisers to malaria eradication and provided nineteen fellowships for training the first cadre of Mexican eradicators in the Venezuelan Maracay School and in a facility of the U.S. Centers for Disease Control and Prevention located in Savannah.

UNICEF's contribution was used for the purchase of vehicles, insecticides, sprayer's equipment, and microscopes.[97] The Mexican government promised to fulfill its financial obligations by using federal and state funds and devoting part of the profits of the lucrative National Lottery. This game—which could be traced to the late colonial period, namely, the 1770s—was controlled by the government and traditionally contributed financially to the construction of hospitals and public health programs.[98] During the years 1955, 1957, and 1958, the share of the Health Secretariat budget devoted to malaria eradication was significant, increasing from 10.6 to 17.5 percent, a portion above any other single health program. This figure was also much higher than the percentage of the health care budget used for malaria control during the period 1951–54 (an annual average of 0.84 percent of the general budget of the Health Secretariat).[99]

The malaria eradication agreement also stipulated that the Mexican government would secure special legislation for the duty-free import of campaign materials and for requiring that political, educational, and health personnel should report "all suspicious fever cases" that might be malaria. A pamphlet explained that a vigorous legislative instrument was necessary because the application of the insecticides and the control of the sick required a drastic intervention in the private lives of citizens—entering their homes to spray and to search for ill people.[100] Namely, the campaign entailed an increased process of medicalization—an expansion of the authority of medical institutions in daily lives and the capacity to control deviance from medical advice.

The Tripartite Agreement was followed by a presidential decree that officially launched the campaign in December 1955. The decree declared malaria eradication a matter of public interest and explained the benefits of eliminating a disease that affected the land where more than half the Mexican population lived. Soper was pleased with these developments. He considered the launching of the Mexican campaign as "undoubtedly one of the most important developments" of the year that "would put pressure on other Latin American countries."[101]

The National Commission for the Eradication of Paludism (Comision Nacional de Erradicación del Paludismo, CNEP) was created a few weeks after the signing of the Tripartite Agreement to carry out the campaign. This new institution replaced the underfunded Department for the Control of Paludism, part of the Board of Epidemiology and Sanitary Campaigns of the Health Secretariat. The new federal health unit was different from other health services of the secretariat. CNEP covered all state entities and enjoyed substantial autonomy under the Public Health Secretariat. It was positioned above the two subsecretariats of the Health Secretariat, which meant that it was only accountable to the secretary of health and to President Ruíz Cortines, who was formally the head of CNEP. As the only health program headed by the president, CNEP was well funded and financially self-sufficient, technically self-contained, and established a rigid hierarchical unit, features considered essential for its efficacy.[102]

A CNEP Executive Board, under the chairmanship of the health secretary, was responsible for general policy and budgetary matters. The board consisted of an executive director, the heads of CNEP's divisions, and representatives of international agencies. The former were all Mexicans and the latter, called "advisers," were foreign, usually Americans. The chief international adviser was Donald J. Pletsch, an expert in entomology from Idaho and director of the PASB office in Mexico.[103] Pletsch had participated before in DDT campaigns for the U.S. Army fighting typhus and malaria in

New Caledonia, the Philippines, and Japan toward the end of World War II. After the War he was employed by the Division of International Health of the U.S. Public Health Service and detached to the International Cooperation Administration. In 1952, he worked for WHO in an international health campaign related to the American political objectives of the Cold War—the control of malaria in Taiwan. After the Chinese revolution of 1949, the pro-U.S. government of the island was recognized by American administrations as the true representative of China, instead of the communist regime of the continent.[104] In 1956, when Pletsch arrived in Mexico, he was regarded not only as a noted international health worker and field malariologist but also as an appropriate leader for the effort. According to one report, he exuded self-confidence and was known as a disciplinarian.[105]

A Mexican executive director, who presided over CNEP's Board, ran the day-to-day operations with the assistance of four staff members called *vocales ejecutivos*.[106] The three main CNEP divisions—administration, operations, and epidemiology—covered specific activities such as training, research, public information, supervision, and logistics. Some years later, CNEP consolidated these functions into four departments, Epidemiology, Field Operations (which included spraying operations), Public Relations (which included training and education of the public), and Administration.[107]

Logistics was entrusted to the army in accordance with the government's intention to make the military an active component of public works. A Mexican general, two colonels, and a group of Army officers worked full time for CNEP training local personnel, drawing detailed maps, and establishing the best routes to reach all villages in the countryside. The Navy cooperated in the spraying operations along the coastal areas.[108] To reinforce the authority of CNEP workers, the defense secretary ordered all provincial military chiefs to fully support the eradication campaign.

The first executive director of CNEP was the bacteriologist José Zozaya, who conducted medical research in nonmalaria fields and directed the Institute of Public Health and Tropical Diseases from 1944 to 1946.[109] He was assisted by Mexican malaria experts such as Manuel B. Márquez Escobedo. When Zozaya experienced an undescribed physical condition that made him unable to take part in the campaign, Márquez Escobedo was immediately appointed "chief administrative officer" of CNEP; but in practical terms, he was the head of CNEP (by 1958, he served as CNEP's director general).[110]

Márquez Escobedo came from a different background than his predecessor. Before becoming head of CNEP, he was director of health for the Federal District, a powerful position in the public health bureaucracy because he administered twenty hospitals and a number of medical and public health centers.[111] These institutions served mostly low-income people of the capital who were not covered by the Social Security program.[112] His leadership style resembled that of Pletsch. A writer described Márquez Escobedo as a "heavy-set, no-nonsense general, who runs the program along semi-military lines."[113] Another important member of CNEP Board was Humberto Romero Alvarez, a Mexican sanitary engineer trained at the University of Michigan, Ann Arbor. Since 1957, he had been chief of spraying operations and, in the early 1960s, he would succeed Márquez Escobedo as head of CNEP.[114]

Another prominent member of the CNEP Board was Luís Vargas. Like Zozaya, he was also a medical investigator, but his research experience was related to malaria. His career symbolized the Americanized Mexican medical scientist distinguished from a former generation of physicians who idealized French medicine. After completing his medical studies at the National University of Mexico City in 1929 with a thesis on malaria, he worked as a researcher at the Hygiene Institute of the Board of Health and attracted the attention of the Rockefeller Foundation fellowship program, which was seeking medical investigators.[115] Being awarded a Rockefeller fellowship enabled him to pursue a master's degree in public health at Johns Hopkins University in the 1930s. Upon his return to Mexico, he worked as an epidemiologist at Downs's Oficina in Morelos, and Vargas studied for a master's degree in biology at the National University. From the 1940s, his interests were concentrated in entomology and on the Mexican *Anopheles*. His commitment to the challenging subdiscipline that studied the malaria vector was revealed when he wrote: "The study of *Anopheles* in Mexico is difficult but fascinating."[116] It is important to note that Vargas underscored the presence of malaria on the Mexico–United States border in an article that was published in a WHO journal a few years before malaria eradication began.[117]

In 1950, when Vargas was head of the Laboratory of Entomology of the Institute of Tropical Diseases, he published a comprehensive study on Mexican *Anopheles* that identified the two main vectors of malaria in the country, *A. pseudopunctipennis* and *A. albimanus*. His study replicated what Russell had done with mosquitoes for the whole world some years before. Vargas admired Russell and was the translator of his main textbook.[118] Vargas's and Russell's works would be widely distributed among Mexican and Latin American health authorities. Vargas's publications in mainstream journals made him the most noted entomologist of CNEP.[119] In 1956 he became director of CNEP's influential Office of Supervision and would remain in that position until 1962, when he became chief of CNEP's Office of Special Studies.

Soper was slightly displeased with the research focus of Mexican eradicators. In a 1956 comment that was surely aimed at Vargas, Zozaya, and the Rockefeller Foundation studies of the 1940s, the PASB director complained that "Mexicans have not yet gotten the idea regarding the eradication of malaria. . . . They are more interested in investigations and studies than they are in antimosquito measures. Experimental therapy is also a predilection."[120] This comment reflected the beginning of a dispute between those who paid more attention to research and supervision, a position that would become stronger in Geneva's WHO, and others who, like Soper, emphasized practical interventions. Soper's position would eventually prevail in the Mexico of the late 1950s. For example, when the four CNEP departments were created, the originally established research board disappeared.[121]

To organize its activities, CNEP divided the whole country in fourteen zones, which were broken down into sectors with a chief for every five sectors.[122] These zones reported directly to CNEP's headquarter in Mexico City, in contrast to the practice of other medical services that reported first to regional health authorities. By 1956, a total of 118 sectors and 567 areas of work had been established, and more than 2,000 health workers were ready to carry out eradication.[123]

An illustration of the characteristics of the fourteen zones and their relationship with number of sprayers and houses during the campaign appears in table 3.1.

After health engineers, entomologists, epidemiologists, and chiefs of fumigation operations, there were a number of clerks, drivers, and sprayers occupying the lower rungs of the staff hierarchy for each zone. Brigades consisted of one chief inspector and four inspectors or sprayers. Each sprayer had to carry with him 15 kilograms of spraying equipment, which included a hand compression sprayer and a suspension of water-dispersible DDT powder. A fashionable and celebrated specialist headed each zone: the malariologist. He coordinated his activities with local governors, medical practitioners, schoolteachers, and local newspapers.

This was the job of a sixty-year-old medical doctor, Gustavo García Carrasco, the head of a zone that included the predominantly indigenous State of Oaxaca, which with its over 35,000 square miles represented the sixth place in the country in terms of territory, with its capital, Oaxaca, located some 310 miles southeast of Mexico City. Born and raised in the city of Oaxaca, he studied medicine at the University of the State and had worked

Table 3.1. Fourteen Working Areas of the Comisión Nacional de Erradicación del Paludismo

Zone	Headquarters	Territory	Number of Inhabitants	Number of Sprayers	Houses Visited
I	Mérida, Yucatán	State of Yucatán, 7 municipalities of Campeche, territory of Quintana Roo	805,438	141	159,687
II	Villa Hermosa, Tabasco	State of Tabasco, 24 municipalities of the State of Chiapas, 2 from Campeche, 20 from the south of the State of Veracruz	881,483	172	193,717
III	Veracruz, Veracruz	The central part of the State of Veracruz, 6 municipalities of the southwest of the State of Puebla, the municipality of Tuxtepec	1,767,521	323	431,811
IV	Tuxtla Gutiérrez, Chiapas	The State of Chiapas with the exception of 24 municipalities of the north that depend on Zone II	859,531	173	196,090
V	Oaxaca, Oaxaca	The State of Oaxaca, with the exception of Tuxtepec, Putla, and Jimiltepec, which belong the first to Zone III and the last two to Zone IX	1,139,311	211	276,437
VI	Ciudad De Valles, San Luís Potosí	The States of San Luís Potosí, Querétaro, and Hidalgo and 30 municipalities of the State of Veracruz	1,160,613	208	269,998
VII	Cd. Victoria, Tamaulipas	The States of Tamaulipas, Nuevo León, and Coahuila	1,508,674	161	254,817

VIII	Puebla, Puebla	The State of Puebla, with the exception of the 6 municipalities of the southwest that belong to Zone III; the States of Guerrero and México, with the exception of the 7 municipalities that belong to Zone X; the State of Tlaxcala and the Distrito Federal	1,005,055	183	240,189
IX	Chilpancingo, Guerrero	The State of Guerrero, with the exception of the 9 municipalities that are part of Zone VIII: 2 municipalities of the State of Oaxaca	1,145,309	208	252,212
X	Morelia, Michoacan	The States of Michoacán and Guanajuato and 22 municipalities of the State of Mexico and two of the State of Jalisco	1,707,921	214	315,828
XI	Guadalajara, Jalisco	The States of Colima, Jalisco, and Nayarit, with the exception of the Jalisco municipalities, situated on the east side of the Santiago River	2,100,849	378	412,719
XII	Aguas-calientes, Aguas-calientes	The States of Aguascalientes and Zacatecas, plus the municipalities of Jalisco located north of the Santiago River	944,453	93	105,576
XIII	Culiacán, Sinaloa	The States of Sinaloa and Durango and those that belong to the south of Baja California and 5 of the State of Chihuahua	1,202,945	163	190,648
XIV	Hermosillo, Sonora	The States of Sonora, Chihuahua, except 5 municipalities that belong to Zone XIII and Baja California Norte	487,954	61	61,700
Total			16,717,057	2,689	3,361,429

Sources: Luís Vargas and Arturo Amaraz Ugalde, "Observaciones sobre la epidemiología del paludismo en México," Salud Pública Mexicana 5 (January–March 1963): 39–51 (the citation here is on 50); and "Integración de sectores y brigadas según medio de transporte, segundo semestre de 1959, 10 de Diciembre de 1959," fondo Secretaría de Salubridad y Asistencia, sección Comisión Nacional de Erradicación del Paludismo, serie Dirección, caja 44, expediente 4.

for the State's Board of Health since the mid-1930s. First, he was chief of the Centers of Hygiene of Villa Hermosa, Tabasco, and Tlapa, working on the control of infectious diseases, mainly smallpox. Due to his efficiency, he received a fellowship for an epidemiology training course in Mexico City. Upon completing his postgraduate studies, he returned to Oaxaca, where he concentrated on smallpox and typhus in the Mixteca region, which covered about a third of the state of Oaxaca, and was marked by dispersed communities that did not receive adequate medical services. He received a Mexican fellowship to study in the School of Maracay, the prestigious antimalaria center in Venezuela. He returned to his home country with the prestigious title of malariologist and worked between 1949 and 1955 in malaria control in the indigenous zones of Chiapas and Tampico. In December 1955, he attained the apex of his career when he was appointed head of CNEP Zone V.[124] As the case of García shows, it was pivotal for the campaign to recruit personnel locally and to train them in Mexico City or abroad. During the period 1955–58, the antimalaria training program trained about fourteen thousand health workers from the capital of the country and from the different malaria zones of the country.[125]

A sympathetic description of the twenty-three-year-old sprayer Pedro Rivas Sosa from Santiago, Tuxtla, illustrates the routine and describes the economic motivations of a health worker who was in the lower ranks of CNEP:

> He liked the job not only because of its importance to the Republic, but because as a member of the staff of CNEP he receives his payment on time. He arrives at the commission headquarters in Tuxtla at seven-thirty each morning, spends half an hour checking his equipment and going over the maps of the territory to be worked in that day with the Chief of brigade, and by eight he is in a Dodge pickup heading for the fields. He works spraying until four in the afternoon . . . and then returns to headquarters, where he spends another hour cleaning his pump and storing DDT into small sacks to be used the next day. . . . He was paid fifteen pesos a day [$1.25], the same amount that he would make on construction work.[126]

The year 1956 was devoted to the organization, training, and equipment of 2,312 sprayers organized in 539 brigades, and to the preparation of 633 vehicles, including jeeps, trucks, six light planes, and boats with an additional 2,000 horses and mules.[127] In the following years, the staff of CNEP would grow significantly; by 1957 it was 3,993, of which 77 percent were sprayers or chiefs of a brigade.[128] They were full-time workers in rural areas, an unusual occurrence in Mexican public health agencies that used to hire personnel who would work mostly in offices located in urban centers. CNEP members' conviction and enthusiasm were remarkable. A Mexican health officer announced with confidence: "If in five years there is but one case of malaria in Mexico we will have failed."[129]

According to an observer of CNEP at the beginning of the campaign, the human and technical resources devoted to malaria eradication were outstanding. His comment also suggests that the upper rank of the bureaucracy received salaries that were higher than those received by inferior health workers: "The administrative facilities are particularly striking. It is always difficult for a government to make a special case for one of the government branches and yet in Mexico the employees of the Malaria Eradication Campaign are getting salaries from 50% to 100% higher than the salaries paid to the employees of other public health branches."[130] In the long run, these and other privileges were counterproductive because they augmented the envy of other health personnel and reinforced the perception that the malaria service enjoyed too much autonomy.

Thanks to UNICEF, during the first months of 1956, eradication equipment was brought into the country and distributed to the points of use. At the same time, CNEP local personnel were recruited and trained. On September 7, 1956, the "initial phase" or pilot program of field-spraying operations began and continued for three months with the hopes of launching a national operation in the following year. During those last months of 1956, 478,871 houses were sprayed in all fourteen zones by motorized, mounted, and mixed (motorized and waterway) brigades. They used about 500,000 pounds of DDT and 15,099 pounds of Dieldrin. The latter more powerful insecticide was especially suited for remote zones where it would be difficult to carry out biannual spraying campaigns.[131] Brigades were required to list and number all houses, fix itineraries, draw maps, and have them codified by specialists.

Two important unexpected difficulties came to light as a result of the pilot program: The total number of houses that had to be visited, numbered, and mapped was slightly higher than expected. Furthermore, it was difficult to establish a definitive "malarious area" because in some places, the disease appeared at different periods of the year and the common practice of self-treatment destroyed evidence of the disease in the blood of individuals. Despite these problems, which would increase in the following years,

Mexican agencies and UNICEF firmly decided to move along with the national campaign, hoping to adjust estimates and solve any problems during 1957.[132] After the pilot project, the Mexican government was enthusiastic about eradication and received numerous complimentary telegrams, letters of gratitude, and exotic proposals from its citizens such as adding homemade magical drugs.[133] In January 1957, CNEP health workers began the gargantuan campaign by spraying more than 3 million houses in Mexico. Although this was an impressive figure, it was short of the ideal that was established initially of 3,370,096 houses.

CNEP carried out eradication with a military-style exactness, with clear chains of command and overconfidence on technological solutions that replicated patterns of mosquito-born disease containment rooted in the early twentieth century, such as the work against the *Aedes aegypti* mosquito of yellow fever.[134] However, there were several important differences. Whereas before, the destruction of mosquito larvae breeding sites was limited to urban centers and the main rural towns, in malaria eradication, the scope was national because of the assumption that all rural houses should be sprayed, and only adult mosquitoes were targeted by the campaign. In addition, malaria eradication established carefully detailed plans that gave a sensation of security. CNEP's plan followed WHO's four-stage design. In Mexico, the timeline was as follows: 1956 for the "preparation" stage, 1957–60 for the "attack" stage, 1961–63 for the "consolidation" stage, and 1964 and onward for the "conservation" stage. If no malaria cases were reported after three years, the disease would be considered permanently eliminated.[135]

The detail was extensive; estimates for each sprayer's daily chores neared 8.6 houses, and the average subsequently increased. The use of DDT was regarded relatively easy because it was used as a powdery water emulsion that could be transported by a health worker and prepared shortly before spraying.[136] During the second year of the campaign, 1958, fumigation reached 3,827,642 houses, and 3,503,297 houses the following year. By then, the number of CNEP personnel also grew to 4,000, of which 2,852 were sprayers or chiefs of brigade.[137] In a confusing statement, a CNEP pamphlet announced that the countrywide project would kill all *Anopheline* mosquitoes within five years, thus halting the transmission of malaria and eradicating the disease from Mexico. The idea was repeated in headlines of provincial newspapers.[138] The statement caused confusion, because the deadline was postponed several times and because the goal changed from the elimination of the mosquito to the elimination of the *Plasmodium,* an important difference that will reappear later in this book.[139]

The CNEP example in Mexico was promptly followed in many of the twenty Latin American republics infected with malaria. By the end of 1957, two countries had eradicated the disease (Chile and the United States), eighteen had begun eradication campaigns (Argentina, Brazil, Ecuador, El Salvador, Guatemala, Haiti, Honduras, Mexico, Dominican Republic, and Venezuela), three had completed plans for converting control malaria projects to eradication programs (Nicaragua, Panama, and Paraguay), and five were considering how to transform their control programs into an eradication campaign (Bolivia, Colombia, Costa Rica, Cuba, and Peru).[140] In the Caribbean, five of the sixteen originally infected islands had eradicated malaria, and malaria eradication was either under way or planned in many other countries.

Mexico's leading role in these efforts is revealed by the fact that between 1957 and 1962, five hundred Latin American malaria eradicators were trained in Mexico, thanks mainly to Pan-American Sanitary Bureau fellowships.[141] As a result, Mexico became, along with Venezuela, the Latin American educational center for malaria eradication. There were two types of training in Mexico. Medical doctors and engineers received a special course of twelve-week duration that included biomedical and epidemiological principles on malaria, and the chief of a sector and of brigades attended more practical and shorter courses that emphasized the adequate use of techniques.

By the early 1960s, CNEP's work in Mexico proved impressive. Between 1957 and 1962, sprayers visited more than 4 million houses, more than 27.2 million spraying operations were carried out, a little more than 6 million blood samples were taken, and 11.2 million pills of antimalaria drugs were used.[142] In the short term, malaria eradication yielded almost immediately an impressive positive impact. During the early 1960s, malaria almost disappeared from the urban areas in Mexico, and the number of deaths caused by the disease was drastically reduced. The campaign freed several areas from the disease such as the cities of Veracruz, Acapulco, and Guadalajara, most of the Gulf of Mexico coast, and the northern area of the country. Another indirect benefit of the campaign was the decrease of dengue and yellow fever transmitted by *Aedes aegypti,* killed by the insecticides because it was a more vulnerable mosquito than the *Anopheles* that liked to live near human beings.[143] The fact that fewer people died of malaria was indeed a remarkable achievement.

Malaria eradication's impact on malaria morbidity is suggested by the official figures, which contrasted a rate of 136.7 per 100,000 inhabitants in

1955 (or 40,591 cases) with the lower rate of 10.2 in 1960 (3,665 cases).[144] In terms of the blood exams, the decline was even more acute. In 1956, 10.09 percent of the blood examined was positive. In 1957, only 3.21 percent was positive; and in 1958, only 0.77. The downward trend continued during the first six months of 1959—to 0.44 percent.[145] By 1960, the fourth year of the campaign, the Mexican authorities suspended partially spraying in thirteen of the fourteen zones under the assumption that eradication was near. Newspapers celebrated the "life-saving intervention" that avoided the death of about "26,000 Mexicans" and spared 600 million pesos of federal resources.[146]

However, these figures should be viewed with caution because methods of diagnosis changed before and after the campaign was launched. Since 1957, laboratory confirmed cases have been considered as malaria cases, whereas before that year, malaria was diagnosed by clinical symptoms, mainly recurrent fever. It seems plausible that although clinical diagnosis and clinicians overstated malaria figures before eradication, after 1957 many malaria cases escaped confirmation because the laboratory facilities were insufficient. Although the U.S. *Manual for the Microscopical Diagnosis of Malaria in Man* was widely distributed, CNEP could not fully implement laboratory facilities and a surveillance system based on blood tests.[147] An indirect proof of the insufficiency of medical registration appeared in 1963, when a health officer admitted that only 50 percent of all death registries in the country were done by physicians and the remaining 50 percent were still done by civil judicial authorities, which in the rural areas "had no capacity to judge the causes of death."[148]

A more serious issue was that the campaign of malaria eradication resulted in diverse regional patterns of results. After the initial spraying operations, the disease was absent in the North but persisted in the South. These patterns paralleled developments in agriculture: Export agriculture and the large landowners of the North made impressive gains, but "primitive" agriculture resisted market pressures. It proved more difficult to eliminate malaria in poor southern indigenous areas such as Oaxaca, Chiapas, and Guerrero—with a territory that was 100 percent considered malarious in 1956—where 75 percent of the population was rural, living standards were low, and commercial agriculture made little progress.[149] As late as 1971, Guerrero reported 8,194 cases of malaria, of which an undetermined proportion were caused by the deadlier *P. falciparum*.[150]

An additional difficulty was that, during its initial years, international and Mexican agencies generated the impression that the main urgency was additional funding and deemphasized research or an examination of the first obstacles that appeared for achieving success. The idea of the need for more funds framed the negotiations between the Mexican government and the donor agencies. For example, an "informal" conversation between Morones Prieto and a PASB officer regarding the "possible contribution" of Mexico to the special malaria eradication fund of the PASB, held in the initial years of the eradication campaign, presented the Mexican secretary of health as a shrewd negotiator. The conversation was narrated by the PASB officer in a confidential letter:

> Dr. Morones Prieto . . . told me that the government of Mexico has received a request from UNICEF to contribute $500,000 for 1958, which represents a substantial increase over the $300,000 that Mexico gave to UNICEF in 1957. After a number of considerations, Dr. Morones told me that, subject to the approval of the President of the Republic, he was prepared to recommend that PASB receive a contribution of $250,000 for 1958, leaving the door open to obtain $500,000 in 1959, which of course would be subject to the approval of the next administration. Dr. Morones was very insistent that this conversation was entirely private and confidential.[151]

Negotiations for additional funds were linked with an "extension" of the Tripartite Agreement that was signed in 1961, when it became clear that the original deadline was unachievable. The so-called problem areas persisted in about 18 percent of the areas previously sprayed, in spite of the use of orthodox techniques. Finally, a new plan and deadline were created in 1961, in which the years 1961–63 would be devoted to eliminating the "problems areas." In 1964 and 1965, active vigilance would confirm the success of the campaign. In addition, the identification of malaria cases was actively sought in all locations, and blood smears were taken in all febrile cases. The cost of the extension was estimated to be 255 million pesos, of which the Mexican government would provide about 60 percent. UNICEF and the PASB agreed with the proposal.[152] Despite the trouble, most health workers and authorities were enthusiastic according to the editorial in a bulletin of the indigenous state of Guerrero published in 1961: "Malaria is ending, an unquestionable truth that must be underlined and announced."[153]

However, before conducting a detailed examination of the final result of the campaign, it is important to first explore how it was embraced at the local level.

The Mexicanization of the Campaign

Mexican and international health authorities oversold the benefits of eradication to secure public support by using various forms of propaganda. The campaign transcended its technical scope, became part of the official "nationalistic" discourse, and even established a relationship with popular culture. According to a 1960 report, 11,167 copies of a comic book, 9,800 copies of the poster titled "Just a Drop of Blood," and 13,250 copies of two more posters were distributed in all malaria zones.[154] The interweaving of propaganda and health education in Mexico could be traced to projects of the 1930s directed by the Health Secretariat and the Secretariat of Education (Secretaría de Educación Pública, SEP) that trained rural teachers working among indigenous populations.[155] This work was also related to the impressive growth of rural schools and the promotion of a "socialist" education in Mexico in the 1930s. A total of 309 rural schools existed in 1922; the number rose to 10,161 in 1935; and the trend continued in 1947, with 13,700, and in 1952, with 16,054.[156] By the 1940s, the goal of educational and health projects in rural areas was to "civilize" and "incorporate" peasants who lived in a subsistence economy into the rest of society. A growing assumption among state officers was that public health and rural education should work together. Moreover, since the revolution, there had been a tradition of portraying rural teachers and physicians as central agents in modernizing the countryside. According to an official publication that celebrated the agrarian reform as one of the main achievements of the 1910 Revolution, "If the future of the motherland . . . is in the hands of the peasant, the future of the peasant is in the hands of schoolteachers and rural medical doctors."[157] By the early 1950s, SEP's unit of school hygiene distributed basic information on child illnesses, administered a few dispensaries, coordinated the visits of physicians to schools, and trained professors in smallpox vaccination.[158]

In 1956, SEP signed an agreement with the Health Secretariat to instruct teachers on how to educate their students and their families about the benefits of the campaign, provide geographical information for spraying operations, identify fever cases, and take blood films.[159] The assistance received by CNEP was crucial because schoolteachers were the largest workforce in the public sector and frequently the only public officers in remote rural villages by the mid–twentieth century. According to an estimate, 150,000 teachers reached about 5 million students and were in contact with

2 million parents. This meant that SEP was a sort of intermediary between the state and about a fifth of the national population.[160]

The combination of educational and health efforts was also a central theme for CNEP propaganda. A poster portrayed a sleepy-headed child in a classroom above the caption: "Students who are sick with malaria do not benefit from schooling." Another antimalaria poster was titled "The Children Are the Hope of Mexico."[161] The caption of an illustration's pamphlet published anticipated any irrational "superstitious" indigenous explanation for the transmission of the disease, stressing scientific authority: Malaria was "only" transmitted by the *Anopheles;* "any other explanation" was "false."[162] Special materials were prepared for rural schools, such as calendars and notebooks with drawings of health workers spraying insecticides.[163] Imaginative schoolteachers organized local contests for the best antimalaria poster, poem, or anthem, and prepared exercises on malaria like drawings of *Anopheles.*[164] Some even went beyond CNEP's mandate and tried to initiate a general sanitation campaign. For example, a letter addressed by the school inspector from Cuicatlan, Oaxaca, to the health secretary, demanded materials for a general campaign of hygiene in rural communities that would encompass malaria eradication but include the control of other diseases.[165]

Initially, CNEP's educational work was carried out by a Health Education Division, which had the following goals: obtaining "active participation" in the campaign of local "key people," such as political authorities, health personnel, schoolteachers, priests, journalists, and administrators of rural estates; and informing or "sensitizing" the public (*sensibilizar*) to gain its acquiescence to spraying and blood sampling.[166] The division also had to report those families that had resisted spraying. In addition to posters and pamphlets, the CNEP Educational Division designed pins, radio spots, leaflets, pamphlets, lantern slides, sonograms, short motion pictures, newspaper articles, and television programs. National cinema stars, such as the comedian Mario Moreno ("Cantiflas")—who represented a smart but impoverished peasant-slumdweller who overcame the challenges of the city and became a symbol for Mexico's popular culture—were recruited to support CNEP's propaganda activities.[167]

In some non-Spanish-speaking regions, bilingual pamphlets were produced. Three audiovisual mobile units performed important work for CNEP in illiterate areas.[168] According to the census of 1960, 37 percent of the national population was illiterate, and the proportion in rural areas reached

52 percent.[169] The use of radio occurred during a period of growth of the Mexican radio industry and of regional broadcasters who repeated programs designed in the capital. The number of commercial radio stations increased from 201 in 1951 to 332 in 1959, while the number of radio receivers grew from more than 2 million in 1952 to more than 3 million in the late 1950s.[170] The campaign's use of films was decisive in the countryside, which built upon the nation's tradition of popular films that were supported by the state and consumed by Mexicans. By the mid-1950s, Mexico produced about one hundred films a year.[171] Films in illiterate areas became powerful means of propaganda, even in remote villages. According to some accounts, movie theaters existed in even the smallest provincial towns, or a screen was usually improvised outdoors to watch films.[172]

A newspaper article from Tabasco celebrated CNEP's propaganda materials because it was carefully crafted as "in the best commercial ads," using phrases that created curiosity, "enthusiasm, and cooperation" in short "convincing hooks."[173] After a few years, these appealing materials caught the attention of different countries, and CNEP received requests for posters and pamphlets from all over the world.

The content of propaganda material matched its volume. Drawings used in posters and pamphlets were done by the excellent artists from the National Lottery, the same institution that provided part of the funding for the campaign.[174] The first 100,000 CNEP pamphlets presented a pathetic figure of a sick Mexican child above a clear message: "Let's finish with *paludism*."[175] Poster slogans also underscored modernization and communal responsibility, such as "National Prosperity without Malaria" and "All [Houses] Must Be Sprayed."[176] Some posters indicated how common people should welcome the sprayers, allow them to spray DDT indoors, signal those who were ill with fevers, and exhibit with pride pins and marks attesting that their houses had been sprayed.[177] Subsequently, posters used messages that strongly appealed to family and nationalist sentiments. For example, the poster "I Am a Patriot" was to be distributed to people whose houses had been sprayed.

The slogans of other posters resonated with the military metaphors typical of international health cooperation during the first decades of the twentieth century: "Paludism Kills, War to Paludism" and "War against Malaria is for Mexico." A reiteration of military euphemisms was explained by a CNEP officer sent to a province, who said that there was a need to unite the whole country because it was in a new kind of war and "the enemy" was malaria.[178] Another pamphlet called on citizens to "expel" the "enemy" from Mexican soil. The cover of a pamphlet gave a new meaning to the term; the "enemy" was not only the mosquito but any person unwilling to allow his or her house to be sprayed.[179] The persistent use of the term "enemy" in CNEP propaganda reveals that military euphemisms were combined with Cold War anxieties. State Department officials also feared that communism could be harbored by apparently "freedom-loving" citizens. Edmund Russell, a historian, studied campaigns of pesticides before and during World War II that interwove public health technology and war euphemisms.[180]

Cold War metaphors and enthusiasms were shared by an American nurse who participated in the campaign in a semitropical small town in Oaxaca. Her comments suggest that some health workers gave their own interpretation to these euphemisms:

> What an exciting fight this could be! To liberate an entire country from malaria! Cold war, hot wars were far away from the U.S. here in the open classroom in Guelatao. This would be our war, a fight to finish war, a constructive war where enemy germs were killed. This was the kind of war to which I could give myself wholeheartedly.[181]

Cold War anxieties were entwined with the entrenched official nationalism that hearkened back to the 1910 Revolution. After 1940, nationalism shed its more militant and anticlerical features in favor of a mild version of populism, a uniformed ethnic mix, and the transformation of rural cultural traits into "folklore" or a tamed and minor subculture of an ideal national identity. The new features validated the state-building efforts of the post–World War II conservative regimes that promoted orderly nonviolent social progress and the assimilation of the indigenous population into the mainstream of Mexican culture and society. Official nationalism emphasized national unity based on the dissolution of what was a multicultural society. Ethnic diversity should undergo a process of cultural homogenization assisted by educational and health services. Inspired by the ideas of José Vasconcelos, a noted intellectual and president of the Mexican Institute of Hispanic Culture in 1948, and by other Mexican intellectuals, the image of an ideal mestizo, the result of a Mexican melting pot, was constructed as the symbol of a full new "race" rather than as a hybrid between Europeans and native Indians.

The practical implementation of the mild official nationalism of the 1950s meant the assimilation of peasants through their participation in the market economy and in health and monolingual educational programs.[182] Radio, television, and school texts carried nationalistic messages that tried to make "citizens" out of peasants and members of indigenous communities.[183] The inauguration of the National Museum of Anthropology, which occurred a few years after malaria eradication was under way, glorified indigenous achievements of the pre-Columbian era but encapsulated ethnic diversity into common national bonds obliterating multiculturalism and social inequalities. The celebration of pre-Columbian cultural achievements was taken as a preamble for the creation of new mestizo identities for the descendants of these cultures.[184]

CNEP's propaganda combined official nationalism with prescribed gender roles and with the traditional glorification of mothers common in predominantly Catholic societies. A poster presented a defiant woman with the caption: "In Defense of My Homeland, in Defense of My Children, War on Malaria."[185] In other instances, women were portrayed as a critical human resource for malaria eradication due to the fact that the first health care providers in poor rural areas were usually mothers. In an article, a female health worker announced her readiness to fight for her beloved family because she already had firsthand experience with malaria. The disease was especially dangerous for pregnant women and children, who were more likely to die than men if they received no prompt attention. The medical use of nationalism also idealized pro-natalist policies.[186] A pamphlet titled *More Mexicans, Better Mexicans* dismissed the concern with overpopulation and underscored the population goals of the Mexican government—to increase the population of the country to have a larger and healthier workforce. According to the publication, a healthier Mexican meant a more capable citizen, a "master of his fate."[187] As a result, malaria eradication was portrayed as an instrument not only for improving the economy and standards of living but also for improving the lot of the Mexican population.[188] According to a pamphlet that asked Mexicans to participate actively in the campaign, malaria eradication was an act of individual, familial, and social "redemption."[189]

The propaganda of malaria eradication also stressed the need for an integral national development aimed at modernizing the poorest regions of the country. The campaign appeared as a technological solution to social backwardness. A newspaper article targeted for "readers of the southeast" of the country underlined regional differences by describing the pathetic situation of peasants who were unable to work their land because of the shaking fevers of malaria. The author wrote, "It is rightly said that while the north works, the southeast sleeps. . . . It is true it sleeps too much, not because it is lazy but because the illness forces him to sleep. . . . By finishing with paludism, the southeast will wake up from its lethargy."[190]

The most fascinating educational materials of the campaign were the free, monthly, usually poor-quality bulletins from some of the fourteen different campaign zones.[191] They introduced the voices of local health workers in official sanitary discourse and contributed to popular metaphors that facilitated popular consent for a state-driven campaign. Originally, CNEP envisioned two types of bulletins, a one-page monthly magazine to indoctrinate the public, and a four-page publication to educate CNEP health workers. The latter would provide instructions on how to request permission from householders, spray their premises, and find possible malaria cases. It will also praise the work of the best health workers. According to official directives, the bulletins could include "humoristic" notes "of good taste." However, the last recommendation was not easy to follow, and authors occasionally used the bulletins to criticize local characters, something that was considered "offensive" by CNEP headquarters.[192]

Eventually, the bulletins took a life of their own and were appropriated by local health workers. Only one type of bulletin was published per zone, combining information for the public and for health workers. Most carried ingenious names, such as *El Chamula,* a name generally given to indigenous people and the name of a town. This was a smart move in a region like Chiapas, home to a large indigenous population and with the third highest rate of malaria mortality among Mexican states, after Oaxaca and Tabasco. In addition, *El Transmisor* alluded to mosquitoes, and *La Cotorra* referred not only to the distinctive crested bird but also to a person who echoes another's words.[193]

The bulletins helped unite, discipline, and give a midterm vision to health workers. According to an article in *La Cotorra,* a "sound morale" was absolutely necessary for each health worker to "feel responsible for their work." Likewise, CNEP advised its sprayers and field officers to behave properly when entering a home and respect their "fellow citizens," because this was the most effective tool to create the much-needed trust and friendship in "the great Mexican family."[194] The bulletins also reinforced the self-esteem of health workers. An editorial titled "Pillar and Giant in the Program" worshiped sprayers as heroes who reached the remotest regions, defying sun and rain with the sole objective of spraying all houses (figure 3.1).[195]

Some publications revealed that local health workers maintained an awareness of subtle ethnic and social differences. For instance, a poem

Figure 3.1. *In the mountains, a pony is better than a jeep. This man looks at home in the saddle, his spraying equipment beside him (1968).*

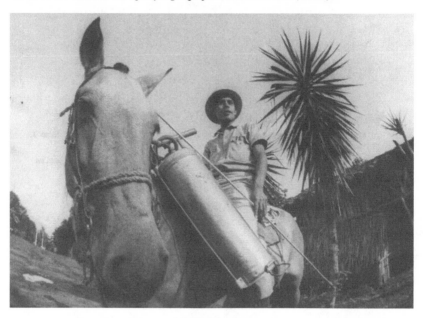

Source: Photograph by Peter Larsen. Courtesy of the World Health Organization Archives.

narrated how a rich señor watched impassively as people in his town died of malaria. His indifference was castigated by a mosquito bite, an outcome that suggested the socially equalizing effects of malaria.[196] According to an editorial in *La Cotorra,* published in the mainly indigenous state of Guerrero, urban and rural people had different perceptions of the disease:

> Perhaps these figures [figures of malaria cases] do not mean anything important to the people of large cities in the nation, but they remind us of dramatic nights in fever, watching the slow end of a child, a wife, or a sibling's life in the hot, dusty, peasant, lands of Veracruz, Chiapas, [and] *Lacandona* forest. . . . They remind us of the misery of households due to the lack of a salary not earned because of disease.[197]

The *Lacandona* people in the state of Chiapas were portrayed as alien from the rest of the country, partially because connecting roads were completed in the early 1950s. According to a study, they were a "tribal group," illiterate, monolingual, with no official services, and living on subsistence agriculture in isolated and scattered huts on common lands where even *ejidos* were nonexistent.[198] The apprehension toward *Lacandona* people appeared in article in the *New York Times* that described them as primitive: "[They] still hunt and fish with bows and arrows and worship their ancient gods."[199]

An important persuasion gimmick used in the bulletins was the rewriting of the lyrics of popular songs and poems that alluded to hygiene. Bulletins included new lyrics for popular *corridos,* a type of Mexican ballad, usually linking daily life with malaria eradication activities. For example *"Corrido a la CNEP"* praised nationalism and prosperity and ended with "death to paludism, death to paludism/and long live my motherland!"[200] The lyrics of another *corrido* by Antonio Bautista y López made an intriguing metaphor between the mosquitoes and the government, and celebrated insecticide spraying:

The *Anopheline* mosquito
ruled more than the government
Its laws, a disaster
made by judges in hell

. . .

¡How beautiful is the spraying!
with DDT or Dieldrin

. . .

Millions of Mexicans
of the paludic zones
have been saved from the *Arcano*[201]
from which *la pelona*[202] comes

. . .

¡War to all slavery!
¡And hurrah for democracy![203]

Poems, usually written by field health workers in their bulletins, tried to create easy-to-remember messages, expressed intense life experiences, or just commented on humorous events. A poem titled "Modern Combat" toyed with military metaphors and the revolutionary legacy of the 1910 Revolution:

The squad that marches to battle
Formerly grasped the rifle.

. . .
Today scientific trappings
Will win victory in combat.[204]

Another poem elaborated by a health worker from Oaxaca repeated the
theme; sprayers were gladiators who "saved" the nation and created the
basis for a prosperous future.[205]

Articles in these bulletins were also an effort to make eradication part of
people's thinking about health care and reflected the changing perceptions
among the population regarding malaria, health, and death. Until then, many
had regarded malaria as an inevitable fact of life that would infect or kill
part of a rural community. As Lomnitz has articulated, the mid–twentieth
century was a period when urban Mexico was banalizing and folklorizing
popular traditions such as Dia de los Muertos and minimizing the perception of death as an unavoidable and frequent tragedy in society. This resulted
in a decline of "death" in the public sphere and placed it in the public imagination at a safe distance."[206] A poem suggested how the campaign chal-
lenged a popular attitude, of resignation to premature death, and tried to
domesticate what used to be a feared life event. The poem ridiculed how
the *Calaca* (death), considered in popular culture a character with will and
malice, felt when malaria was brought under control:

Death, very indignant
at seeing everybody happy said
"I'll take them, I'll take them"
flapping her arms around. . . .

I'll take them altogether
Before an earthquake comes,
They are leaving me jobless, these
The paludism guys. . . .

The *Calaca* is surprised

And dives into the abyss

When visiting this Zone
And not finding Paludism.[207]

As this poem suggests, malaria eradication percolated into expressions in popular culture. Another example was a love letter from "an anonymous malariologist" that twisted romanticism with underlined technical terms familiar to a textbook of malaria eradication:

The most emotive *notification* of my feelings came when your eyes like *infected Anopheline* nail me in an impressive form; producing an emotional *paroxysm* that made the miracle of *sensitizing* my *resistant* and *feverish* heart. It was then when I understood the existence between your life and mine as a *coordination* as profound as the powder of *DDT* and *water.* It would be useless for you to *investigate.* . . . Convince yourself that my love is *positive.* Understand that my love is integral and does not require evaluations. . . . Yours.[208]

Besides the imaginative use of propaganda by field health workers, another dimension of the popular Mexicanization of the campaign was its use of lay volunteers. The recruitment of volunteers was a fundamental grassroots component of the Mexican campaign, and they exceeded what international agencies expected.[209] Referred to as "hygienic education honorary auxiliaries" (*auxiliares honorarios de educación higiénica,* AHEH), they were also known as "notifiers," due to their responsibilities of identifying malaria cases. They were also in charge of recruiting supporters of antimalaria work in communities with approximately one hundred inhabitants, and of creating related Educational Action Groups (Grupos de Acción Educacional) that appointed a president and requested propaganda materials from Mexico City.[210] The AHEHs received a diploma from the secretary of public health and a toolkit with epidemiological forms, lancets, cotton, alcohol, plates, and some drugs—all marks of prestige. They periodically visited houses to inform people about the campaign, to identify fever cases, and to take blood samples.

Each notification post was run by a member of CNEP who had a zone of influence sustained by an AHEH. Notification posts were established in every locality with five hundred inhabitants or more, and if possible, in smaller ones where malaria cases existed. Overall, it was a tightly knit network spread all over the malarious areas of the country. During 1959, this case-finding network consisted of 31,407 notification posts established in 13,684 localities, with information on 21,877 of the 4,252 localities in the malarial area of the country.[211] Frequently, notifiers provided first aid and

Figure 3.2. *A teacher in the village of Calotmal explains malaria to his class,
showing how blood samples are taken and then examined in the laboratory
(1962).*

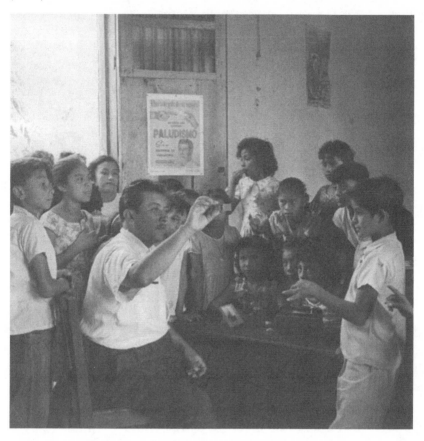

Source: Photograph by Paul Almasy. Courtesy of the World Health Organization.

practiced traditional medicine, assuming that there was no contradiction between the use of these methods and the techniques of Western medicine. An
important change in the original design of malaria eradication, to which the
AHEHs contributed, was the decision to administer medicines to fever patients from the beginning. In a culture that perceived treatment, rather than
prevention, as a symbol of medical concern, this decision consolidated the
AHEHs' authority. Likewise, it was an appropriate way to build trust and

overcome the population's reluctance to take the bitter antimalaria drugs, which had secondary effects.[212]

The AHEHs led the effort to find feverish cases and take blood samples from individuals who had recently suffered from recurrent fevers. The AHEH covered a large proportion of localities scattered all over the Mexican territory. By mid-1958, there were already 23,388 AHEHs, and more than 56,000 in 1961. In the mid-1970s, the AHEHs still existed, and many praised their work as key to the official health system.[213] The bulletin of the Yucatán zone, a Maya area, included in one of its 1962 issues an article about an AHEH named Olegario Cime, a primary schoolteacher in two towns within the Camino Real de Campeche. His house proudly exhibited the number CNEP had assigned him and an emblem reading: "Notification Post." The fifty-year-old Cime was a native of the region where he lived, spoke Maya, had suffered from malaria, and was the father of seven children. Many schoolteachers became AHEHs. They could read and write, were influential in the community, and could check if there were cases of malaria in the families through the children. The community knowledge from AHEH volunteers allowed linking an international health campaign to local motivations (figure 3.2).[214] They developed a sense of ownership, and they adapted the meanings and technologies brought by international health. These AHEH volunteers' intense work often expressed feelings of solidarity and compassion under adversity and a search to meet the fundamental aspirations of the poorest: relieving pain, enabling work, protecting loved ones, delaying death.

The bulletins also illustrated how the work of the AHEHs became a testing ground between different cultures, official nationalism, and health propaganda. It was precisely at this crossroads of malaria eradication and the indigenous culture where the limitations of the campaign became evident. These local responses to the campaign will be analyzed in the following chapter.

4

Local Responses

The local reception of the antimalaria campaign by provincial physicians and rural populations in Mexico was diverse, complex, and sometimes inconsistent. It did not follow a systematic pattern nor propose an alternative public health perspective. On the contrary, the local reception was contradictory, uneven, and spontaneous. It revealed diverse, and sometimes entrenched, notions of health and disease that were not taken into account in metropolitan and governmental designs of malaria eradication. To explain these responses, I have organized this chapter into four sections describing these topics: first, the health education efforts of the National Commission for the Eradication of Paludism (Comisión Nacional para la Erradicación del Paludismo, CNEP); second, the criticism of two medical anthropologists at the beginning of malaria eradication in Mexico; third, the reactions to the campaign of a provincial doctor, who almost singlehandedly revealed inadequacies in malaria eradication; and fourth, the scattered objections and protests of indigenous leaders and communities.

Intercultural Challenges

The CNEP authorities devoted some attention to challenges of its cross-cultural health activities, health communication, and health education in a culturally diverse environment. These activities were never prominent because it was assumed that indigenous people would be pleased and thankful when malaria rates were reduced as a result of malaria eradication. Although there were a few unsystematic attempts to establish a bridge between rural communities and official health care institutions, it is relevant

112

to review their main characteristics and limitations besides what has been already mentioned about the Division of Health Education in a previous chapter.

One of the challenges of malaria eradication was the existence of several languages other than Spanish. The most common indigenous languages were Náhuatl, Maya, Zapoteco, and Mixteco, all frequently spoken in the Southeast of the country. In Tabasco, a health worker complained about the lack of a map showing the distribution of ethnic groups and dialects spoken in the area.[1] A report on health education from the chief of a zone that made up Guerrero, an area occupied by four different ethnic groups—Mexica, Mixteco, Tlapaneco, and Amuzgo—which comprised about 200,000 individuals, complained as late as 1962 of the lack of a map indicating the location of ethnic groups and of their languages and the proportion of people who used them. (It is interesting to note that in the copy of this report studied for this chapter, this section was underlined and had a question mark written in the margin by a health authority, a probable indication that the task was difficult.)[2]

A high CNEP officer who perceived native languages as a "barrier" to the campaign emphasized that it was hard to find good translators. According to this officer, some people feared that information given to "foreign" medical doctors or their translators would be used to "exploit" them or "charge" them for services. In a country where the state was the overwhelming force for social projects, the notion that physicians working on a government project would not be "charged for any of the services provided" appeared—according to a report—as something impossible.[3] An indication that citizens were aware of these problems is the fact that CNEP received proposals to overcome language barriers. For instance, a local savant from Apipilhuasco, Veracruz, offered, in exchange for a small salary, to recruit indigenous translators for "Otomi, Azteca, Tepehue, and Totonaco"— regional "tongues"—because in some towns, "nobody spoke Spanish."[4]

The linguistic challenges of malaria eradication and its relationship with the varying reception of the campaign is illustrated by the $100,000 "Dieldrin Study Project," developed between 1956 and 1957 by the Pan-American Sanitary Bureau (PASB), the Shell Chemical Corporation, and the Mexican government. Although the program was formally designed to assess the effectiveness of insecticides on absorbing rural mud walls and reached no definitive conclusions, it also addressed the cultural challenges of malaria eradication.[5] The study was conducted by teams of Mexican and American experts that included a "public relations" unit—a euphemism for health educational work—in three climatic malarious villages, Acapulco, Puebla, and Oaxaca. According to the final report, in general, people were very friendly and allowed the health workers "to enter their homes twice a month to make the tests."[6]

However, the report showed that local reception varied. For example, in Acapulco, the best area in terms of socioeconomic development, "the people . . . with few exceptions, have been very cooperative. . . . Often candy is given to the children and a few pictures are made. . . . We feel that our public relations are excellent."[7] In Puebla, a rural area close to the standards of living of Acapulco, the team also encountered a favorable reception and was willing to expand its public relations obligations by providing transportation, money, and medicines, praising babies, and listening to accounts of good and bad health. For instance, on one occasion a health worker became the proud godfather of a baby.[8] In Oaxaca, the ancestral home of the Zapotec people, which was inhabited by several ethnic groups with different dialects, the "public relations" approach confronted its limitations. The troubled work in the poor and remote highland village of Santa Ines Yatzechi, with 914 inhabitants, was explained by "fact that the population speaks only Zapotec and with very few exceptions we could not communicate with the inhabitants except in the crudest way."[9]

CNEP paid some attention to linguistic diversity and designed pamphlets, records, and posters in at least four different indigenous languages.[10] Assistance was also provided by the Summer Institute of Linguistics, a modern missionary Protestant organization active in Mexico since the 1930s, which trained American linguists in Oklahoma to preach, study, and translate the Bible into numerous native languages. The North American Institute, which had sound experience in producing the first dictionaries and grammars for many of these languages, published bilingual pamphlets for malaria eradication.[11] However, the problem of language incommunication could not be solved only by the amount of bilingual propaganda material produced. One of the limitations of malaria eradication's educational campaign was its assumption that the diffusion of scientific information would induce rational behavior. On the contrary, in a number of towns, despite Western medicine propaganda in posters, pamphlets, radio, newspapers, and movies, self-medication, traditional medicine, and distrust of Western medicine persisted.

As a result, the educational goal of malaria eradication became encouraging people to conform to house-spraying and blood-sampling requirements. A CNEP education officer described his work as providing information to rural communities so that people "will gladly cooperate in all the work to be carried on."[12] Compliance as a goal appeared clearly in a 1957 meeting of the PASB and the heads of the antimalaria services of Mexico, Central America, and Panama. Carlos Alvarado, the PASB officer in charge of eradication—and later head of the Malaria Division of the World Health Organization (WHO)—explained the compulsory characteristics of educational work. According to Alvarado, eradication did not seek changes in the population's lifestyle but instead tried to make them understand the need to spray their houses, provide blood smears, take medication, inform the authorities about feverish cases, and follow all the instructions of health officers.[13] Moreover, he believed that temporary mobile units would suffice to provide education.[14]

The prescriptive style and limitations of propaganda materials in Mexico are illustrated in the records of a meeting between CNEP officers, schoolteachers, and indigenous leaders of El Nayar, Aguascalientes, of which only a small percentage could read Spanish. A debate on the best poster for the area resulted in an image of an Indian dressed in the area's typical costume with a caption in the native language asking: "Are you suffering from shivers and colds? . . . Let your house be sprayed."[15] A similar direction appeared in a bilingual pamphlet designed for a Huasteca's town, in San Luís Potosí, that recreated an imaginary dialogue between a sanitarian and a peasant. At a given moment, the health worker convincingly argues: "If you have a sick person at home . . . I will extract a tiny drop of blood and take it away. . . . And if there is disease, a doctor will come and will give him medicine, but right now I will give him two or three pills. . . . The doctor will not charge you anything because he is paid by the government to treat all the poor" (figure 4.1).[16] The ideal peasant's response appeared to follow a script: "Hum! . . . OK."

Paternalistic and charitable bilingual propaganda could not solve the challenges of intercultural health care. Linguistic diversity became a persistent issue in the South, where there were many local dialects and languages, not only because it made health communication and education more difficult but also because indigenous languages were looser and more flexible in naming people, objects, and illnesses. A health officer from Mexico City who visited the towns Zinacantecos and Chamulas in Chiapas complained that it was not easy to identify malaria cases because many Indians spoke only their native language and understood little Spanish, and many individuals had different names and no identity papers.[17]

A similar linguistic challenge for CNEP came with the use of the Spanish

Figure 4.1. *A little Mexican girl gives a sample of her blood for a test (1962).*

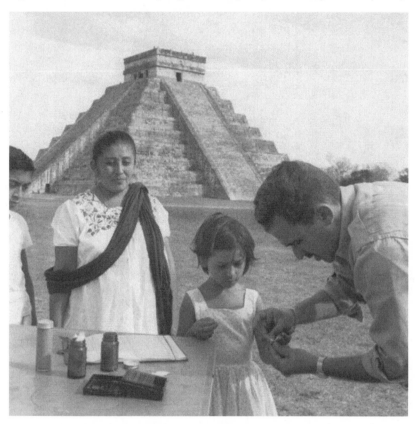

Source: Photograph by Paul Almasy. Courtesy of the World Health Organization.

word for malaria, *paludismo,* which was a French-inspired term used by the Mexican medical elite, who were not interested in symptoms per se but in connecting a series of symptoms with a specific medical entity with a unique biological origin and mode of transmission. Orthodox medical thought derived from a tradition of "discovering" and naming discrete entities with a unique biological origin that could produce a pattern of predictable clinical symptoms. Using a scientific name was also parallel to validating a body of technical knowledge segregated from lay knowledge and only comprehensible by experts. In using the very name *paludismo,* CNEP strengthened the term imported by the medical elite from the early twentieth century. And thanks to Paul Russell, WHO's Malaria Expert Committee developed a whole vocabulary for health workers—a guide to malaria terminology that would define and standardize precise concepts and indicators.[18]

In contrast, indigenous people and even provincial municipal officers used about thirty different Spanish and indigenous terms to name malaria.[19] These terms usually reflected an understanding of illness as several symptoms that might have a life of their own and could be imposed upon the body by various agents. It was hard to make *paludismo* the hegemonic name for the disease. Various names persisted during the 1960s, partly because the percentage of civil death records certified by a physician remained low in the southern indigenous areas of the country until 1970.[20]

Even CNEP's limited attempts to reach out to indigenous cultures with anthropologists were tainted with the functionalist notion of "assisting" indigenous ethnic groups "in their transition" to the non-Indian world. An agreement was signed in 1956 between CNEP and the Instituto Nacional Indigenista toward this end. Initially, this work was concentrated in Oaxaca, the Mexican state with the most speakers of indigenous languages, and it later extended to other southern rural areas.[21] Although the institute, which was created in the late 1940s as part of the design of the leftist pre–World War II president Lázaro Cárdenas, initially emphasized the teaching of practical skills over a Spanish literary education, after the war it accommodated the conservative administrations that ruled Mexico.[22]

By the mid-1950s, the Instituto Nacional Indigenista was concentrating on "instilling" modern cultural values for the "incorporation" of rural populations, which was carried out through education, hygiene, and social programs that tried to change "backward" customs and lifestyles located "outside" the money economy and the political system.[23] The institute's "Integral Planned Acculturation Program" in the southern zone of the country included four "coordinating centers." The most important of these was the Tzeltal-Tzotzil Center, with headquarters in San Cristobal de las Casas and influence over 100,000 indigenous people who spoke dialects of Maya. These centers established schools, medical posts, and agricultural experimentation fields and trained bilingual lay *promotores* as advocates and intermediaries for new customs and official campaigns.[24] They were designed as tools to promote development and integration with the rest of the country, provide new economic opportunities, and defend the inhabitants of poor villages from the exploitation of urban centers.

The sanitation work of these centers included the construction of latrines, immunization campaigns, and maternal care services, and followed the acculturation pattern of other government activities. In a pamphlet published in 1955, the Instituto Nacional Indigenista explained that one of its main goals in public health was

> to change the concept of etiology of diseases among indigenous communities. Generally these believe that illness is not the result of a natural process but results from magical causes. . . . This magical concept . . . is the main reason why no hygienic precautions are taken and that the Indians . . . have no faith in scientific medicine.[25]

In addition, these centers used DDT from the early 1950s. For example, in 1951 the Tzeltal-Tzotzil Center's DDT spraying "benefited" more than 10,000 people, and by 1955 the number had grown to 62,000.[26]

Educational authorities also reinforced the acculturation work done by CNEP and the Instituto Nacional Indigenista. For the Secretaría de Educación Pública, national cultural integration would be achieved by teaching Spanish to Indians who were monolingual in an indigenous language.[27] Educational, medical, and Indigenista activities were part of a larger state-supported cultural nationalism projected to Westernize the native rural communities through a process of de-Indianization. The project entailed an intense but nonforcible cultural diffusion process, namely, the spread of Western and biomedical cultural elements as the best tool to modernize rural indigenous communities rapidly and create an educated, healthy, and politically mobilized citizenry. Ultimately, their mission was to induce cultural change and to reinforce what was contemplated as an inevitable trend: the emergence of a single mestizo national culture—in short, to *Mexicanize* the indigenous population. In the eloquent words of one director of the Instituto Nacional Indigenista who worked in Chiapas, the goal was "to make Mexicans of all the Indians of our country."[28]

CNEP linked assimilation to the promotion of a racialized version of malaria. Indigenous peoples were often perceived as disease carriers, and their culture was seen as an obstacle to health progress. The role played by anemia, a typical clinical symptom of malaria, was overemphasized to explain the traditional "apathy," "fatalism," "indolence," and even "depressive character" of rural people. This conceptualization of the disease coincided with a tradition of subtle racial prejudice in Mexico that portrayed Indian workers as inherently lazy, stupefied by alcohol, and even thieves whose reckless behavior validated close supervision and exploitative working conditions.[29] In addition, for medical doctors and field officers of CNEP, malaria eradication was a tool for the expansion of Western medicine in rural areas. An illustration of this notion is a 1959 report that emphasized as one of CNEP's achievements "the defeat of peasant skepticism regarding malaria."[30] This phrase was framed to underline the dismissal of infectious diseases as an inevitable fact of life and the emergence of a new popular trust in medical science. A few years later, a CNEP officer stressed that a persistent system of "rural penetration" was an important achievement of the campaign.[31] It is important to mention that although Western medical assimilation was the hegemonic trend, health workers occasionally avoided an outright disapproval of peasants' traditional curative practices.[32]

CNEP criticized traditional medicine as a primitive and superstitious cultural trait that would be brushed aside by the campaign. The campaign aimed to discount and disparage local beliefs about disease causality. Little attention was given to the fact that a variety of shamans, midwives, and diviners had a long tradition and were widespread in rural Mexico.[33] Malaria eradication was also understood as the "eradication" of traditional and domestic healing practices and the validation of the "supremacy" and rationality of Western medicine. According to a Mexican health officer, the eradication campaign involved forcing people to leave behind atavistic lifestyles, "prejudices and superstitions . . . strongly rooted in the rural milieu," as well as heterodox healing systems.[34]

An inherent contradiction of the medical process of acculturation and assimilation was that CNEP had to gain compliance for measures that were difficult to realize for many peasant families. A poster placed on the doors of houses the day before they would be sprayed instructed dwellers to place all furniture, pictures, and lightweight objects away from the walls, provide the sprayer with about 10 liters of water to mix with the insecticide, and prevent their animals from eating the insects that died from insecticide spraying. In addition, it was expected that the peasants, during the week following spraying, would sweep the floors, burn the waste, and not wash, grate, or paint the walls.[35] This measure was difficult to follow because many houses lacked sprayable surfaces (e.g., reed walls) and many families slept outside the house in the summer and constructed rooms after spraying.

In some cases, medical acculturation failed because CNEP's educational activities confronted resistance from people who distrusted government officers, disliked their houses being sprayed, or questioned the request to give blood samples to foreigners. In addition, popular resistance was due to the overlooked fact that insecticides were also toxic to people and to their domestic animals. However, CNEP minimized resistance. In 1958 it proudly announced as an achievement the small number of houses unwilling to be sprayed: 2.9 percent during the first half of that year and 2.7 percent in the second semester.[36] Although it is hard to quantify the magnitude of resistance, scattered reports suggest that these claims were exaggerated and that all forms of resistance (to spraying or blood sampling) were as high as 10 percent. Some CNEP health workers linked resistance to their negative perception of the indigenous population. They believed that peasants lived in a state of indolence and a could-not-care-less state of mind regarding malaria eradication. One health worker's letter complained about a community that was against "the good that we pretend."[37]

A complaint made by a CNEP field officer after the campaign had been under way for five years vividly illustrates the challenges of malaria eradication educational work. According to the officer, "despite many efforts," little had been accomplished with respect to the "enthusiasm of the people" in favor of the campaign; though people complied with CNEP, full support was still lacking.[38] The challenges of cross-cultural health care reflected in the linguistic gaps and obstacles described above became the cornerstone of anthropological comments and critiques against a campaign implemented from above.

Anthropological Critique

During the late 1940s and the 1950s, a new subdiscipline of anthropological research—sometimes called applied anthropology, and later better known as medical anthropology—developed in Mexico and in the United States.[39] The origins of this subdiscipline can be traced to the valuable work of the American George Foster, a professor of anthropology at the University of California, Berkeley, and the Mexican Gonzalo Aguirre Beltrán. They did not disapprove outright of all aspects of traditional medicine, and they truly believed that it was possible to identify, examine, and overcome the challenges faced in introducing Western culture and medicine in indigenous cultural settings. They also believed that anthropological techniques could facilitate better communication with indigenous cultures, gain the trust of peasants, and integrate ethnic minority groups into mainstream society. Their ultimate goals were to persuade rural people that Western medicine and personal hygiene were better than traditional and domestic medicines and to identify cultural and social factors of resistance to medical programs in rural areas.[40] In sum, their work was that of culture brokers.[41]

Foster was able to convince U.S. government officers that these ideas were sound and practical for bilateral programs and to carve an academic niche for this version of anthropology, a discipline that used to emphasize only field and theoretical work.[42] Foster had been a consultant to bilateral public health programs since the late 1940s. In 1951, as a member of the Institute for Social Anthropology of the Smithsonian Institution, he began to work with the Health Division of the Institute of Inter-American Affairs, the first permanent bilateral organization of the United States in the region, to analyze the relationships between culture and public health innovations with the aim of facilitating medical change.[43] According to Foster, the successful development of public health programs required social scientists to fulfill the role of an enlightened educator: "After the most practical public health program for a given country or area is determined, the people must be convinced that the program is really good for them, that it is in their interest to adopt the new and abandon the old."[44]

Accordingly, work was designed under the assumption that adequate educational programs could overcome the cultural and psychological resistance to Western medicine. Foster believed that these programs were pertinent because health interventions coming from outside the rural communities were not always self-validating—even if they produced objective improvements—and the people's perception could oppose the intervention both before and after it occurred. In addition, he believed that international public health agencies could improve their work. He even attended, as an adviser to the U.S. delegation, a WHO Health Assembly, and he allegedly was an informal public health student of Henry van Zile Hyde, the official American representative to WHO.[45]

Besides developing his own valuable research for years in Tzintzuntan, in Central Mexico, Foster's Institute for Social Anthropology recruited and funded a few American and Mexican anthropologists in Latin America. These included some of the first American medical anthropologists working in the region, such as Richard Adams in Guatemala, Charles Erasmus in Colombia, Ozzie Simmons in Peru, and Kalervo Oberg in Brazil.[46] Particularly notable among them was Isabel Kelly, a young anthropologist from California who had lived and worked in Mexico for many years, at least since the late 1930s.[47]

Although most of Kelly's publications focused on archaeology, she was also interested in midwives and traditional medical practices. An indication of her identification with the country and her intention to settle there was that she taught anthropology in Mexico and purchased a few thousand square meters of land and a bamboo house in the countryside.[48] She also marveled at the people and landscape encountered in her fieldwork. One one occasion, after complaining about logistical challenges for her research, she wrote: "But the country is WONDERFUL."[49] In a comment that reveals the importance that she, as well as Foster, gave to language, she added in the same letter: "The village where we are to work has one mestizo woman and her two adolescent offspring. Otherwise the population is exclusively To-tonac. Not one woman speaks Spanish, and among the men, only those un-der ca. 30 years. I've left duffle on the spot, have arranged provisionally with interpreters; and to boot, have bought 6 Totonac dictionaries."[50]

To a smaller degree than some Americans victims of the Red Scare of the early 1950s, Kelly had to endure part of the Cold War. During this whole period in Mexico, she was a research associate, with no salary, of her alma mater, the Department of Anthropology at Berkeley. Suddenly, in 1951 she received letters from university authorities demanding, first, an anticom-munist "oath of allegiance" to the Regents of the University and, second, a similar oath for the State of California. The latter implied her willingness to defend, if necessary by force, the security of California. Apparently, the Red-baiting tactics of Senator Joseph McCarthy had made these oaths stan-dard practice in some American universities. For American nationals living outside their country, it meant registering affidavits with local notaries and U.S. embassies. Although she regarded the request as unconstitutional, she signed the first letter under protest. Her response to a university authority illustrates her discomfort: "I can think of no one less likely to have com-munist leanings than myself."[51]

Moreover, Kelly ridiculed what was ridicule: "The whole business is so idiotically futile. If anyone were really engaged in subversive activities, he'd be the first one to perjure himself."[52] Kelly refused to sign the second oath and manifested her opposition by demanding that her name removed from the roster of the Department of Anthropology. However, she envi-sioned that "if, some time in the future, the skies is clearer, I'll come trot-ting back to the family circle."[53] The appreciation felt from colleagues who had mixed feelings is suggested by an excerpt of a letter by the chair of the department written shortly after the matter was resolved with her removal from the department:

Kelly has held an appointment as research associate without salary in the Department of Anthropology for many years. During this period of time she has been resident during the whole or most of each year in Mexico. She has made a number of outstanding and significant contributions to the culture history of western Mexico. . . . In addition, she has been a notable benefactor of the [Berkeley] Museum of Anthropology.[54]

Starting in 1953, Kelly began to collaborate with Héctor García Manzanedo and the Mexican Health Secretariat on rural projects.[55] Their work was inspired by Kelly's professor and colleague, George Foster. García Manzanedo was an officer of the Public Health Experimental Studies Bureau, an organization in the Health Secretariat supported by the Rockefeller Foundation. Kelly and García Manzanedo's work was not easy, because Mexican medical doctors frequently jealously maintained a legal monopoly on practicing medicine and condemned indigenous healing practices as nonsensical and primitive. The doctors tried to enforce this monopoly with a series of regulations enacted in the capital and the main urban centers.[56] However, the work of applied medical anthropologists was facilitated by the emergence of anthropology as a valid field of higher education and professional advice in Mexico following the creation in 1946 of the National School of History and Anthropology, where Kelly taught.[57]

Shortly after the inception of malaria eradication, García Manzanedo and Kelly prepared a critical report that opposed malaria eradication's totalizing approach, given Mexico's indigenous diversity.[58] Their relationship with government institutions and the framework of applied anthropology made their criticism mild and subtle. They argued that while the campaign took into account a number of technical and geographic factors, it overlooked an essential issue: the great diversity of indigenous languages. This issue was particularly important in the South, due to the fact that the diverse ethnic groups, who lived in malarious areas such as the Tehuantepec Isthmus, the Yucatán Peninsula, and the Quintana Roo territory, spoke a variety of languages, dialects, and subdialects.

This linguistic diversity was more intense in some regions. For example, in Oaxaca, a region that had the highest rate of malaria mortality among the Mexican provincial units and a rural population of 75 percent in 1960, there were fifteen different language groups, among which the most important were the Zapoteca, Mixteca, Nazateca, Trique, and Chinanteca.[59] According to García Manzanedo and Kelly, although the majority of the rural population spoke Spanish (over 19.2 million), 1.6 million spoke Spanish along with an indigenous language, and 795,069 people were monolingual in a native language.[60] The latter two figures were taken from the census of 1950, which defined ethnicity as the use of a "native tongue" and was commonly related to illiteracy.

Initially, García Manzanedo and Kelly used linguistics as an indicator of ethnicity ambivalently, something common among anthropologists at the time. However, they also stressed the existence of 19.2 million rural people, most of whom had some command of Spanish but were part of an indigenous culture. According to a 1957 estimate the figure represented more than 60 percent of the nation's population. In this emphasis, Kelly and García Manzanedo went beyond a restricted linguistic indicator and suggested that even those with a command of Spanish would not understand the campaign.[61] León Portilla, a renowned Mexican anthropologist, criticized the narrowly language-based ethnic definitions used in the Mexican censuses of 1950s and 1960. He believed that many more individuals living in the countryside and urban slums should be registered as Indians, because even if these individuals no lónger used an Indian language, they still maintained an indigenous lifestyle that consisted of cultural traits such as communal life; a diet based on corn, chile, and beans; sleeping on mats; and wearing *huaraches* (a shoe consisting of a sole fastened by straps to the foot).[62]

García Manzanedo and Kelly also criticized malaria eradication's assumption that rural life was static—that people were sedentary and lived in one house. This assumption was crucial for biannual spraying operations, because it was believed that people would continue sleeping for at least a year in the same house that held the residual powers of the insecticide. The authors of the critical report underscored that on the contrary, human life in rural areas was dynamic—involving migration, nomadic tribes, religious pilgrimages by peasants from Oaxaca and Chiapas to festivities in Guatemala, the building of new houses, and the construction of temporary houses. A 1960 survey of over 2.5 million Mexican dwellings showed that 41 percent of them had been partially or totally altered within the six-month intervals between spraying.[63] Some of these houses corresponded to the different plots of land cultivated at different times of the year by a peasant family, something that made it difficult to spray these places of residence when the owners were absent.[64] A related issue was that in some jungle areas of Mexico, people were accustomed to sleeping outside during the hot months of the summer.

García Manzanedo and Kelly considered the attention given to health education as insufficient. Along with other applied medical anthropologists, they believed that medical programs in the rural areas made few or inadequate attempts to explain and adapt scientific messages about the origin and transmission of infectious diseases to indigenous communities. Their report suggested increasing the number and training-days of bilingual sprayers, the abilities of health educators, and the recruitment of priests and school-teachers for malaria eradication.[65] In addition, they noticed an even more serious fact: In many rural localities, there were few health entities supporting malaria eradication. A so-called National Coordinated Services—supposedly created to link antimalaria work with other non-antimalaria programs of the Health Secretariat and of the Social Security program in rural areas—was underfunded and lacked personnel.[66] Regarding contamination produced by insecticides, they briefly stated their preoccupation with the fact that DDT killed not only mosquitoes but also hens, bees, and other domestic animals, something that would damage the peasant families' diet, for they obtained eggs, meat, and honey from these insects and animals.

The most interesting criticism by García Manzanedo and Kelly was that malaria eradication did not take into account indigenous concepts regarding blood, the body, and fevers.[67] For many indigenous communities, "fever" could be a disease in itself, and many different fevers were believed to exist.[68] Peasants explained the origin of malaria as the result of magical harm, sudden temperature changes like bathing in cold water after working in the sun, eating unripe fruits, and sleeping on the floor. Fevers were treated with medicinal plants, by rubbing sick bodies with alcohol, and by drinking rue tea mixed with lime juice or strong alcoholic beverages.[69] A popular treatment was to take infusions of bitter herbs to "extract the cold" or to "scare" the patients. Mosquitoes were an inconvenience, like bothersome house-flies, and received popular names like *mollote* in Oaxaca, but not a menace; and according to a study, indigenous people did not feel compelled to destroy them. A common measure was to produce smoke to move them away.[70] According to a report of the malaria work done in the national Oil Camps, workers did not distinguish between the mosquitoes that transmit malaria and other mosquitoes and demanded a campaign against all flying insects.[71]

The human body itself constituted another area of conflict. According to the campaign's principles, blood samples had to be obtained to confirm the presence of *Plasmodium,* but peasants were usually afraid to give away their blood.[72] García Manzanedo and Kelly signaled that it would not be easy to obtain blood samples from some indigenous groups and even from acculturated mestizo populations. For medical doctors, blood was just a liquid component of human anatomy that could reveal the secrets of a microscopic world. But for Indians, on the contrary, blood had had mystical, religious, and historical meanings since the pre-Columbian period. For example, blood was essential in the heart sacrifices practiced in pre-Columbian Mexico for divination, preparation for war, the inauguration of temples, the "renewal" of nature, and the "recreation" of the social order.[73] Indigenous communities in central Mexico and Central America practiced ritual blood-letting and burned blood-spattered media to establish direct communication with celestial supernatural beings. Many centuries later, blood was still used in rural Mexico in religious offerings and was given by traditional healers to sufferers from anemia and malnutrition.[74] In some rural parts of Chiapas and Oaxaca, endemic diseases such as onchocercosis, characterized by partial or complete blindness among highlanders, were taken as divine punishment, whereby vampires sucked the blood of people and made them lose sight.[75]

Blood smears were also feared in rural Mexico in the 1950s because the loss of a vital nonregenerative fluid was believed to produce permanent weakness, to create sterility in men or women, and to make people prone to illnesses perceived as more menacing in rural areas than the Evil Eye. In addition, the intrusion of foreign objects into the body, such as the sharp stabs used for pricking fingers, was also taken as a cause for sickness.[76] In fact, during the campaign, some individuals evaded blood examination, and in a few cases even forbade other members of their family to comply.

Likewise, blood sampling was feared because blood was typically used to cause poisoning. Drawing blood in order to obtain laboratory information played with recurrent rumors that poor people were being assessed before being destroyed. An unfounded rumor that indigenous blood was sold to "the Americans" was consonant with the fear that prevailed in societies with acute inequalities where the poor harbor fears of losing their most precious goods and people to outside forces. In other cases, according to García Manzanedo and Kelly, Indians could not understand why health workers took blood from them and thereby weakened them if they were concerned about their health, so blood sampling was perceived as contrary to medical treatment and healing.

The emphasis on blood sampling by malaria eradicators also reconfigured the process of diagnosing malaria. Before the campaign, provincial physicians relied on clinical symptoms such as recurrent fevers to identify the disease. A less intrusive medical examination was accepted and even appreciated by rural people. With malaria eradication, the existence of *Plasmodium* in the blood was taken as the only definitive evidence of malaria.

Health workers magnified the menacing presence of the parasite concealed in natives to postulate the need to test, treat, and control symptomless individuals, something difficult to grasp for an indigenous culture in which the notion of apparently "healthy" individuals carrying disease was an oxymoron. Medical doctors emphasized the scientific fact that many infected people living in areas where malaria was endemic could have parasites in their blood while displaying no outward symptoms of malaria for days because symptoms could appear about fifteen days after the infected mosquito bite. This scientific notion was also in opposition to the popular perception of the disease, which associated it with acute pain and the physical inability to work. Many lay people did not regard it as possible for a person to be ill if he or she felt well or if mild symptoms of a disease did not prevent work.[77]

Another area where the indigenous body and Western medicine conflicted was the use of drugs. Many antimalaria medicines made the skin yellow and produced nausea, a temporary inconvenience for medical doctors but a sign of alarm for peasants. This fact had been noticed shortly before the campaign began. An editorial written by an anthropologist who had lived three years in a malarious area was published in the journal of an Indigenista institute based in Mexico. He complained that the need to constantly use drugs in "infested zones" was "annoying and uncomfortable," with their prolonged effects and reactions.[78]

García Manzanedo and Kelly's report revealed the tensions during the campaign between different meanings of disease, fevers, and human blood. These tensions were not resolved during the campaign. Malaria eradicators—and the few state-supported rural health services organized by the Social Security system and the Health Secretariat—could overcome peasant resistance, but indigenous beliefs about malaria usually coexisted uneasily with the policies of government health services. Though Western medicine was eventually integrated as a resource for some conditions, traditional medicine and its less complicated and expensive practices survived. As a result, traditional healing persisted, and different versions of medical pluralism developed. In addition, the disdain by medical doctors for traditional medicine and indigenous culture persisted.[79] In 1972 a medical publication in Oaxaca described one of the local ethnic groups, the Triques, in the following terms: "The Trique Indians belong to one of the less culturally developed groups. They had miraculously and stubbornly survived adverse conditions. As with other indigenous groups, the evolution of their culture appears arrested. As if encroaching on themselves was the best self-defense, . . . the Triques have been a turbulent, distrustful, belligerent indigenous group."[80]

In their report, the anthropologists confessed that they did not have a solution for the cultural mismatches they described. For them, it was not possible to provide a universal prescription for such a large and ethnically diverse area. They simply indicated the campaign's lack of flexibility and truly expected that some changes would be made. The lack of specific advice also suggested the hegemonic position of CNEP and the limited room for alternative paths during malaria eradication. In addition, Kelly was unable to follow up on this criticism. By the end of 1957, she had left Mexico to become part of an anthropological project promoted by the U.S. government in Bolivia.[81]

Despite the fact that García Manzanedo and Kelly never received an official response and that their report's main recommendations were not followed, the personal impressions of a WHO officer made some years later in Mexico coincided with the anthropologists' perspectives. The officer noticed that the "crisis" of Mexico's malaria eradication program in the so-called "problem areas" (where the campaign made little progress despite the implementation of adequate technical interventions) occurred more intensely in the territory occupied by indigenous communities, namely, in Morelos, Oaxaca, Guerrero, Michoacan, and Puebla. He even compared maps of "the Indian areas and the 'problem areas'" and found to his surprise "that these were extremely similar. In fact, when placed one above the other, the areas corresponded exactly."[82]

Yet not every medical doctor acquiesced to CNEP's authority and orders. Some provincial physicians questioned not only the manipulation of health education as a tool for imposing technical interventions disliked by the community but also the scant regard for the collateral toxic effects of malaria eradication. These questions were raised clearly by the provincial doctor José Villalobos.

A Provincial Doctor Rebels

At the end of 1956, José Villalobos, a physician living in Juchipila, Zacatecas, was visited by local CNEP health workers, who asked for his help in convincing peasants to open their houses to DDT sprayers. Because opposition to spraying had been strong, and sometimes armed, the CNEP workers sought the support of Villalobos, a locally respected physician. Although he initially provided some help, he eventually became a vocal critic against malaria eradication and DDT. To frame his opinions, it is important to present his background.

Villalobos graduated from the Medical School of Mexico City, a public higher education institution created during the colonial period and the most prestigious of the approximately fifteen medical education centers in his country. His official degree was "doctor of medicine and surgery" (*médico cirujano*).[83] Toward the end of his studies, he served in a compulsory social service program aimed at counteracting the maldistribution of physicians that made medical students spend about a year in rural locations in addition to their six-year course. Since 1936, President Lázaro Cardenas and the Mexican health authorities had embarked upon a program of rural medicine consisting of sending pregraduate physicians to rural sections instead of allowing them to serve in city hospitals. This was done with the hope that many of them would later set up their offices in provincial towns instead of large urban centers. Between 1936 and 1943, 2,400 medical students went to rural locations from the National University alone, and about 400 from smaller medical schools.[84] This partially helped to end the lack of medical services in remote villages. Although there are no provincial indicators, the national rate of physicians per population was low; it amounted to 1 per 2,029 in the mid-1950s, when the international standard was half that figure.[85]

Many rural villages suffered from a scarcity of physicians, because the best jobs were concentrated in the cities.[86] Villalobos fulfilled his rural service obligation, supported by a small stipend from the Health Secretariat in Jalpa, a rural town of about 32,000 inhabitants located in Aguascalientes near Juchipila. As was typical with other medical students serving in the same program, he used this experience in the thesis he was required to complete before being granted a degree. His thesis, which emphasized malaria and other illnesses, followed a canon of sociomedical description that was less attractive for students who pursued an American-style degree and thus usually submitted a thesis describing laboratory experiments or quantitatively recorded hospital observations. Instead, Villalobos's thesis exhibited a holistic approach, examining the geography, roads, climate, education, and garbage disposal of Jalpa.[87] He concluded with some recommendations, such as encouraging more health education using "colorful posters" for rural schools, the establishment of a rural hygiene center (which he was willing to head), more intense immunization programs, training midwives in obstetrics, and educating mothers on the benefits of breastfeeding over using artificial milk.

After graduating in 1952, Villalobos established his medical practice in Juchipila, near where he had lived during the research for his medical thesis. Only two other university-trained doctors lived in town. Like other provincial doctors, he became familiar with a vast array of medical conditions, such as malaria, typhoid fever, and trichinosis. More important, he knew how to earn the peasants' trust. He was especially proud of how he had saved a family suffering from rabies transmitted by bats. Although he had very little free time and resources, Villalobos installed a modest laboratory in his office and performed some medical research, which was published in newspapers rather than the academic journals preferred by elite Mexican medical researchers. An examination of his writing reveals not a "scientist" by the standards of the time but a flamboyant writer who combined basic medical knowledge, common sense, and extravaganza. It was perhaps this combination that made him bold enough to be open and heterodox in his medical thinking.

When Villalobos was approached by the CNEP officers requesting help, he in turn asked them blunt questions that they could not answer. Two were related to migration patterns and the housing conditions of rural people: "A large percentage of the rural population does not live in houses. They live in huts, cabins, and even caves. Huts have many openings in their walls. . . . Who will control the migration of workers from malaria to nonmalaria areas, and back?"[88] In fact, according to the census of 1950, only 41 percent of the rural population lived in homes made of mud, a material known to provide some protection from mosquito bites if sprayed with insecticides. In places such as Oaxaca, more than 75 percent of the rural population lived in homes (*jacales*) made of nonmud materials such as sticks.[89] In addition, peasants' homes did not follow hygienic rules, partially because of their misery, and had only one room for cooking, sleeping, and storing goods. The government did not provide safe water and garbage disposal systems in rural areas, with the exception of major towns. Overcrowding was marked in Oaxaca, where 73 percent of rural families lived in homes where the healthy and the ill shared one single room.[90] The coexistence of healthy and sick family members in the same room made malaria transmission more frequent. Even in houses made of mud or more solid materials, precarious doors and unprotected windows eased transmission.

Despite his questions revealing the inadequacy of the campaign in relation to the social conditions prevailing in rural areas, Villalobos initially collaborated with CNEP. He even went out to the fields with the sprayers in 1957. However, after that year, he began to denounce malaria eradication.

His first criticisms were directed against insecticides that not only eliminated the *Anopheles* but also bees, butterflies, mice, and many hens. In a dramatic account that resonates with the environmental concerns that became popular in the United States during the early 1960s, he wrote: "Spring has arrived and so have swallows, but . . . their eggs . . . were left dead in their nests." As a provincial doctor who knew the people in his town relatively well, it was even more serious to see that after the second insecticide spraying cycle, the peasants looked pale, weak, and tired, and two-thirds of schoolchildren presented a stubborn version of conjunctivitis that was resistant to the usual medical treatment. The illness relapsed in some cases after it was apparently cured. According to Villalobos, this was a result of careless sprayers applying insecticide not only on walls, doors, and furniture but also in children's and adults' hair, in drinking water wells, in storage areas, and on cattle forage. Sometimes they even bathed dogs and cats with DDT.[91]

To make matters worse, according to Villalobos, sprayers risked their lives in an effort to overcome any resistance. They occasionally drank a glass full of insecticide in front of unbelieving peasants to prove that the substance was not harmful. Safety recommendations on the use of masks, rubber gloves, and aprons as protective clothing, which appeared on the pump labels or which sprayers received during training, were not followed. Others just ignored the fact that DDT was poisonous. Scientific studies on pollution show that insecticides could be absorbed through the skin, especially in hot climates, were unknown because they had appeared later in international scientific journals to which sprayers had little access. Furthermore, the scientific consensus that emerged on DDT—as a persistent organic pollutant that built up in animal tissues and impaired reproduction in wildlife; was especially toxic for domestic animals, predatory birds, and fish; and could damage the human nervous system—only developed fully in the mid-1960s and outside Mexico. Other factors also increased the risks of contamination for health workers, such as poor storage conditions and bad labeling of DDT containers or labeling that could not be understood by sprayers, sometimes because of a lack of proper training or illiteracy. However, there was little regard for the bioethical dimensions of health work. Another indication of this trend is that starting in the early 1960s, "human bait"—literally, "volunteers" who were allowed to be bitten by mosquitoes during the night— was regularly used by CNEP to study the bite rate of mosquitoes.[92]

Environmental pollution produced by insecticides affected humans in numerous ways. According to Villalobos, after the third spraying, flies, mosquitoes, cockroaches, wasps, scorpions, spiders, and bedbugs did not die. On the contrary, they were larger in size and became real pests. An unforeseen event was that insecticides increased the resistance of these insects. In fact, scorpion bites were a medical concern in Mexico and prompted a number of medical studies. According to a study that covered the period 1940 to 1958, scorpion bites produced significant mortality among children in the Eastern rural areas, including Oaxaca.[93]

Besides DDT, Mexico also sprayed Dieldrin, an insecticide that was highly toxic to humans, domestic animals, and poultry, as well as an ideal means for building up resistance in insects. Approximately 400,806 kilograms of Dieldrin were sprayed between 1957 and 1958 before it was discontinued in 1958. Although this amount was lower than the 4.4 million kilograms of DDT used in those same years, Dieldrin was the main cause of insecticide poisoning of sprayers. Officially, by 1960 only seventeen cases of intoxication among Mexican sprayers were officially reported.[94]

According to Villalobos, pollution also affected livestock and small animals. There was a decrease in milk production, many cows had miscarriages, most hens died, and not a single cat survived. His own cat died in his hands vomiting blood. Upon careful examination of his pet's corpse, Villalobos found its liver swollen, confirming his suspicions of severe toxicity. The cat's death most likely came when it licked its contaminated fur. It is interesting to note that after a few years, the sprayers had to deal with the pejorative nickname of "cat killers" in several regions of Mexico.[95] A Latin American malaria expert noticed that Dieldrin was killing so many cats in eradication campaigns that rats were becoming a serious difficulty.[96]

Other provincial people noticed, as had Villalobos, the differing effectiveness between the first and subsequent spraying operations, partly due to the increased resistance of mosquitoes. Pollution produced a number of courteous requests from middle-class individuals addressed to the president of Mexico, going above CNEP, which was a signal of a growing lack of confidence in the health authorities in charge of malaria eradication. For example, the representative of an insurance company of Huixtla from highland Chiapas complained to the president that the "liquid" used against malaria in the second year did not kill mosquitoes, as had the first spraying, when "we did not see any mosquitoes, cockroaches, and other insects." In contrast, he denounced the fact that "now chicken, cats and other animals die . . . but the mosquito remains . . . It is said that the first spraying was good because it was done by the *gringos*."[97] This comment suggests a distrust of health authorities and their techniques and a suspicion that some dishonest sprayers were diverting the genuine DDT to make profits on the side. Some middle-class provincial homeowners accounted for similar predicaments and asked to exempt their homes from spraying.[98] Others urged the health authorities to return to traditional and less harmful malaria control measures, such as using petroleum in swamps to kill the larvae (a measure discredited by eradicators because it was typically done in malaria control, namely, before malaria eradication begun).[99] The title of a 1957 article in a town in indigenous Guerrero suggested discredit: "Mosquitos Laugh Off DDT."[100]

Villalobos's actions did not follow the polite tone described above. He traveled to Aguascalientes, a larger town of about ninety-three thousand inhabitants with a number of patients he had been treating with "marked anemia, pre-hepatic jaundice, and conjunctivitis" that he believed were produced by the toxic effects of spraying. However, he received a cold reception and subsequently traveled alone to Mexico City to discuss pollution with the CNEP authorities. He had a three-hour meeting with Donald J. Pletsch, the PASB technical adviser in chief in Mexico, to whom he complained bitterly about malaria eradication. Villalobos remembered from this interview that Pletsch kept on asking the same question: "Then, are you against the Anti-Malaria Campaign?" This insistence suggests that loyalty to CNEP was above any other consideration. His response: "I would not be a doctor if I were against the campaign," which reveals the little room for dissent as well as a human contradiction. He also added that his opposition was to the way in which "they"—CNEP workers—pretended to eradicate malaria.

The dialogue with Pletsch did not yield any positive results for Villalobos. He returned home discouraged and isolated. He later declared that the fourteen critical newspaper articles against CNEP he had been publishing in provincial and national newspapers such as *El Heraldo de Aguascalientes, El Excelsior,* and *El Universal* had landed him in jail for a few months in 1958. It was not clear what the charges against him were, but it seems that he was considered subversive and fastidious by the authorities. The short time he spent in jail also suggests that he was not perceived as a menace by the authorities and that his position was probably rare among medical doctors.[101]

Villalobos managed to attract some attention from regional authorities. A letter from the Bishop of Zacatecas thanked Villalobos for his report on the dangers of DDT to malnourished people who eat food sprayed with the insecticide. The Bishop's letter in the Archive of the Health Secretariat is attached to a note written by Villalobos informing the Bishop of a letter containing seven hundred signatures of people from Jalapa who were convinced that the CNEP "[wants] to finish us off."[102] A similar popular perception that public health's ultimate purpose is to eliminate the poor has been found by other studies on colonial and postcolonial countries with societies marked by acute economic inequalities and anxieties of mutual distrust between elites and the population at large.[103] Although Villalobos was able to get the bishop's attention, the bishop was not persuaded by Villalobos's claims, and no action was taken by the Catholic Church authorities against malaria eradication.

The Mexican doctor must have felt isolated even among his peers when voicing his interpretation of the impact of DTT pollution on human beings. He thought there was a relationship between the patients he looked after and "viral mutations due to environmental changes." Although his interpretation remains mysterious and unpacked, he claimed to know about the subject thanks to two scientific articles that appeared in American journals. One of them dealt with virus mutation for vaccination but had nothing on environmental pollution. He also thought that the increase in cancer cases was a consequence of the insecticide's pollution. Later on, he found other information that validated his claims—in two articles that appeared in what was regarded as a symbol of U.S. cultural imperialism: the Spanish version of *Reader's Digest.*

Despite Villalobos's unconventional means of legitimizing his heterodox scientific opinions and his lack of explanation of the content of these opinions, it is important to underscore his hybrid rejection of an American donor-driven campaign by using sophisticated scientific journals and a U.S. magazine.[104] In addition, his ideas were not totally uncommon at the time. Many of the antipesticide activists of the 1960s supported the idea that poisonous elements in insecticides produced cancer. (The contemporary scientific consensus on DDT as carcinogenic in humans is not definitive; nor there is any definitive evidence that the insecticide affects human reproduction.)[105]

Despite his isolation, Villalobos refused to give up. Inspired by his eclectic readings and heterodox viewpoints, he prepared a paper for the Mexican Congress of Public Health, held in 1960 in Hermosillo, Sonora, with a completely neutral name: "Some Data on the Loss of Viral Specificity (Mutation) Observed in the Rural Population of the Mexican Republic and Its Determining Factor." To counter specialists' criticisms, Villalobos noted that "all works are generally presented with a bibliography but there is none in this one," referring to his paper. The statement reflects the little regard he had for academic rules common among the scientifically trained leaders of CNEP. Attending this event also gave him a chance to leave the province, where his alarm calls were not heeded, and after the meeting he moved to Mexico City, his family's place of residence. Also at this time, he sent a discordant telegram to another academic meeting, that of the United States–Mexico Border Public Health Association, with headquarters in El Paso, which also took place in Hermosillo: "CNEP goes against the laws of nature, decimating useful species . . . and enormously increasing malnutrition in the rural milieu. . . . An urgent and serious investigation is needed."[106]

Although the health authorities never agreed to have public discussions with the few physicians such as Villalobos who opposed the malaria eradication campaign, his criticism resurfaced in the early 1970s, when it was evident that eradication had not achieved its target and when the assimilation assumptions of applied medical anthropology had eroded. Encouraged by the populist presidency of Luís Echeverría (1970–76)—which promised more democracy, subtly stimulated a critique of the traditional homogenizing cultural role played by the Instituto Nacional Indigenista, and proclaimed a renewed interest in meeting the needs of disadvantaged citizens—Villalobos sent a letter to the health authorities.

A senior CNEP executive member responded to Villalobos's letter with a report downplaying the document, saying that it was just one of the few nonrelevant cases of resistance and criticism of provincial physicians. According to the report, the origin of the criticism of these doctors was animosity. Some private doctors were considered uncooperative by the health authorities because they were losing their traditional malaria patients and were being displaced from the powerful positions they enjoyed in remote locations by official health programs. According to CNEP, it was just an illustration of resentment produced by the displacement of empirical clinical knowledge by scientifically based public health knowledge. The report, which was used only for internal purposes, recognized some mistakes, such as the fact that sprayers swallowed insecticides and the little attention paid to migration patterns.[107] With regard to the relation between the toxic effects of insecticides and Villalobos's unexplained "viral mutation," a concise but definitive sentence dismissed Villalobos's idea as unscientific. The report sought to avoid a public debate because it regarded the potential dissemination of such a discussion as "extremely harmful" for malaria eradication. In this way, Villalobos received a response where some mistakes were recognized, albeit never in public.[108]

The case of Villalobos illustrates the tension between the health authorities and some provincial doctors during malaria eradication. His opposition was more visible because his university training gave him some credibility, he had access to local and national newspapers, and his criticisms were somewhat rare in Zacatecas, where malaria was not a dramatic issue. According to an estimate for the period 1949–53, this state had a malaria mortality rate slightly above 18 per 100,000 inhabitants, far below the national average of 89.[109] Although Villalobos's opposition to the malaria eradication campaign appears isolated but prominent, less visible but more acute and widespread resistance can also be found in some peasant villages.

Indigenous Resistance

On August 16, 1959, a few years after the malaria eradication campaign was implemented, Marcial Matías Velasco and a brigade of DDT sprayers entered Quiotepec, located in a region known as Cuicatlán, an enclosed lowland in the northern hills of Oaxaca that separate Zapoteca territory from Mexico's central and eastern zones. Quiotepec was a village of about 105 houses where the primary language was a unique form of Chinanteco, Spanish was virtually unknown, and people lived on subsistence farming. Surprisingly to Matías Velasco, CNEP health workers encountered adamant resistance to their work from villagers who had previously accepted DDT spraying. People broke their propaganda, rose menacing wood sticks, and shouted vociferously: "Fucking bedbuggers. . . . Go to hell with your bullshit. . . . My house will not be sprayed. . . . First I will burn it to see it with more bedbugs."[110]

This complaint about bedbugs referred to the disgusting brownish flattened ovoid insects with small wings, known by scientists as part of the order of *Cimex* and called in Spanish *chinches,* that usually appear to arise from nowhere. Their sudden proliferation was a dangerous inconvenience because these blood-feeding insects are usually active during night; move quickly over floors, walls, and ceilings; can survive for a long time without a blood meal; are parasites on humans, chickens, and occasionally domesticated animals; and leave a foul odor from oily secretions. To make matters worse, the insect's bite leaves an inflamed itchy red welt and their reproduction rate is rapid—they can complete development in as little as a month, producing three or more generations a year.

Apparently, the villagers were convinced that the spraying teams knew about the poisoning effects of the insecticide and the proliferation of DDT-resistant bedbugs. Although the transmission of pathogens to humans by bedbugs is unlikely, an understandable concern in Quiotepec was that just like the *Anopheles,* they could transmit a disease. The very next day, Matías Velasco returned to the village and requested full backing from the municipality's president, the highest local officer, and the schoolteacher, even though municipalities had little power and resources in that rural location.[111] Despite his energetic call, no one appeared. Even the local notifiers about the spraying excused themselves by saying that their lives were in danger with the radical opposition to malaria eradication of the villagers.

After searching the huts of Quiotepec, Matías Velasco found Manuel Correa, the principal municipal officer, who explained that people believed that DDT, known as the "dust" (*polvo*), contained *chinches'* eggs, and that spraying merely increased the bedbug population with no beneficial effects. He accused the CNEP authorities of deceiving them by sending a useless insecticide and suggested a radical change in the campaign: to eradicate bedbugs instead of *Anopheles.* Matías Velasco and the sprayers paid little attention to what they perceived as illogical and unsound explanations and tried to spray Correa's house. Even that could not be done. The municipal officer cursed the CNEP workers and impeded the spraying attempt.[112] Shortly thereafter, the CNEP workers tried to spray a few more houses in the village, achieving little success. Eventually, only 25 of the town's 105 houses were sprayed.

A few days later, a higher CNEP authority visited the town again. Correa demanded to see a decree signed by the Government of Mexico that specifically said that the people of Quiotepec had to allow their houses to be sprayed with DDT. Although the CNEP officer readily presented the presidential antimalaria decree of 1956, the evidence was unconvincing to the municipal officer, because he thought it referred to Mexico in general but not to the specific location where he lived. More aggressively, Correa refused to sign a document put forth by the health workers, in which he accepted his opposition to the health authorities and accused the CNEP workers of being part of a government conspiracy against poor peasants; his refusal was adamant: "What you want is solely to fuck (*chingar*) the people, as always has been done by the government." In a more sober tone, he confessed that his opposition also came from his fear of being killed "by the Indians" if he helped CNEP.[113] His repeated use of the strong curse-verb "*chingar*"—literally, "to rape"—had a special connotation because it was linked to an official intervention that appeared intolerable.

Again and again, CNEP resorted to the authority of the federal government in cases of open resistance. For example, in Guerrero, where opposition to spraying had been stern in some areas, a mid-1966 leaflet began with this warning signed by the Health Secretariat: "By Presidential decree, your house will be sprayed with insecticides." Moreover, health workers relied more on this kind of authority to enforce their recommendations.[114] Another indication of the need to persuade people to comply with malaria eradication was the emergence in the late 1960s and early 1970s of a number of posters and pamphlets with titles that reveal a need to overcome distrust and find consent, such as "The sprayer; your friend," "Open the door of your house," "Just one drop of blood," and "The notifier will help you."[115] Yet despite the propaganda used by CNEP, the resistance of some municipal rural authorities persisted.[116]

In other locations, village dwellers believed that careless and dishonest spraying teams were loosing or diverting genuine DDT and substituting it with an inferior product. Similar examples of suspicion that the insecticides used in some localities were of a lower quality, defiant opposition to spraying because of bedbug infestation, and even attacks on the spraying brigades occurred in Cuicatlán, Oaxaca, and Morelia.[117] In the indigenous state of Guerrero, the CNEP authorities recognized that unscrupulous sprayers have been requesting food or payment from peasants.[118] These incidents were similar to previous indigenous rejections of sanitary campaigns, such as smallpox vaccinations.[119] The headline of a provincial newspaper echoed these concerns: "Mosquitoes Laugh at DDT."[120] An American nurse who worked in Oaxaca in the 1950s ironically registered in his memoirs an entrenched belief in Cuicatlán that "bedbugs climbed up legs of chairs, fell from beams. I learned that the whole canyon was infested with bedbugs. The spraying against malaria had not touched a whisker on their bodies."[121] The concern with bedbugs made people in some places wash or replaster their walls after the sprayers were gone, or contravene CNEP recommendations and sleep outdoors to avoid bedbug attacks. For CNEP officers, all these actions nullified the effects of the insecticide.[122]

Initially, CNEP had little to say with regard to bedbugs and denied a relationship between the pest and DDT.[123] According to health officials, the insecticide did not increase the population of *chinches*—it only took them out of their hiding places. The medical explanation was that as an irritable insecticide, DDT increased the "mobility" of bedbugs, thereby giving the impression of an increased infestation. For CNEP, bedbugs could easily be eliminated with good sanitation and domestic measures such as disinfectants, filling the fissures in the walls, applying kerosene to surfaces where the bugs rest, such as window frames and cracks in walls, and general house cleanliness.[124] Contrary to what the official propaganda said repeatedly at the beginning of the campaign, health officers affirmed that malaria eradication's ultimate goal was to eliminate the *Plasmodium,* not the *Anopheles.* Moreover, these and other insects would still exist.[125]

Years later, scientists discovered that popular complaints were right. After a few years of DDT spraying, bedbugs developed resistance, as did many other insects. A similar situation developed in the United States as well. According to an imaginative American popular writer, DDT was guilty for creating "Frankenstein" insecticide-resistance mites and other pests just for the sake of "benefiting the agricultural chemical industry."[126] In time, bedbug infestation became a critical issue in Mexican malaria eradication, causing delays, an increase in the working days needed for spraying operations, and a discrediting of the whole health intervention. Even the hygienic emphasis of CNEP was useless because, unlike cockroaches that feed on filth, the level of cleanliness has little to do with most bedbug infestation. As a result, openly or silently, some people refused to cooperate with sprayers in measures such as empting houses or providing water for spraying.

In 1962, Luís Vargas, the most noted scientist in Mexican malaria eradication, decided to intervene. He launched a project to determine how best to deal with bedbugs, and he trained entomologists to identify and control them. The task was difficult because warm human dwellings were a suitable habitat for bedbugs, and because these insects could be transported on clothing or hide in bedding and furniture. CNEP's unpreparedness and naive perspective on this matter were evident a few years later, when Vargas published a paper in which he described bedbugs as a serious complication of only a "public relations" nature; in other words, something that might be resolved with educational programs and dissemination of "scientific" information.[127] During the middle and late 1960s, the popular and medical challenges of malaria eradication became more intense. At the same time, the political climate that sustained the international health campaign in the first place also changed.

A Campaign in Decline

Since 1960, Mexican and international malaria eradicators had resorted to a euphemism to minimize the conundrum encountered by the campaign: "problem areas." After four years of intensely covering the country with residual insecticides, the attack phase of eradication ended, and "control" was almost complete—but only in three-quarters of the original malarious area. This was an unexpected outcome, because the original design had promised to advance the whole country to the last phase of "consolidation" by that time, a stage at which there would be no infected *Anopheles* and no feverish cases harboring *Plasmodium* in their blood. Surprisingly, transmission persisted in pockets of the remaining "problem areas," where transmission had not been interrupted and spraying had to be maintained. Although there was no thorough examination of the nature of the problem, most medical reports emphasized that problem areas were mainly technical and localized, and naturally tended to decrease.

However, shortly thereafter, Mexican "problem areas" expanded. According to health experts, the main cause was resistance of *Anopheles albimanus* to DDT and Dieldrin. At almost the same time, Dieldrin resistance was reported from *Anopheles pseudopuntipennis*. As a result, residual insecticides were partially ineffective for the two main vectors in the country.[128] To make matters worse, some species of *Anopheles* were able to penetrate DDT-sprayed houses made of sticks, bite their sleeping residents, and escape without having picked up a lethal dose of insecticide. "Erratic behavior" was the new euphemism encapsulating in medical terms the unexpected fact that undermined one of malaria eradication's main assumptions—that a mosquito would rest on its victims' walls.[129] Another technical difficulty was that frequent use of insecticides eroded a pump's nozzles. Some sprayers either delivered too much insecticide and their operations become grossly wasteful, or they sprayed too little and failed to cover walls with sufficient insecticide.[130]

Anopheles resistance to insecticides began in the southeastern corner of Chiapas, near the Guatemalan border, in an area recently converted to pesticide-addicted commercial cotton cultivation that helped to build up resistance among the *Anopheles* and received a significant number of migrants from northern Guatemala, the poorest region in this Central American country.[131] Since the 1960s, Central America had become a booming market for pesticide manufacturers and commercial cotton agriculturalists, who often allowed chemicals no longer used in industrial countries because of their toxic impact on the environment.[132]

To make matters worse, Guatemala had intense malaria in its rural areas, its health services were precarious, and its malaria eradication program lagged behind Mexico. Malarial areas increased in Chiapas because of the indiscriminate use of DDT and pesticides in Central American agricultural systems, an increased migration of Guatemalan peasants to the South of Mexico, and deforestation to open up new rural areas for development projects.[133] The number of Guatemalan immigrants grew during the 1970s and early 1980s. An illustration of the relevance of the Guatemala-Mexico border was that since the 1970s, more than half of malaria cases in the state of Chiapas—which accounted for about 60 percent of Mexico's southern frontier—occurred in Mexican municipalities located next to the Guatemala border.[134]

As a result, starting in the mid-1960s, Chiapas, sections of Oaxaca, and successive parts of the country, where it was hoped that malaria was ending, were "lost" by malaria eradicators. Malaria reestablished itself, usually with an initial low but persistent transmission, and whole areas had to be placed back under "attack," which meant a return to total coverage spraying. The increase in the total number of malaria cases is illustrated by these figures: 11,700 cases in 1961, and 16,700 in 1963.[135] Most of these cases were found in scattered small rural localities of fewer than 500 inhabitants with poor communications systems and little information on what was happening in the rest of the country.[136]

To confront these challenges, CNEP developed a few pilot programs that used a more frequent spraying schedule, lapsing every four instead of every six months; intense treatment called a "radical cure," which consisted of daily supervised doses for recurrent fever cases; closer surveillance of blood samples; and strict house-to-house searches for feverish individuals. The loosely implemented rule established at the beginning of the program that required health workers to take preventive pills twice a week was more rigorously enforced. In an effort to intensify treatment in remote villages where people had little experience with Western medicine and little reason to adhere to an extended treatment regime, CNEP personnel stayed close to patients for the fourteen days required for the daily dose of primaquine, the drug used to treat and prevent *vivax* malaria in "radical cure" programs.[137]

One pilot project was called the Collective Plan of Antimalaria Treatment (Plan de Tratamientos Colectivos Antipalúdicos, PTCA), which was implemented in Pochutla, in southern Oaxaca, a region of about 1,400 square miles where steep narrow valleys constituted a formidable barrier to communications and prevention.[138] The name of the plan was considered a contradiction because it combined an emphasis on community-based prevention and individual treatment, two stages that usually are separated in public health thinking. PTCA visited 727 towns and treated 75,000 individuals with primaquine pills. By 1963, more than 92,000 Mexican patients had received primaquine.[139] In addition, the plan of Individual Responsibility (Responsabilidad Individual Antimalarico, PRIAL) was launched in areas of the state of Morelos, in which fieldworkers were responsible for the supervision and recovery of specific feverish cases within their area of work. Again, treatment appeared to be more important than the former emphasis on prevention that had prevailed when malaria eradication emerged.

PRIAL also suggested that fieldworkers were to be blamed for the failures of the campaign, a trend that would intensify.[140] CNEP began to criticize "loose fieldwork" as a "major administrative issue" and notifiers as always useful, accurate, or productive. One common accusation from CNEP headquarters was that sprayers and notifiers did not obtain useful blood smears.[141] Part of the problem came from the rapid training that they had received and from the lack of CNEP methods to test films on the spot that required sending blood samples to regional laboratories.

Intense "radical" treatment was the source of new resistance in Oaxaca because primaquine produced nausea, dizziness, and allergic reactions. The drug was not indicated for people suffering from rheumatoid arthritis, and it caused vomiting and stomach cramps if overdosed. Furthermore, unfounded popular rumors magnified the more harmful collateral effects of the drug.[142] To confront such resistance, local political and religious authorities requested that the entire population cooperate with the program. A general letter addressed to the population supported the program in terms that stressed the traditional paternalism coming from the state and indicated that there was some popular suspicion of the health authorities: "Do not distrust us! Your government would never give you something that might harm you."[143]

Toward the mid-1960s, the complications faced by the Mexican campaign intensified and the enthusiasm of Mexican politicians and of international and national public health leaders began to wane. The initial impression that "problem areas" or merely technical and administrative problems were the main causes of the campaign's shortcomings became problematic. From a social perspective, other socioeconomic problems pointed out by García Manzanedo, Kelly, and Villalobos came to the fore and became more salient, such as rural misery; the primitive construction of rural houses with numerous openings, which allowed mosquitoes to enter and exit freely; temporary shelters built in different farm fields; and nomads and migrants who moved from areas where the malaria program was beginning to areas in "consolidation."[144]

An important political factor was the tradition of discontinuity, namely, a lack of consistency in public health work. When malaria declined, complacency ensued. It was hard to persuade people, particularly politicians and young health workers who had never experienced the havoc of malaria outbreaks, to continue the fight for something that was no longer perceived as an emergency. Local politicians thought it was exaggerated to maintain a strict eradicationist discipline when epidemic outbreaks no longer occurred. According to some medical doctors, this posture was similar to that of a careless patient who, having received an antibiotic prescription for more than one week, abandoned it after a few days when the fever began to subside.

An obstacle for the continuity of malaria eradication was the fragmentation of the public health system. In many rural areas, there were no permanent medical organizations and few professional health personnel capable of sustaining antimalaria activities once the sprayers were gone. The rural population was scantly supplied with hospitals, public health care centers, and rural medical posts, and in some regions there was no health service of any kind.[145] The eradication program lost legitimacy among urban inhabitants when accidental malaria cases, produced by contaminated blood transfusions in hospitals, appeared in the cities.[146] Alarmingly, "transfusion malaria" occurred in urban residents who had never traveled to the countryside. Although the number of cases was minimal, the event revealed a crack in the public health system: Little was or could be done to screen blood donors, who frequently came from poor areas and who ignored or concealed their illnesses because they were often motivated by financial gain. Sometimes one of the few commodities they could sell was their own blood. A Mexican medical expert "confessed" in 1962 that because parasite density in an infected donor may be very low, an adequate laboratory test to screen blood stored in hospitals for *Plasmodium* was unavailable.[147]

After its inception in 1955, the Tripartite Plan for malaria eradication was relaunched by the United Nations Children's Fund (UNICEF), the PASB, and the Mexican Health Secretariat. A new beginning was planned for 1963, when some experts insisted that eradication was still possible, such as Paul Russell, who edited the second edition of his *Practical Malariology* in that year.[148] The 1963 five-year plan of intense attack and surveillance set 1968 as the new deadline. An innovative, effective method that was implemented tailored diverse programs to the different ecological and epidemiological zones of Mexico. According to the new plan, two financial limitations of prior efforts were the small economic resources and the fact that the Mexican government spent much more than was originally expected compared with the international agencies, approximately 70 percent of the total cost of the campaign. In the 1963 plan, the campaign's cost was estimated at 748.3 million pesos, but almost half the budget had to be obtained from abroad. Trying to overcome the difficulties and disillusionment because the initial targets were not reached on the foreseen dates, the plan presented a dilemma: "either to continue with insufficient budgets during a still not defined number of years, not spraying the areas appropriately . . . or the necessary sums are gotten."[149] The necessary amount of money was never obtained, causing disappointment.

By 1966, the Mexican malaria program was judged by international health officers to be in a state of stagnation, and even to be deteriorating in some areas. The Chilean Abraham Horwitz, the new director of the Pan-American Health Organization—the Pan-American Sanitary Organization, PASB, had changed its name in 1959 to Pan-American Health Organization—tried to "save" a program in a "dead end."[150] That same year, the hopes for malaria eradication were dashed by a malaria epidemic outbreak of 33,000 cases in Paraguay.[151] Two years later, the international reputation of the program was further discredited when more than 1 million people in Sri Lanka (Ceylon) contracted malaria.[152]

The World Health Assembly of 1969 in Boston reversed malaria eradication and approved a resolution that established a tense coexistence between control and eradication.[153] A resolution titled "Re-examination of the Global Strategy of Malaria Eradication" blamed, with no clear organizing principle, unforseen socioeconomic, financial, administrative, and operational factors, and the inadequacy of the basic health services, as the reasons for the failure of malaria eradication.[154] According to new malariologists based in Geneva, one of the main reasons for the change was the notion that eradication without the previous creation of rural health services was impossible. They correctly discerned that the dismissal of research by leaders of eradication, such as Fred L. Soper, was one of the causes of the campaign's failure. Their criticism suggested an erroneous assumption in international public health: developing countries had been perceived in the original design as places where knowledge elaborated abroad just waited to be implemented. Some provincial CNEP officers agreed with the opinion of Geneva. In October 1966, the chief of Zone IX, which comprised the state of Guerrero, lamented that for the past few months there had been no epidemiological investigations in the most critical areas because of a lack of personnel, and he complained that unfortunately he did not have a good idea of what was going on in localities previously reported as having malaria cases.[155]

According to a WHO officer, a new "comfortable" assumption was that while there were technical reasons for the difficulties in malaria eradication, the primary cause of the program's failure was the lack of a complete, continuing health service infrastructure that could reach every household and remain in place.[156] This idea was contrary to the initial design, which had envisioned malaria eradication as an entry point for the creation of these services. It would take a number of years and a new generation of public health workers to elaborate a different model for building public health services.

WHO's decision was accepted by multilateral and bilateral health agencies but was questioned by developing countries trying to maintain loyalty to this largest single international health cooperation activity.[157] At the Boston assembly, the delegate from Brazil criticized the inherent contradiction and hesitation of WHO policymakers, and defiantly asked to stick with the military metaphors used at the beginning of the campaign: "Malaria eradication was spoken of in military terms. . . . Are we at war with malaria or not?" A sarcastic representative from Costa Rica held not the *Anopheles,* but rather the population and the "ministries of finance," responsible for the growing "resistance," and lamented that WHO could not convince them to maintain their support for eradication.[158] A different delegate from a developing country found fault in the changes in Cold War priorities, because in the late 1960s, donors and agencies were more interested in the conquest "of outer space" than malaria eradication.[159] This reference alluded to an emphasis on the space race between the Soviet Union and the United States over the priorities of developing countries during a period of increasing "peaceful coexistence" between the superpowers. These and other comments indicate that an organized turn to control was never fully implemented and therefore explain why the new strategy was ineffective. Mexican and Latin American governments interpreted the agreements as a signal to relax their fight against the disease.[160]

In 1970, against all odds, a resilient CNEP made an effort to relaunch malaria eradication with a new six-year plan. By that year, malaria was reported in 58 percent of the whole country, a proportion close to that which existed before eradication began in the mid-1950s. Although only 49,000 cases were recorded, the true figures were estimated by experts to be at least four times higher. The chief focuses of the disease were, first, locations along the Gulf of Mexico, including the Yucatán Peninsula, where about 10 million people lived; and second, the Southern Pacific coastal areas. The new campaign involved the intensive use of DDT, and new insecticides such as the toxic organophosphate Malathion (more expensive to produce than DDT) and Hexachlorocyclohexane, a manufactured chemical also known as HCH.[161] Malathion later made a bad reputation for itself because it caused numbness, headaches, tremors, nausea, abdominal cramps, blurred vision, difficulty breathing, and a slow heartbeat, along with debilitating sprayers' immune systems. HCH also had harmful side effects such as dizziness, headaches, and seizures.[162] The fact that DDT and other pesticides began to be produced and sold by the Mexican government, especially for commercial agriculture, played a decisive role in the decision to continue with eradication. This was first done by a company called Guanos y Fertilizantes de Mexico (GUANOMEX), later known as Fertilizantes Mexicanos (FERTIMEX), which became a state-owned monopoly for producing seed, fertilizers, pesticides, and insecticides.[163] Starting in 1970, different zones of CNEP were receiving and using the DDT produced by the Mexican companies.[164]

As a result of these factors, malaria work ceased to be "glamorous," and donors lost all enthusiasm for eradication. In the late 1960s, UNICEF abandoned malaria work in Mexico, and the country continued malaria eradication solely with the support of the Pan-American Health Organization, WHO, and the U.S. Agency for International Development (USAID).[165] A book on the history of UNICEF held that this agency had "psychologically abandoned" malaria eradication in many parts of the world due to waning government support and because insecticides were being used excessively.[166] Other international organizations, such as USAID and WHO, also tried to forget about eradication without a complete assessment, just as one would rather forget a dream turned into a nightmare. The abandonment of the campaign after the lengthy deployment of such massive human and financial resources became an embarrassment to many Latin American governments and agencies, and malaria work ceased to be mentioned.

Three more factors explain the decline of malaria eradication from multilateral and bilateral agencies' agendas: the accusations that health campaigns contributed to overpopulation, the widespread denouncement of the contaminating effects of insecticides, and the retirement of the old guard of malariologists. The World Bank led the way in blaming malaria eradication for igniting a population explosion in developing countries with its concomitant pressure upon subsistence resources and national economies. The World Bank's president, Eugene Black, endorsed a book titled *Does Overpopulation Mean Poverty?* questioning the role played by "miracle drugs and insecticides" in the decline of infectious diseases within a context of high birthrates and poor living conditions.[167] A table in the book titled "How Much Does the United States Government Spend Each Year on Health Programs in the Underdeveloped Countries?" blamed malaria eradication for absorbing more than 38 percent of all nonmilitary foreign aid.[168] Leaders of industrial countries followed, augmenting the fear that in the near future, developing countries would have to confront Thomas Malthus's prediction that increased poverty was unavoidable unless fertility rates were reduced.[169]

Some American medical journals joined the neo-Malthusian chorus and warned about the dangers of overpopulation for national security. Best-selling books like *The Population Bomb* by Paul Ehrlich, a distinguished professor of population studies and biological sciences at Stanford University, which went through more than twenty editions from 1968 to 1971, blamed DDT for contributing to an international disaster.[170] A Johns Hopkins University professor who considered overpopulation "the most serious problem we face today" was more blunt: "A contributing factor . . . is the control of malaria and other diseases. Withdrawal of DDT would reinstitute one natural check on the human population."[171]

Latin American, and particularly Mexican, population growth—the result of reduced infant mortality and unchanging birthrates—was considered acute by international agencies, more intense than in any other developing region of the world, and this played a central role in the "overpopulation debates."[172] Mexico's population was expanding rapidly, almost entirely from natural increase, because immigration was negligible, at an annual growth rate of 3.1 percent between 1950 and 1975—the highest proportion in Latin America. In addition, Mexico City was becoming the largest city on the continent and a megametropolis with 11.9 million inhabitants by the mid-1970s.[173] An unexpected population effect of malaria eradication was its contribution to urbanization. Before the 1950s, dwellers from the highlands, who were usually free of malaria but experienced acute attacks if they were infected in the lowlands, were "fearful of the wet, tropical climate of the coastal areas" partly because of "malaria and other diseases."[174] This fear disappeared with the elimination of malaria from urban areas. A 1970 indicator of the growing importance of the cities is that the shares of the urban and rural populations that year were almost the opposite of those in 1950 (respectively, they were 58.7 and 41.3 percent in 1970 and 42.2 and 57.8 percent in 1950).[175] Furthermore, between 1930 and 1960, Mexico City nearly quadrupled its inhabitants to almost 6 million.[176] The migratory process increased after the early 1950s due to the confluence of factors such as urban industrialization and the crisis of agriculture. This process transformed Mexico from a country where half the population lived in rural areas into one where most people lived in urban areas.

WHO, the Pan-American Health Organization, and other international health agencies were slow in responding to these attacks. According to Symonds and Carder, UN agencies, especially WHO, delayed their participation in the "overpopulation debates" of the early 1960s.[177] Initially, multilateral agencies regarded the question of overpopulation as a "technical" issue of interest only to demographers. In 1965, Donald Pletsch, the former representative of the PASB in Mexico, who was then working in malaria eradication in Ethiopia for USAID, responded to this concern in a letter to the editor of *Science,* using a metaphor with a classical theme of the Cold War, namely, atomic weapons; he noted that "no workers on the Manhattan Project could have done more soul-searching than many of us engaged" in malaria eradication. He also responded to the objection that eradication was counterproductive, stating energetically that malaria eradicators were saving lives and avoiding the recurrence of epidemics.[178] It was only in 1967 that a reorganization of the United Nations accommodated the increasing demand for population services by creating a Population Division and emphasizing the need for government policies on fertility control. Two years later, this division became the basis for a larger organization—the United Nations Fund for Population Activities (UNFPA). Placed under the United Nations Development Program, the UNFPA shifted population recommendations from demography to development.[179]

Some Mexican and Venezuelan malaria eradication leaders such as Vargas and Arnoldo Gabaldón resorted to old arguments to defend the antimalaria campaign, claiming that eradication contributed to a general decline in mortality and to an increase in life expectancy and the amount of healthy labor power available for productive work in developing nations.[180] The Mexican and other Latin American governments, physicians, and intellectuals initially rejected the idea of controlling population growth because of their Catholic roots, on the one hand, and because they believed that one of the main development questions of their countries was underpopulation, on the other.[181]

DDT came under harsh attack by environmentalists after the publication of Rachel Carson's *Silent Spring* in 1962, which became a turning point for the public perception of damage caused to the environment by industrialization in the United States.[182] A number of studies followed that proved that DDT polluted the environment; killed fish, birds, and several small animals; and was dangerous to human beings in large amounts. The insecticide was blamed for the decline in the North American population of the bald eagle, the emblem of the United States, and of the peregrine falcon, one of nature's most beautiful birds of prey.[183] These negative perceptions about the consequences of the massive use of insecticides resonated with Villalobos's idea about the danger of modern medical technology: Sometimes the cure was worse than the disease.

For the Food and Agriculture Organization of the United Nations (FAO), a UN agency devoted to agricultural development and based in Rome, maintaining the insecticide's production was important because it accounted for more than half the insecticides used for crop protection in developing countries. The agency believed it was a sound method to fight not only malaria but also hunger.[184] In 1969, FAO's biannual conference alerted developing countries not to follow what was becoming a growing trend in the United States and Western Europe: a wide curb on DDT and other insecticides in crops.[185] A WHO officer concurred: "It was preferable to live in fear of cancer in old age than to die in infancy (from malaria)."[186] Leading scientists such as the biochemist Philip Handler, president of the National Academy of Sciences, subscribed to these opinions. In 1971, he published an article in *Science* lamenting the "appalling exaggerated statements" made by scientists advocating a total ban on DDT.[187] To soften the international opposition, FAO and WHO promoted the so-called "integrated pest control system," which endorsed the proper, restricted, and safe use of insecticides and examined the use of natural enemies to insects that transmitted diseases. The debate on the advantages and limitations of DDT would continue for years to come.

In 1972, two years after the establishment of the U.S. Environmental Protection Agency, DDT was the first pesticide the agency banned in the United States. Similar decisions were made simultaneously by Canada, the United Kingdom, Sweden, and Norway. In the same year, the United Nations sponsored the first major international conference on environmental issues in Stockholm and created the United Nations Environment Program, with headquarters in Nairobi. This new multilateral agency had the mandate to achieve a scientific consensus on environmental issues and encourage "sustainable development," which meant improving the standards of living of poor nations without destroying their environments.[188]

Because of the increasing cost of producing and testing insecticides, their production declined in the United States. However, they were still exported—in 1971, more than 22 million pounds of DDT were purchased and shipped abroad, and 11.3 million pounds were exported in 1973.[189] During the 1970s, as multilateral agencies avoided a definitive decision on DDT, chemical corporations were not held accountable, and massive quantities of toxic pesticides not used in the United States were dumped for sale in poor countries. Pesticides that had been banned in the United States were exported to other countries and applied to agricultural exports. Often these countries had few regulations, unsafe practices, and improper or useless labeling because final users were illiterate. When the United States imported the pesticide-bearing crops, what has been called a circle of poison was complete; consumers in America were exposed to invisible poisons, despite the existence of domestic regulations prohibiting them. This resulted because of the cultivation of contaminated agricultural products in developing countries and their consumption as food imports in developed countries.[190]

During the period 1972–75, more than 14,000 poisonings and a few deaths from pesticides were recorded in the cotton plantations of Central America, due to the indiscriminate use of pesticides.[191] In the following years, WHO recognized that the number of fatal and nonfatal accidental poisonings by pesticides among agricultural workers in developing countries had increased dramatically.[192] Even in the early 1980s, however, the malaria authorities in the Mexican Health Secretariat dismissed the perils of contamination. Although the classic work of Carson had been available in Spanish since 1964, thanks to a translation done in Spain, environmental concerns evolved slowly in Mexico in the late 1960s and early 1970s.[193] A director of CNEP wrote that he would always like to protect species in danger of extinction such as the bald eagle but that he had to give priority to the children that suffer from malaria and thus supported malaria eradication, saying that it confronted the contamination of houses by *Anopheles*.[194]

Another dimension of the retreat of malaria eradication was that experienced health officers began to leave malaria eradication services and were not replaced. The Pan-American Health Organization's commitment to eradication was less intense after 1959, when Soper retired from the organization. Russell also withdrew from an active career, and Marcolino Candau retired from WHO in 1973. Like Soper, Candau expressed his opposition to new antimalaria policies quietly and in a low voice.[195] Maurice Pate, UNICEF's executive director, died in 1965 and was replaced by Henry R. Labouisse, who had a greater interest in community development projects. Only Gabaldón publicly criticized WHO and the new international policies to control malaria.[196] A paper presented at a symposium organized by the New York Academy of Medicine by the British scientist Leonard Bruce-Chwatt, who was a supporter of the old guard, lamented the perception of malariologists as "sorcerer's apprentices," unable to control the forces they unleashed.[197] An anecdote illustrates Soper's detachment, isolation, and longing for better days. In 1972, one of his disciples visited him and had the following awkward conversation: "He looked at me with his piercing eyes and asked 'How are things doing?' I replied 'Bad!' and he asked me 'Who will be our ally?' I said 'Malaria'—and he almost hugged me because this was the answer he expected."[198] It seemed as if malaria eradication had really eradicated the leading malariologists.

By end of the 1960s, malaria eradication seemed hopeless, and international funding rapidly dwindled. USAID ended its annual contribution to the Pan-American Health Organization's Special Malaria Fund in 1970, a decision that led to the restriction of several national programs[199] The American bilateral agency—with the full support of President Lyndon Johnson—had a greater concern about overpopulation and began to emphasize the promotion of family-planning programs and birth control in developing nations. An article based on the response of Latin Americans to the new emphasis on fertility control over any other health program questioned the population bomb–defusing official policies: "Perhaps the burdens of the space race, hot and cold wars, and the development of nuclear facilities were causing the United States to look to solutions cheaper than economic development."[200] An editorial in *The Lancet* had a self-explanatory title: "Epitaph for Global Malaria Eradication?" Other articles in mainstream journals questioned the whole eradication approach.[201] In 1974, a brokenhearted new director general asked WHO's Executive Board: "Was malaria eradication a foolish enterprise? Where, when and how did the program go wrong?"[202] A WHO officer described the atmosphere at the end of the malaria campaign and the new priorities emerging at international health agencies: "[In the late 1960s] . . . WHO and many countries were struggling to face the implications of the failure of malaria eradication. . . . And the long knives were out looking for . . . scapegoats to blame."[203]

Starting in the mid-1960s, WHO began to insist on better mechanisms for malaria's continuous assessment and surveillance, and it criticized the "autonomy" of malaria eradication services from local health services. This idea was contrary to the original design, which envisioned self-contained antimalaria units. In a new and idealistic policy, antimalaria programs should transform themselves to work not in isolation but as part of a national development plan for basic health services in rural areas.

Mexican health workers, partially impressed by the new international public health policies, began to look more deeply into the distribution and roles of basic health services in rural areas. A tense meeting between CNEP and other rural public health agencies in 1965 was an indication that the lack of coordination among rural health services was a problem in Mexico, particularly in the rural areas.[204] It proved difficult to coordinate segments of a fragmented public health system with their own tradition and leaderships. The health authorities in Oaxaca also complained four years later that the effort was "absolutely insufficient" and wondered if the country should unify its public health system, as had been done by Sweden, the United Kingdom, Chile, and the USSR.[205] Even in the 1970s, when the Mexican health authorities that attempted to enforce the new WHO malaria decision in their country found that local services did not favor integration with the rest of the rural services, they preferred to continue with antimalaria work "as a vertical structure." According to the health officers of Mexico City, this reaction was provoked more by the fear of losing privileges and power than by an expected effectiveness of vertical work in public health.[206]

The Cold War political context that initially validated malaria eradication was also vanishing. "Modernization theory" was criticized by a Latin American school of development that argued that it was ethnocentric because the "past" of their nations did not resemble the "past" of the United States.[207] These and other critics also questioned Cold War modernization models and believed that increased commercial ties with industrial countries and foreign bilateral assistance from the United States would increase dependency rather than the development of poor nations.[208] Development programs launched from abroad, or from capital cities, were blamed for concentrating on the most "modern" and commercial areas of a country and ignoring its "backward" regions. The Mexican sociologist Rodolfo Stavenhagen argued that there was really no opposition between modern and traditional poles—as modernization models assumed—but both were part of the same process whereby the powerful elites of these groups worked together to keep the population oppressed.[209]

Mexican anthropologists also criticized the modernization model for its authoritarianism, refused to follow the "taming" goals of applied anthropology, criticized the manipulation of their discipline by official programs, and claimed that so-called cultural "indigenous obstacles" were an official tool for blaming the victims that obliterated the social roots of rural poverty. They also rejected the notion of a single "mestizo culture" unifying all Mexican ethnic communities, and instead they envisioned a pluralistic culture that would respect the autonomy and idiosyncrasy of indigenous minorities.[210]

Latin American and international antiestablishment movements criticized traditional "modernization" programs such as the Alliance for Progress and questioned the validity of the claim that the United States was a model to be followed by developing nations. According to some authors, the Alliance had "lost its way" because the United States was afraid of the Latin American left taking over the program. Cumbersome local bureaucracies were also blamed for this result.[211] Even American government officers recognized the shortcomings of the program, but they argued that it failed because of the selfishness of Latin American entrepreneurs and oligarchs who were unwilling to reinvest their profits to improve the living conditions of the indigenous population.[212]

President Johnson stalled the Alliance for Progress partly because he was immersed in the war in Vietnam and domestic headaches such as the unfulfilled demands of the civil rights movement and his troubled attempts for to create a "Great Society." Starting in the mid-1960s, U.S. foreign policy commitments to Latin America were reduced. During Johnson's two terms, the U.S. government shoved aside bilateral programs and returned in practical terms to unilateralism with regard to many developing countries. In Latin America, the change was made clear in 1964, when Marines landed in the Dominican Republic to overthrow a regime that was accused of becoming communist. This was the first overt intervention in the region in fifty years and a symbol of the impossibility of continuing with the Alliance for Progress. The official end of the program came in 1973, when the Organization of American States disbanded the permanent committee created to implement the alliance.

Malaria was related to these international political, economic, and cultural developments. During the 1960s, the United States slowly but steadily suffered a reemergence of the disease. In 1959, fewer than 50 cases of malaria were registered in America. It was estimated that during the mid-1960s, nearly 10 percent of American soldiers experienced malaria during the Vietnam War. In 1967 alone, there were 2,669 cases of malaria among returning Vietnam veterans as well as 146 civilian cases in the continental United States.[213] By 1970, the figure rose to 4,239 reported individuals, mostly soldiers who had never before been exposed to malaria. The repatriation of infected soldiers to the U.S. mainland brought the danger of importing drug-resistant strains of *Plasmodium* to areas where *Anopheles* still existed. According to a military history of the Vietnam conflict, malaria was the leading cause of medical disability. U.S. Army physicians quietly expressed their concern with the failure of traditional drugs to protect troops against *Plasmodium falciparum* malaria and shifted to mefloquine, a potent replacement developed at the Walter Reed Army Institute of Research. After a few years, that drug also was not effective enough. The U.S. Army was also preoccupied about its inability to convince private pharmaceutical firms to undertake research to discover new antimalaria drugs because, as a spokesperson for one company stated, it made little sense to produce costly pharmaceuticals for a disease that was mainly prevalent in countries with "people who cannot afford shoes," much less costly drugs.[214]

Although malaria was not the main cause of the defeat of the U.S. Army in Southeast Asia, the impact of the disease is a little-studied factor in this defeat. Though American doctors could not fully protect their troops, the disease posed little danger for the Vietnamese, who had some immunity because they had been exposed to it since childhood and had relied on an ordinary sweet wormwood called *Artemisia annua,* a medicinal plant also known as *qinghaosu* (which was especially effective against *Plasmodium falciparum* and had been used for decades in Asian countries to treat malaria and hemorrhoids). The Vietnamese authorities appealed to their allies, the Chinese, who were interested in reassessing plants used in traditional medicine, to develop new antimalaria drugs. In 1970, Chinese medical scientists extracted *Artesimin,* the active ingredient of the plant, and developed a new antimalaria remedy. This efficient antimalaria medicinal plant was kept secret by the Chinese and Vietnamese for a few years so it was unknown to the Americans and the rest of the world.[215] In addition, transfusion-transmitted malaria began to appear in American hospitals, affecting an unprepared civilian population. Although the number appeared insignificant—twenty-six cases of transfusion-induced malaria were reported from 1972 through 1981—its appearance caused great preoccupation among medical doctors, and it was suspected that it was underreported; namely, only a small proportion of episodes was officially recorded.[216]

Despite the lack of support from the United States and international health agencies, the Mexican health authorities persisted with malaria eradication during the 1970s.[217] They became convinced that abandoning such a great medical enterprise would mean wasting an important investment already made in health personnel and ideals of development. They also became convinced that their determination and stamina would extend the limited gains of eradication and overcome the shortcomings of the program, namely, the need to change rigid structures and the increasing cost of the operations. CNEP continued during the 1970s, but most of its budget went to fieldwork, equipment and supplies became scarce, and little was done to investigate the diverse ecological and epidemiological conditions of the disease. During the 1980s, CNEP lost 30 percent of its personnel because of resignations, voluntary retirements, and transfer to other public health programs.[218] Less was done to research the social and cultural dimensions of malaria, change traditional educational programs, and sensitize health workers to the culture of rural people. With fewer financial resources, no increase in personnel, rusting equipment, and decreasing morale among health workers, the work of the notifiers was weakened, and the visits of health personnel to motivate them and provide them with material became sporadic.

A significant difficulty for malaria eradication in Mexico was the demands of CNEP's fifteen different labor unions, a powerful lobby that was unwilling to eradicate malaria after the mid-1960s because of the assumption that it would eliminate the work of its members and they would lose the autonomy and special allowances gained when the service was created.[219] The CNEP unions demanded permanent appointments and higher salaries during the late 1960s, a conflictive period between the Mexican health sector and the government marked by a number of physicians' strikes. According to Gabaldón, who was by the early 1970s the most noted Latin American malariologist, the original announcement that the malaria service would be disbanded after the achievement of eradication undermined the morale of health workers, who were less than thrilled about having a temporary occupation.

In an attempt to save the program, Gabaldón suggested that the health authorities create a permanent health unit against mosquito-borne diseases on the basis of the malaria eradication services and devote more resources to research and fixing what might have been incorrect. Unfortunately, his advice was not followed.[220] By the late 1970s, CNEP still survived, but 90 percent of its budget went to payrolls, little to fieldwork, and none to research, and 70 percent of CNEP vehicles were out of order. According to a report, administrative routine prevailed, and the 5,000 CNEP health workers had the lowest morale.[221] What had previously been the most important unit of the Health Secretariat was in a state of decay, not knowing exactly what its future held.

In addition, what was left of the political commitment to malaria eradication was undermined by new political priorities. After 1970, with the election of a new president, Luís Echeverría, the Mexican political authorities began to echo the international concern over the "excessive" population growth of the country, then approaching 60 million inhabitants. In 1970, a regional conference on population, the first of its kind in Latin America, was organized by the most prestigious institution of higher education in the social sciences, El Colegio de Mexico. The meeting was under the auspices of the International Union for the Scientific Study of Population, the UN

Economic Commission for Latin America, and the Centro Latinoamericano de Demografía. They received funding from the Inter-American Development Bank, USAID, the World Bank, the Social Science Research Council, and the Rockefeller Foundation.[222] In the wake of the event, a few Latin American government officers and scholars rejected traditional pro-natalist policies and promoted birth control as the cornerstone of new "population policies." In 1973, President Echeverría revised the population law and initiated family-planning programs to limit population growth.[223] This decision was a departure from the pro-natalist policies implied in malaria eradication.

During the 1970s, Mexico also went through an erosion of the political and economic context that had stimulated malaria eradication in the first place. Examples of this erosion were the stagnation of the Mexican agricultural sector in the 1970s, the beginnings of an economic crisis that exploded in 1982, the clash between university students and the government that can be traced to the protesters gunned down by the Army at the Plaza de Tres Culturas in the Tlatleolco section of Mexico City in 1968, and the emergence of guerrillas in Guerrero in the late 1960s led by Lucio Cabañas, a schoolteacher-turned-revolutionary who was hunted down by the military in 1974.[224] Although these were mostly middle-class movements, they drew attention to larger social and political ills such as intolerable authoritarianism, the worsening of rural poverty, growing urban underemployment, and Mexico's skewed distribution of wealth, which strained the basis of popular support for the governments of the Partido Revolucionario Institutional (Institutional Revolutionary Party). These events also underscored the fact that the Mexican miracle boom initiated in the late 1940s was ending. President Echeverría attempted to regain popular support by repairing relations with the university students, reorienting federal policies toward the poorest segments of the population, nationalizing the mining and electrical industries, redistributing private land in some states, and opposing, albeit verbally, the U.S. foreign policy in the region.

A letter addressed to the new Mexican president and signed by the leaders of an indigenous community reveals that popular distrust of malaria eradication persisted in the early 1970s. This document is also an example of how individuals and communities considered public health not as the right of any citizen but as a limited resource that could be obtained from or blocked by a paternalistic authority. The letter was written by peasants from Cosolapa, Oaxaca, in a broken-Spanish style that demanded the end of malaria eradication because it was just a waste of money for the Mexican nation and a loss of useful time and we are sorry that our nation has been fooled with [the idea] that with this powder paludism will end. . . . Not even medical doctors realize what is paludism; paludism has several causes:

1. Bad nutrition
2. The person is working and goes for a bath or receives rain. . . .
3. When someone drinks too much water before eating. . . .
4. When the patient is cold and then the fever gets into him. . . .

Since this powder arrived, all the peasants are losing. All the chickens and hens, the pigs and even the dogs and cats. . . . The brigades come. . . . They don't care about spilling in the water or in the food, is this fair? And if there is a very sick person, they do not care, they spray him, . . . and they threaten us if we oppose, they take us to jail, is this good? No, Mister President, you must stop all the brigades and save our nation and we Mexicans will be grateful to you who knew how to look after your children.[225]

CNEP's brief response was to order the local authorities to provide the correct information and give "advice" to those who had signed the letter under the assumption that, as in the case of Villalobos, it was just a matter of poor "public relations."

From the late 1970s on, Mexican and international health leaders became convinced that there was no "magic bullet" in the work against malaria. Instead, antimalaria activities needed to attack many fronts and adapt to diverse ecologies and cultural contexts. Furthermore, they demanded the creation of permanent rural health services tied to significant improvements in the living conditions of the rural poor.[226] As a 1970s Mexican medical evaluation correctly suggested, "Prospects to eradicate malaria cannot be examined outside the context of the country's overall development problems."[227] By the early 1980s, a malaria researcher recognized the wisdom of indigenous objections to the campaign from individuals who could not understand why malaria should be selected for elimination "rather than poverty, hunger, or other diseases."[228] It's interesting to note that a similar idea was expressed at the beginning of the campaign by a municipal authority of a village in Oaxaca that requested work against endemic diseases and environmental sanitation.[229]

A new international health perspective, later called Primary Health Care, emerged, which stressed the importance of antimalaria health workers first understanding the living conditions and culture of recipients, using

acceptable and inexpensive technology, and which promoted the active participation of local leaders in the design and implementation of comprehensive health programs. In the mid-1980s, WHO published a technical report
that promoted malaria control as an intrinsic part of Primary Health Care.[230]

It was not easy to produce an orderly withdrawal of sprayers and malariologists from former health policies and reorient them to a new perspective.
The Mexican health care unit in charge of malaria maintained its vertical
characteristics and limited its activities to treating the sick, reducing transmission, and distributing a chemical larvicide. Little was done with regard
to vector control, the removal of inadequate water systems in rural areas,
or the eradication of rural poverty. Not only had the dreams of eradicating
malaria vanished, so had those of controlling it. Individual treatment became the main response to the disease.[231] In epidemiological terms, malaria
in Mexico, as in other Latin American nations, returned to a similar condition, albeit not as serious as the one of the first half of the twentieth century.
The rural poor resigned themselves to accepting malaria as an unavoidable
part of life. Their ability to dodge or overcome malaria infection, as well as
other illnesses, became part of a strategy for a *culture of survival.*

A precedent for this culture of survival was the deeply rooted human
dimension infused in the local responses to malaria eradication in Mexico,
the criticisms of provincial private doctors such as Villalobos, the questioning of insider anthropologists such as García Manzanedo and Kelly, and
even the indigenous resistance to the toxic effects of insecticides. All these
activities suggested the existence of a holistic effort to understand the cultural dimension and local dynamics of health and disease. Furthermore,
they proved that the local appropriation and adaptation of any international
health campaign was crucial to its success.

5

Conclusions: The Return of Malaria and the Culture of Survival

This chapter briefly recounts Mexico's recent experience with malaria and examines contemporary international health programs aimed at controlling the disease. It also offers conclusions stemming from the lessons learned from malaria eradication efforts in Mexico that are useful for other developing nations dealing with the scourge of the disease. It underlines the limitations of a "vertical," technologically driven eradication program and its legacies in the rural population. The emphasis of international health cooperation on sanitation from above and the transference of modern technologies and foreign experts could gain the commitment of national political and medical authorities but failed to convince fully provincial leaders, doctors, and communities. An unsuccessful short-term intervention facilitated a partial return of the disease and contributed to a limited understanding of international public health work. This understanding undermined the efforts to control malaria, disengaged community participation, and sustained a popular belief that the poor have to survive the perils of endemic and epidemic diseases by themselves.

Mexico's Recent Experience with Malaria

Since the mid-1980s, there have been periodic outbreaks of malaria in Mexico. In 1982, the number of malaria cases was estimated at more than 20,000 (most of them in the southeastern part of the country); and three years later, an epidemic outbreak resulted in more than 140,000 cases.[1] There was a slight decrease in 1988, when the number of registered malaria cases in the whole country was 116,230.[2] However, data for the state of Oaxaca in the

1980s illustrate an unrelenting and tragic trend: A total of 5,861 malaria cases registered in 1978 meant a rate of 258 cases per 100,000 inhabitants for the whole state. By 1984, the number of cases and rate had respectively grown to 17,375 and 684. Four years later, in 1988, the 28,852 malaria cases in Oaxaca represented a rate of 1,089 per 100,000 inhabitants, and 25 percent of the cases in the whole country (which had a much lower rate of 140 per 100,000). In addition, malaria was the fourth-highest cause of morbidity in Oaxaca, after respiratory diseases and two types of diarrheal disease. The situation was also becoming critical in other southeastern states, such as Chiapas and Guerrero, which in 1988 respectively had 18,922 and 17,062 cases, representing rates of 751 and 667 per 100,000.[3]

At the same time, the capacity of the country's public health system to respond to this challenge was curtailed by medical unemployment, economic crisis, severe recession, and mounting foreign debt.[4] During the 1980s, the paradox of overpopulated medical schools but few positions for medical doctors—especially in the rural areas—became acute and hindered anti-malaria activities. The number of medical schools had increased from fifteen in the mid-1950s to fifty-seven in 1983. At the same time, only a fourth of medical school graduates could expect a permanent job, and the number of unemployed physicians was estimated at 40,000.[5] To make matters worse, the government still discriminated against the practice of traditional and domestic medicine in general, and this type of medicine was separated from the rest of the official public health system.[6]

Although malaria rates fell by the end of the decade, in 1995 it was estimated that 47,505 Mexicans lived in malarious areas. The malaria situation was more dramatic in Chiapas and Oaxaca, where transmission was more frequent and higher than in the rest of the country.[7] Fortunately, since 1982 no malaria-attributable deaths and few cases of the Chloroquine-resistant, pernicious, and deadly *Plasmodium falciparum* strain have been reported in the country. According to the U.S. Centers for Disease Control and Prevention, the number of reported malaria cases was to 3,819 in 2003, for which *P. falciparum* accounted for only 1 percent.[8] Although the eradication campaign did not achieve its objective, its spin-off benefits should not be forgotten. Malaria ceased to be a major cause of morbidity in Mexico, and geographical medical reconnaissance produced the first maps for many remote areas that were later used in other health campaigns.

Yet some of the inequalities and old, counterproductive techniques persisted. No malaria transmission occurred in the major urban and tourist centers of the country. In particularly at-risk states, such as Chiapas, transmission was concentrated in rural areas, and DDT continued to be the weapon of choice.[9] Other poisonous pesticides were used in commercial agriculture with the hope of bringing higher yields, but they also negatively affected the health and environment of rural people. In addition to these problems, Mexico must face the increment of migrants from neighboring Guatemala and other Central American countries, where malaria was more widespread. For example, in 2004, according to an estimate from the U.S. Centers for Disease Control and Prevention, there were more than 57,000 malaria cases in Guatemala, making up more than 40 percent of the cases reported for the Mesoamerican region.[10]

Only after international pressure was applied did Mexican government officials and FERTIMEX—the state-owned producer of DDT—begin to restrict and ban some pesticides and insecticides. One of the most acute cases of pesticide poisoning occurred in the mid-1970s in Lagunera in northern Mexico, where 847 people were affected and 4 died.[11] Mexico did not stop using DDT altogether for malaria control until 2000. A year later, an international agreement on organic pollutants—the first global treaty seeking to ban an entire class of chemicals used in agriculture—was signed in Stockholm by more than ninety countries, including Mexico and the United States.[12] Nine organic pollutants were banned outright, but DDT still was placed in a secondary category calling for a gradual phaseout.

During the past few years, a number of medical doctors and international experts have tried to bring back DDT for malaria control, creating a controversy with environmental scholars and activists, who had reemphasized the insecticide's contamination effects. These doctors and experts have argued that the risks of DDT to human health have not been scientifically confirmed, that the reemergence of malaria is strongly correlated with the decreasing number of houses being sprayed with DDT, and that DDT remains the most effective technique for malaria control.[13] The scholars and activists have correctly counterargued that there are diverse techniques available to fight malaria that do not rely on DDT and that developing countries should first address their other basic health needs, such as safe water systems, adequate diets, better housing, and more medical services.[14] However, in September 2006, the World Health Organization (WHO) decided to recommend the safe and correct use of indoor residual spraying of DDT to reduce malaria transmission. According to WHO, what should be banned is the use of insecticides and pesticides in agriculture because it causes environmental and human harm and builds up *Anopheles* resistance.[15] However, the possibility of its "safe" use in poor rural areas is still being questioned, and some environmental advocates maintain their strong opposition to the insecticide.

These developments have been parallel to the emergence of new international antimalaria perspectives. A Global Malaria Control Strategy was adopted by WHO and the Pan-American Health Organization following a major 1992 conference of health ministers in Amsterdam. The strategy placed more emphasis on the early diagnosis and adequate treatment of human cases rather than on vector control. It also emphasized the need for preventive and protective measures and for strengthening local human capacities.[16]

On the basis of the Global Malaria Control Strategy, an important program called Roll Back Malaria was launched in 1998 as part of a global partnership between WHO, the World Bank, the United Nations Children's Fund (UNICEF), and the United Nations Development Program. The program's goal is to cut the world's malaria burden in half by 2010.[17] Initially, the program recognized some of the failures of malaria eradication. Although, in the program's original design, the practice of dipping bed nets in pyrethroids was not promoted as the single most effective technique, it ended up fulfilling the role of former magic bullets such as the insecticides and drugs often used in the 1950s. In addition, since the turn of the twenty-first century, great hope has arisen that an antimalaria vaccine will appear as a new high-technology solution. The first vaccine can be traced to the work of the Colombian medical scientist Manuel Patarroyo, who produced important but unconvincing evidence in the late 1980s. In 1997, the U.S. National Institute of Allergy and Infectious Diseases launched a ten-year research plan for malaria vaccine development, and it remains confident that a vaccine will soon be found.[18] In the following years, great hope was placed in new medicines because previous antimalarials are useless in many regions due to drug resistance. Among these medicines were Artemisinin Combination Therapies—recommended by WHO since 2001 where the life-threatening parasite *Plasmodium falciparum* is the predominant infecting species—whose origins can be traced to the medicinal plant used in Southeast Asia by Vietcong soldiers during the Vietnam War.[19]

In 2000, a Global Fund to Fight AIDS, Tuberculosis, and Malaria was created at the Group of Eight industrial countries meeting in Okinawa as a public-private partnership that included WHO, the World Bank, non-governmental organizations, government agencies, and companies' representatives. In addition to receiving aid from the governments of the major industrial countries, the Global Fund is also supported by the Bill and Melinda Gates Foundation.[20] Some of the Global Fund's documents appeared to be critical of the one-sided vertical malaria eradication campaign and to place a greater emphasis on the transformation of the so-called contextual determinants of malaria, a concept that entails a marked betterment of living conditions in rural areas, greater access to health services, health supervision of population movements, and a readiness for sudden changes in global climate to ease the proliferation of the *Anopheles* mosquito.[21] However, much of the Global Fund's valuable effort is concentrated on AIDS and tuberculosis. Its grants for antimalaria work only accounted for 26 percent of the total between 2002 and 2005.[22]

Although malaria is no longer the main killer in most countries in the Americas, seventeen of the twenty-three North, Central, and South American countries or territories reported cases of malaria in 2001, and 293 million people (almost 36 percent of all the continents' inhabitants) still live in areas with some risk of malaria transmission. Although Brazil has most of the American continents' malaria cases (388,658 of the 960,000 reported in 2001), the disease is still a major concern in Mexico.[23] Moreover, it is a health challenge for the entire developing world, which each year suffers an estimated 1 million deaths and 500 million infections.[24] The great majority of these cases occur in Sub-Saharan Africa.

The Lessons of Malaria Eradication: Patterns of Vertical Health Programs

The Mexican malaria eradication story suggests at least four patterns in disease-oriented vertical programs. First, there has been a tendency to assume that success gained in a specific region can be applied effectively anywhere. This was especially problematic, because the achievements that preceded worldwide malaria eradication came mainly from islands in the Pacific, the Mediterranean, and limited areas in Brazil and Venezuela. These early attempts at malaria eradication received massive amounts of aid, were run by the military, or presented limited difficulties because they occurred in medium-sized areas or were aimed at eradicating a specific species of *Anopheles* (as Fred Soper did in Brazil).

Malaria was eliminated in the United States during the 1940s and 1950s by versatile projects such as the New Deal's Tennessee Valley Authority, which combined environmental sanitation to reduce mosquito breeding areas, such as building dams and drainage projects; the elimination of the adult *Anopheles;* intense health education; and traditional control methods.[25]

The authority was also part of a comprehensive effort that included build-ing a navigable waterway, flood control, reforestation, and the agricultural development of the region. The overall objective was not only to eliminate one disease but also to pull an economically depressed region out of back-wardness.[26] In addition, the malaria infection rate was already in decline, and parasitic transmission was tenuous in the southern United States. Sim-ilarly, some Latin American countries with limited resources and personnel managed to control malaria during the 1940s by combining changes in so-cial and environmental factors. However, these rich national experiences be-came irrelevant for international experts of the 1950s, because the "prom-ise" of new technologies seemed to be more effective.

The belief that it was possible to eradicate malaria anywhere using the same techniques was based more on the conviction of a transnational net-work of brilliant people and bilateral and multilateral agencies than on em-pirical experience. Thus, malaria eradication became a belief system, a "gospel"—or, in the words of some of its advocates, a "doctrine"—and many lessons of the past were conveniently forgotten.[27] Eradication also reinforced the expectations that the use of new techniques and methods would rapidly solve a disease problem, instead of building public health systems and educating people for health and development, which usually took more time and effort.

Second, the vicissitudes of the malaria eradication campaign in Mexico suggest that malaria and other widespread infectious diseases are not only natural realities needing adequate technological solutions but also socially and economically sustained realities requiring a social and a political re-sponse. In view of the cultural constraints the campaign encountered, the three assumptions of the success of the campaign (technical feasibility, economic benefits of eradication over control, and government political sup-port) clearly appear to be insufficient. There was a growing tension between overconfidence in medical technology and cultural challenges that could not be solved. Many Mexican and Latin American health officers struggled between, on the one hand, the convenience and limitations of vertical-specific disease programs, and, on the other hand, community-supported or horizontal approaches. The main problem with this tension is that it absorbs the attention of health workers in short-term efforts, leaves little room for self-criticism, and undermines the construction of unified and flexible pub-lic health systems, as well as the complementary coexistence of diverse perspectives such as vector control and environmental sanitation. It also undermines the possibility of public health leaders and health workers becoming actors among the political forces that define what should be done. Local actors and cultures ultimately determine the success of an international health intervention.

A third important lesson is that there was an assumption that all the information needed was available. No attention was paid to the need for more research or to history as an illuminating reality. Moreover, when things went wrong in international health cooperation, there was a repeated tendency to forget the challenges and move on to something else. Less attention was given to reinforcing local research capabilities and maintaining a historical perspective of the achievements and limitations of prior efforts. As a result, one of the shortcomings of national and international health institutions was their inability to deal with past policies; consequently, the process of dismantling malaria eradication was not fully completed, evaluated, and assimilated by international, national, and local health agencies and practitioners. Partly for this reason, there have been problems of territoriality, a lack of flexibility, and fragmentation between health programs.

Fourth and finally, the main cultural legacy of a technically oriented malaria eradication campaign was that there was little understanding of the nature and aims of public health work. The military format and the aim for "perfection" in public health that the campaign embraced do not work in the long run. Although they might discipline donors and health workers for a while, they fail to engage the public at large. Public health is by nature an "imperfect" social arena. Moreover, a public health program should not be an instrument of narrow political interests, which is what happened when policymakers pursuing Cold War imperatives tried to use the malaria eradication campaigns of the 1950s as a political tool. The legacy of narrowly based societal and political support was clear in the reinforcement of what I have called a *culture of survival* and *privileges of poverty* in health work in Mexico and other Latin American countries that embraced malaria eradication. Many poor people in these countries sincerely believe that public health work is merely a temporary or partial response to emergencies and only involves the provision of insecticides, vaccines, drugs, and hospitals. The malaria eradication campaign assumed that people were passive recipients of its efforts. Moreover, this limited understanding of public health was usually the only health-related demand of Latin American politicians and international agencies. Ephemeral and isolated health activities have the negative effect of reinforcing short-term expectations for public health work. In addition, the limited use of health education and the use of euphemisms such as *canalización* connote that the givers know what is best for the receivers and that the real aim of public health authorities is limited to the compliance of populations.

The *culture of survival* means that poor people are accustomed to struggling to gain access to state programs and foreign aid, to relieve pain, to delay death, and to protect their loved ones. The *privileges of poverty* refers to the situation in which powerful national elites and international agencies control the distribution of limited resources, which become an enormous source of power in a context where health care resources are scarce. In combination, the culture of survival and the privileges of poverty reinforce inequity, dependency, and passivity. Health work is portrayed and perceived as a short-lived and low-valued activity.

It is important to keep in mind these historical lessons of malaria eradication in order to improve antimalaria work in developing countries. In sum, these lessons are the fact that universal and "perfect" solutions do not exist; the need for holistic, persistent, and flexible approaches to develop a popular culture of malaria prevention, vector control, and treatment; and the relevance of the history of public health to illuminate health policy. In addition, the history of malaria eradication provides a remarkable example of underdog Mexican volunteers and critics making extraordinary humanitarian efforts to adapt an international health campaign to their local conditions.

By examining these lessons of the history of malaria eradication, health workers can learn how to break the vicious circle between a culture of survival and the privileges of poverty. Making local adaptations a priority, enhancing community participation in the design of health care programs, improving health workers' appropriation of techniques, and transforming what donors decide can be the beginning of a more inclusive theory and practice of local, national, and international public health cooperation that encourages self-reliance and dramatically challenges the social conditions that recreate malaria.

Notes

Chapter 1. Introduction: The Burden of an Infection

1. See Socrates Litsios, *The Tomorrow of Malaria* (Karori, N.Z.: Pacific Press, 1997), 13; and A. J. Kennel, ed., *Malaria* (London: Wellcome Trust, 1991), 3.

2. David A. Warrell and Herbert M. Gilles, eds., *Essential Malariology,* 4th ed. (London: Arnold, 2002); Jeffrey D. Sachs and Pia Malaney, "The Economic and Social Burden of Malaria," *Nature* 415 (2002): 680–85.

3. On history and public health, see Enrique Perdiguero Gil, Josep Bernabeu Mestre, Rafael Huertas García, and Esteban Rodríguez Ocaña, "History of Health: A Valuable Tool in Public Health," *Journal of Epidemiological Community Health* 55, no. 9 (2001): 667–73.

4. Herbert M. Gilles and David A. Warrell, eds., *Bruce-Chwatt's Essential Malariology,* 3rd ed. (London: Arnold, 1993).

5. Luís Vargas, "Malaria along the Mexico–United Sates Border," *Bulletin of the World Health Organization* 2, no. 4 (1950): 611–20.

6. Oswaldo Jose da Silva, "Malaria Eradication in the Americas," in *Infectious Diseases: Their Evolution and Eradication,* ed. Aidan Cockburn (Springfield, Ill.: Charles C Thomas, 1967), 309–30.

7. W. G. Downs, "History of Epidemiological Aspects of Yellow Fever," *Yale Journal of Biology and Medicine* 55 (1982): 179–85.

8. Margaret Humphreys, *Malaria: Poverty, Race, and Public Health in the United States* (Baltimore: Johns Hopkins University Press, 2001).

9. See Randall M. Packard and Paulo Gadelha, "A Land Filled with Mosquitoes: Fred L. Soper, the Rockefeller Foundation, and the *Anopheles Gambiae* Invasion of Brazil," *Parassitologia* 36 (1994): 197–213.

10. The Japanese invasion of the Dutch East Indies in 1942 cut off the primary world source of quinine. U.S. research and explorations in the Amazon helped to develop Atabrine. See William H. Taliaferro, "Malaria," in *Medicine and the War,* ed. William H. Taliaferro (Chicago: University of Chicago Press, 1944), 55–75; C. W. Hays, "The United States Army and Malaria Control in World War II," *Parassitologia* 42, nos. 1–2 (2000): 47–52; and R. J. Joy, "Malaria in American Troops in the South and Southwest Pacific in World War II," *Medical History* 43, no 2 (1999): 192–207.

11. Oswald T. Zimmerman and Irvin Lavine, *DDT: Killer of Killers* (Dover, N.H.: Industrial Research Service, 1946).

12. The United Nations Relief and Rehabilitation Administration was established in November 1943 when forty-four Allied nations signed an agreement to coordinate the relief of victims of war through the provision of food, clothing, and medical services. See George Woodbridge, *UNRRA: The History of the United Nations Relief and Rehabilitation Administration,* 3 vols. (New York: Columbia University Press, 1950); and Darwin H. Stapleton, "A Lost Chapter in the Early History of DDT: The Development of Anti-Typhus Technologies by the Rockefeller Foundation's Louse Laboratory, 1942–1944," *Technology and Culture* 46, no. 3 (2005): 513–40.

13. Wallace Peters, *Chemotherapy and Drug Resistance in Malaria* (London: Academic Press, 1970), 5.

14. A general history of malaria is Gordon Harrison, *Mosquitoes, Malaria and Man: A History of the Hostilities since 1880* (New York: Dutton, 1978). A study of malaria in the United States before eradication is Humphreys, *Malaria*. For a general study of the World Health Organization, see José A. Nájera, "Malaria and the Work of WHO," *Bulletin of the World Health Organization* 67, no. 3 (1989): 229–43. The 1994, 1998, and 2000 special issues of the journal *Parassitologia* evince the growing interest in malaria among historians: "Malaria and Ecosystems: Historical Aspects—Proceedings of a Rockefeller Foundation Conference, Como, Italy, 18–22 October 1993," *Parassitologia* 36, nos. 1–2 (1994): 1–227; "Strategies against Malaria: Eradication or Control? Proceedings of a Conference, Annecy, France, April 17–26, 1996," *Parassitologia* 40, nos. 1–2 (1998): 1–246; and M. J. Dobson, M. Malowany, and D. H. Stapleton, "Dealing with Malaria in the Last Sixty Years: Aims, Methods and Results," *Parassitologia* 42, nos. 1–2 (2000): 3–7.

15. This relationship was noticed in Harry Cleaver, "Malaria and the Political Economy of Public Health," *International Journal of Health Services* 7, no. 4 (1977): 557–79.

16. See Nils Gilman, *Mandarins of the Future: Modernization Theory in Cold War America* (Baltimore: Johns Hopkins University Press, 2003).

17. "Statement of Otis E. Mulliken, Officer in Charge of Social Affairs, Office of International and Social Affairs, Department of State, 9 February 1956," in *The United States and International Health: Hearings before a Subcommittee of the Committee on Interstate and Foreign Commerce, House of Representatives, 84th Congress, February 8 and 9, 1956* (Washington, D.C.: U.S. Government Printing Office, 1956), 33–34.

18. See Theodore M. Brown, Marcos Cueto, and Elizabeth Fee, "The World Health Organization and the Transition from 'International' to 'Global' Public Health," *American Journal of Public Health* 96, no. 1 (2006): 62–71; and Anne-Emanuelle Birn, *Marriage of Convenience: Rockefeller International Health and Revolutionary Mexico* (Rochester: Rochester University Press, 2006).

19. James Stevens, "Welcoming Address," in *Industry and Tropical Health: Proceedings of the First Tropical Health Conference Sponsored by the Harvard School of Public Health, 8–10 December 1950,* ed. Industrial Council for Tropical Health (Boston: Harvard School of Public Health and International Council for Tropical Health, 1950), 11–15.

20. See John Lewis Gaddis, "The Emerging Post-Revisionist Thesis on the Origins of the Cold War," *Diplomatic History* 7 (1983): 171–90. The term "Cold War" is attributed to the journalist Walter Lippmann and his book *The Cold War: A Study in U.S. Foreign Policy* (New York: Harper & Brothers, 1947). New studies of this period include

Rana Mitter and Patrick Major, eds., *Across the Blocs: Cold War Cultural and Social History* (London: Frank Cass, 2004); Michael Kort, *The Columbia Guide to the Cold War* (New York: Columbia University Press, 1998); Martin J. Medhurst, ed., *Cold War Rhetoric: Strategy, Metaphor and Ideology* (East Lansing: Michigan State University Press, 1997); and Melvyn P. Leffler, "The Cold War: What Do 'We Now Know'?" *American Historical Review* 104, no. 2 (1999): 501–24.

21. Some examples are Ed Odd Arne Westad, ed., *Reviewing the Cold War: Approaches, Interpretations, and Theory* (London: Frank Cass, 2000); Richard Saull, *Rethinking Theory and History in the Cold War: The State, Military Power, and Social Revolution* (London: Frank Cass, 2001); Elaine McClarnand and Steve Goodson, eds., *The Impact of the Cold War on American Popular Culture* (Carrollton: State University of West Georgia Press, 1999); and Peter J. Kuznick and James Gilbert, *Rethinking Cold War Culture* (Washington, D.C.: Smithsonian Institution Press, 2001).

22. See Jessica Wang, *American Science in an Age of Anxiety: Scientists, Anticommunism and the Cold War* (Chapel Hill: University of Carolina Press, 1999); David A. Hounshell, "Epilogue: Rethinking the Cold War; Rethinking Science and Technology in the Cold War; Rethinking the Social Study of Science and Technology," *Social Studies of Science* 31, no. 2 (2001): 289–97; and Thomas C. Lasman, "Government Science in Postwar America: Henry A. Wallace, Edward U. Condon and the Transformation of the National Bureau of Standards, 1945–1951," *Isis* 96 (2005): 25–51.

23. See Scott Lucas, *Freedom's War: The American Crusade against the Soviet Union* (New York: New York University Press, 1999); and Kenneth A. Osgood, "Total Cold War: U.S. Propaganda in the 'Free World,' 1953–1960" (Ph.D. dissertation, University of California, Santa Barbara, 2001).

24. Ben Thomas Trout, "Political Legitimation and the Cold War," *International Studies Quarterly* 19, no. 3 (1975): 57–60.

25. See Richard Barnet, *The Giants: Russia and America* (New York: Simon & Schuster, 1977).

26. Patience A. Schell, "Nationalizing Children through Schools and Hygiene: Porfirian and Revolutionary Mexico City," *The Americas* 60, no. 4 (2004): 559–87.

27. Ana María Kapelusz-Poppi, "Physician Activists and the Development of Rural Health in Postrevolutionary Mexico," *Radical History Review* 80 (2001): 35–50; and Ana María Kapelusz-Poppi, "Rural Health and State Construction in Post-Revolutionary Mexico: The Nicolaita Project for Rural Medical Services," *The Americas* 58, no. 2 (2001): 261–83.

28. E.g., David Arnold, ed., *Warm Climates and Western Medicine: The Emergence of Tropical Medicine, 1500–1900* (Amsterdam: Rodopi, 1996); David Arnold, *Colonizing the Body: State Medicine and Epidemic Disease in Nineteenth-Century India* (Berkeley: University of California Press, 1993); Warwick Anderson, "Postcolonial Histories of Medicine," in *Locating Medical History: The Stories and Their Meanings*, ed. Frank Huisman and John Harley Warner (Baltimore: Johns Hopkins University Press, 2004), 285–306; and Michael Worboys, "Tropical Diseases," in *Companion Encyclopedia in the History of Medicine*, ed. William F. Bynum and Roy Porter (London: Routledge, 1993), vol. 1, 512–36.

29. See Randall M. Packard, "No Other Logical Choice: Global Malaria Eradication and the Politics of International Health in the Post-War Era," *Parassitologia* 40, nos. 1–2 (1998): 217–29; Randall M. Packard and Peter J. Brown, "Rethinking Health, Development and Malaria: Historicizing a Cultural Model in International Health,"

Medical Anthropology 17, no. 3 (1997): 181–94; Randall M. Packard, "Malaria Dreams: Postwar Visions of Health and Development in the Third World," *Medical Anthropology* 17, no. 3 (1997): 279–96; and Socrates Litsios, "Malaria Control, the Cold War, and the Postwar Reorganization of International Assistance," *Medical Anthropology* 17, no. 3 (1997): 255–78.

30. A partial list includes Christopher Abel, *Health, Hygiene, and Sanitation in Latin America c.1870 to c.1950* (London: Institute of Latin American Studies, 1996); Marcos Cueto, ed., *Salud, cultura y sociedad en América Latina* (Lima: Instituto de Estudios Peruanos, 1996); Diego Armus, ed., *Disease in the History of Modern Latin America: From Malaria to AIDS* (Durham, N.C.: Duke University Press, 2003); and Gilberto Hochman and Diego Armus, eds., *Cuidar, controlar, curar: Ensaios históricos sobre saúde e doença na América Latina e Caribe* (Rio de Janeiro: Editora Fiocruz, 2004).

31. See Anne-Emanuelle Birn, "Wa(i)ves of Influence: Rockefeller Public Health in Mexico, 1920–50," *Studies in the History and Philosophy of Biological and Biomedical Sciences* 31, no. 3 (2000): 381–95; Marcos Cueto, ed., *Missionaries of Science: The Rockefeller Foundation and Latin America* (Bloomington: Indiana University Press, 1994); and Christopher Abel, "External Philanthropy and Domestic Change in Colombian Health Care: The Role of the Rockefeller Foundation, ca. 1920–1950," *Hispanic American Historical Review* 75, no. 3 (1995): 339–76.

32. Some works are Diana Obregón, *Batallas contra la lepra: Estado, medicina y ciencia en Colombia* (Medellín: Banco de la República de Colombia, 2002); Marcos Cueto, *The Return of Epidemics: Health and Society in Peru during the 20th Century* (Aldershot, U.K.: Ashgate, 2001); Jaime Benchimol, *Dos micróbios aos mosquitos: Febre amarela e a revolução pasteuriana no Brasil* (Río de Janeiro: Editora Fiocruz, 1999); and Marta de Almeida, "Combates sanitários e embates científicos: Emílio Ribas e a febre amarela em São Paulo," *História, Ciências, Saúde—Manguinhos* 6, no. 3 (2000): 577–607.

33. Julyan G. Peard, *Race, Place, and Medicine: The Idea of the Tropics in Nineteenth-Century Brazilian Medicine* (Durham, N.C.: Duke University Press, 1999); Nancy Leys Stepan, *"The Hour of Eugenics": Race, Gender, and Nation in Latin America* (Ithaca, N.Y.: Cornell University Press, 1991).

34. Steven Palmer, *From Popular Medicine to Medical Populism: Doctors, Healers, and Public Power in Costa Rica, 1800–1940* (Durham, N.C.: Duke University Press, 2003); David Sowell, *The Tale of Healer Miguel Perdomo Neira: Medicine, Ideologies, and Power in the Nineteenth-Century Andes* (Wilmington, Del.: SR Books, 2001).

35. Paul Farmer, *AIDS and Accusation: Haiti and the Geography of Blame* (Berkeley: University of California Press, 1992); Charles L. Briggs and Clara Mantini-Briggs, *Stories in the Time of Cholera: Racial Profiling during a Medical Nightmare* (Berkeley: University of California Press, 2003); Richard Parker, ed., *A AIDS no Brasil, 1982–1992* (Rio de Janeiro: ABIA, 1994).

36. Disease eradication, namely, the total elimination of a disease from the face of the earth, has been and still is a matter of debate. Eradication attempts have been few and have achieved mixed results (the only illness that has been wiped from the globe is smallpox). See Louis Williams Jr., "Malaria Eradication: Growth of the Concept and Its Application," *American Journal of Tropical Medicine and Hygiene* 7, no. 3 (1958): 259–67; Aidan Cockburn, "Eradication of Infectious Diseases," *Science* 133 (1961): 1050–58; Walter Dowdle and Donald R. Hopkins, ed., *The Eradication of Infectious Diseases* (New York: John Wiley & Sons, 1998); Paul Greenough, "Intimidation, Coer-

cion and Resistance in the Final Stages of the South Asian Smallpox Eradication Campaign, 1973–1975," *Social Science and Medicine* 41, no. 5 (1995): 633–45; Perez Yekutiel, "Lessons from the Big Eradication Campaigns," *World Health Forum* 2 (1981): 465–90; and C. V. Brown and Gustav J. Nossal, "Malaria, Yesterday, Today, and Tomorrow," *Perspectives in Biology and Medicine* 20, no. 1 (1986): 65–76.

Chapter 2. Global Design

1. European researchers established the biological facts on malaria transmission in the late nineteenth century. See David A. Warrell and Herbert M. Gilles, eds., *Essential Malariology,* 4th ed. (London: Arnold, 2002).

2. "Resistance of Insects to Insecticides," *Chronicle of the World Health Organization* 8, no. 3 (1954): 397–400.

3. Wallace Peters, *Chemotherapy and Drug Resistance in Malaria* (London: Academic Press, 1970), 6.

4. "Intervention of Eugene Campbell," *Mutual Security Appropriations for 1959, Hearings before the Subcommittee on Appropriations House of Representatives, 85 Congress, 2nd Session, Subcommittee on Foreign Operations Appropriations* (Washington, D.C.: U.S. Government Printing Office, 1958), 1198, record group 287, National Archives, Maryland (hereafter NA).

5. Murray Morgan, *Doctors to the World* (New York: Viking Press, 1958), 3. The phrase "the war on malaria is a race against time" also appears in "Report on the War against Malaria," *New York Times,* January 24, 1960.

6. The terms "communism" and "slavery" appeared in 1950 in a report prepared by the State and Defense departments and cited by Sergio Aguayo, *Myths and [Mis]-perceptions: Changing U.S. Elite Visions of Mexico* (San Diego: Center for U.S.-Mexican Studies at the University of California, 1998), 42.

7. See Martin J. Medhurst, ed., *Cold War Rhetoric: Strategy, Metaphor and Ideology* (East Lansing: Michigan State University Press, 1997).

8. James Whorton, *Before Silent Spring, Pesticides and Public Health in Pre-DDT America* (Princeton, N.J.: Princeton University Press, 1975), 249.

9. See Lewis W. Hackett, *Malaria in Europe: An Ecological Study* (London: Oxford University Press, 1937), 282–320.

10. For an analysis of Cold War foreign policies, see "Introduction," in *America's Foreign Policy 1945–1976, Its Creators and Critics,* by Thomas Parker (New York: Facts on File, 1980), pp. ix–xxvi. On Dulles, see Richard H. Immerman, ed., *John Foster Dulles and the Diplomacy of the Cold War* (Princeton, N.J.: Princeton University Press, 1990); and Michael A. Guhin, *John Foster Dulles: A Statesman and His Times* (New York: Columbia University Press, 1972).

11. According to one author, the "main goal of the U.S. foreign policy from 1945 to 1976 was the containment of communism"; Parker, *America's Foreign Policy,* ix.

12. The first issue of the *Bulletin* appeared in 1939. "The Department of State, 1930–1955: Expanding Functions and Responsibilities," *Department of State Bulletin* 32 (1955): 470–77.

13. The Bureau of Inter-American Affairs was divided into three offices: South America, Middle America (which included some Caribbean countries), and Regional Affairs (which dealt with the inter-American system and its agencies and events). Roy

Rubottom was assistant secretary of state for inter-American affairs between June 18, 1957, and August 27, 1960, and Francis O. Wilcox was assistant secretary of state for international organization affairs from July 28, 1955, to January 20, 1961. See U.S. Department of State, *Principal Officers of the Department of State and United States Chiefs of Mission, 1778–1990* (Washington, D.C.: U.S. Government Printing Office, 1991), National Archives Library (hereafter NAL), 25.

14. Townsend Hoopes and Douglas Brinkley, *FDR and the Creation of the U.N.* (New Haven, Conn.: Yale University Press, 1997).

15. The most important UN agencies besides WHO were the Food and Agriculture Organization (FAO), the International Labor Organization (ILO), and the United Nations Education, Scientific, and Cultural Organization (UNESCO). "Table I United States contributions to international organizations from fiscal years 1956 funds." In Department of State, *American Foreign Policy, Current Document, 1956,* Department of State Publication 6811 (Washington, D.C.: U.S. Government Printing Office, 1959), 1432–33. Only in the 1970s, the U.S. Congress limited American contributions to 25 percent of the budget of UN agencies.

16. Henry Cabot Lodge, "12th Anniversary of United Nations," *Department of State Bulletin* 37 (1957): 768.

17. Francis O. Wilcox, "International Organizations: Aid to World Trade and Prosperity," *Department of State Bulletin* 37 (1957): 749–54.

18. International Cooperation Administration, *Technical Cooperation in Health* (Washington, D.C.: International Cooperation Administration, 1956), 5; found at National Library of Medicine, Bethesda, Md. (hereafter NLM).

19. Francis O. Wilcox, "World Population and Economic Development," *Department of State Bulletin* 42 (1960): 860–67; the citation here is on 864.

20. "Appendix V: Priorities in International Technical Assistance Health Programs, Joint Statement by the Public Health Division of the Foreign Operations Administration and the PHS and the Children's Bureau of the US, Department of Education and Welfare," in *The United States and International Health: Hearings before a Subcommittee of the Committee on Interstate and Foreign Commerce, House of Representatives, 84th Congress, February 8 and 9, 1956* (Washington, D.C.: U.S. Government Printing Office, 1956), 92–95, record group 287, NA.

21. Christopher Osakwe, *The Participation of the Soviet Union in Universal International Organization: A Political and Legal Analysis of Soviet Strategies and Aspirations Inside ILO, UNESCO and WHO* (Leiden: A. J. Sijthoff, 1972).

22. "Intervention of the Polish Delegate," in *Official Records, Second World Health Assembly,* World Health Organization (Geneva: World Health Organization, 1949), 105–6.

23. Intervention of Wilcox, *Mutual Security Appropriations for 1957, Hearing before the Subcommittee of the House of Representatives, 84th Congress, 2nd Session, Subcommittee on Foreign Operations Appropriation* (Washington, D.C.: U.S. Government Printing Office, 1956).

24. Wilcox, "International Organizations."

25. David McK. Key, "World Security and the World Health Organization," *Department of State Bulletin* 31 (1954): 616–18.

26. Howard A. Rusk, "Promotion of World Health Essential in Fight on Reds," *New York Times* January 13, 1952.

27. During Eisenhower's two administrations, the number and importance of U.S mines, plantations, and business operating in Latin America grew. U.S. direct investment in Latin America increased from $4.4 billion in 1950 to $7.5 billion in 1960; see Samuel

Baily, *The United States and the Development of South America: 1945–1975* (New York: Franklin Watts, 1976), 69.

28. "Justification for the Point Four Program in the Other American Republics— FY 1952, Paper Prepared in the Department of State, Washington, 31 January 1951 [Secret]," in *Foreign Relations of the United States, 1951: The United Nations, the Western Hemisphere,* ed. Frederick Aandahl (Washington, D.C.: U.S. Government Printing Office, 1979), vol. 2, 1041–46.

29. Joseph S. Toner (executive secretary, Foreign Operations Administration), "Statement for the Senate Foreign Relations Committee on Fiscal Year 1956: Bilateral Technical Cooperation and Development Assistance Programs proposed for Latin America, 16 May 1955," folder: Latin America, year: 1955, record group 469, entry 1948–55, box: 14, NA.

30. Harlan Cleveland, Gerard J. Mangone, and John Clarke Adams, *The Overseas Americans* (New York: McGraw-Hill, 1960), 3, 70, 89, 102, 103.

31. "Table I: United States Contributions to International Organizations from Fiscal Year 1956 Funds," in *American Foreign Policy,* by U.S. Department of State (Washington, D.C.: U.S. Government Printing Office, 1957), 1432–33.

32. The statement appears in a newspaper article related to Dulles's visit to Peru attending the inauguration of the new president, Prado y Ugarteche, "Peru's New Chief and Dulles Meet," *New York Times,* July 28, 19561.

33. A report of the meetings of the committee appears in International Cooperation Administration, *Technical Cooperation in Health* (Washington, D.C.: International Cooperation Administration, 1961), 417; found at NLM.

34. Roy R. Rubottom, "Economic Relations between the U.S. and Latin America," *Department of State Bulletin* 37 (1957): 536–40; the citation here is on 536. On economic ties between the U.S. and Latin America, see Ben H. Thibodeaux, "The Role of Economic Cooperation and Technical Assistance in Our Foreign Policy," *Department of State Bulletin* 35 (1956): 808–12; the citation here is on 811. There was a growth in State Department officers assigned to Latin America; by 1955, 110 in Washington and 1,125 individuals located in Latin America (in comparison, the staff in 1930 was 22 and 312, respectively). See "The Department of State," *Department of State Bulletin,* 484. On U.S.–Latin American relations during the Cold War, see Peter H. Smith, *Talons of the Eagle: Dynamics of U.S.–Latin American Relations* (New York: Oxford University Press, 1996); Stephen Rabe, *Eisenhower and Latin America: The Foreign Policy of Anticommunism* (Chapel Hill: University of North Carolina Press); Joseph S. Tulchin, "The United States and Latin America in the 1960s," *Journal of Interamerican Studies and World Affairs* 30, no. 1 (1988): 1–36; and Max Paul Friedman, "Retiring the Puppets, Bringing Latin America Back In: Recent Scholarship on United States–Latin American Relations," *Diplomatic History* 27, no. 5 (2003): 611–36.

35. Roy R. Rubottom Jr., "Economic Interdependence in the Americas," *Department of State Bulletin* 36 (1957): 732–35; the citation here is on 733.

36. "Justification for the Point Four Program in the Other American Republics."

37. In "Department of State, INR Files, Secret, National Intelligence Estimate, "Latin American Attitudes towards the U.S. 2 December 1958," *Foreign Relations of the United States, 1958–1960, American Republics,* Vol. 5 (Washington, D.C.: U.S. Government Printing Office, 1991), 60–77; the citation here is on 77.

38. See Chris Tudda, "Reenacting the Story of Tantalus, Eisenhower, Dulles and the Failed Rhetoric of Liberation," *Journal of Cold War Studies* 7, no. 4 (2005): 3–35.

39. "Wilcox Intervention," *A Review of the Relations of the U.S. and Other American*

Republics, Hearings before a Subcommittee on International Affairs of the Committee on Foreign Affairs, House of Representatives, 85th Congress, 31 July 1958 (Washington, D.C.: U.S. Government Printing Office, 1958), 99, record group 287, NA.

40. See Peter W. Rodman, *More Precious Than Peace: The Cold War and the Struggle for the Third World* (New York: Charles Scribner's Sons, 1994).

41. By 1958, communist parties were legal in five Latin American countries (Argentina, Bolivia, Ecuador, Mexico, and Uruguay). Roy R. Rubottom Jr., "Communism in the Americas," *Department of State Bulletin* 38 (1958): 180–85. See also Robert Jackson Alexander, *Communism in Latin America* (New Brunswick, N.J., Rutgers University Press, 1957).

42. "Statement of Secretary Dulles," *Department of State Bulletin* 30 (1954); and "Intervention of International Communism in the Americas," *Department of State Bulletin* 30 (1954), 419–26; the citation here is on 421.

43. Stephen C. Shlesinger, *Bitter Fruit: The Untold Story of the American Coup in Guatemala* (New York: Doubleday, 1982). Dulles said after the events: "We here in the Americas are not immune from that threat of Soviet communism," in "The Spirit of Inter-American Unit, Address by Secretary Dulles, Made at Caracas, 4 March 1954," *Department of State Bulletin* 30 (1954): 379–83.

44. "Statement of Dulles," *The Mutual Security Act of 1954, Hearings before the Committee on Foreign Affairs House of Representatives, 83rd Congress, April, May, June 1954* (Washington, D.C.: U.S. Government Printing Office, 1954), 5, record group 287, NA.

45. Dwight D. Eisenhower, "Toward Mutual Understanding among the Americas," *Department of State Bulletin* 42 (1960): 471–86. Latin American governments often complained that Europe received significant U.S. economic assistance. The United States felt that this complaint was unfair because the needs of devastated Europe were larger and because Latin America prospered during the war. See "Guatemala Highlights Latin American Ills," *New York Times,* June 27, 1954.

46. Chester Bowles, "Why Foreign Aid?" *Department of State Bulletin* 48 (1963): 777–84; the citation here is on 781.

47. The Kennedy administration expected about $80 billion in investment to come from Latin American governments. "Alianza para el Progreso, address by President Kennedy, 13 March 1961, Washington, D.C.," *Department of State Bulletin* 44 (1961): 471–74.

48. Wymberley DeR. Coerr, "Forces of Change in Latin America," *Department of State Bulletin* 44 (1961): 251–55; the citation here is on 255.

49. Roy R. Rubottom Jr. "The Goals of United States Policy in Latin America," *Annals of the American Academy of Political and Social Sciences* 342 (1962): 30–41; the citation here is on 31.

50. Roger S. Leeds, "The Origins of the Alliance for Progress: Continuity and Change in the U.S. Policy toward Latin America" (Ph.D. dissertation, Johns Hopkins University, 1976).

51. Acting Secretary Chester Bowles, "Foreign Aid: The Great Decision of the Sixties," *Department of State Bulletin* 43 (1961): 703–9; the citation here is on 709.

52. Adolf A. Berle, "Alliance for Progress versus Communism," *Department of State Bulletin* 43 (1961): 763.

53. See Thomas W. Zeiler, *Dean Rusk: Defending the American Mission Abroad* (Wilmington, Del.: Scholarly Books, 2000); Dean Rusk, "The Alliance for Progress in

the Context of World Affairs," *Department of State Bulletin* 46 (1962): 787–94; Kimber C. Pearce, *Rostow, Kennedy and the Rhetoric of Foreign Aid* (East Lansing: Michigan State University Press, 2001); and Michael E. Lathman, "Ideology, Social Science and Destiny: Modernization and the Kennedy-Era Alliance for Progress," *Diplomatic History* 22, no. 2 (1998): 199–229.

54. Walt W. Rostow, "Guerrilla Warfare in the Underdeveloped Areas," *Department of State Bulletin,* August 7, 1961, 233–38; the citation here is on 236.

55. See Walter W. Rostow, *The Stages of Economic Growth: A Non-Communist Manifesto* (Cambridge: Cambridge University Press, 1960); and Rostow, "The Alliance for Progress," *Department of State Bulletin* 50 (1964): 496–500.

56. "RF 55129 Mexican American Cultural Institute, 9-30-1955," Rockefeller Foundation archives (hereafter RFA), record group 1.2., series 323, box 28, folder 195, Rockefeller Archive Center (hereafter RAC).

57. The process began during World War II. Between 1942 and 1948, the Institute of Inter-American Affairs provided 500 fellowships to Latin American health professionals to study at American universities. Institute of Inter-American Affairs, *Cooperative Health Programs of the U.S. and Latin America* (Washington, D.C.: Health and Sanitation Division of the Institute of Inter-American Affairs, 1948), 19. New York Academy of Medicine. During the academic year 1956–57, 40,666 foreign students and 1,153 visiting foreign scholars studied in the U.S. George Meany, "Cooperation in Science, Culture and Education," *Department of State Bulletin* 37 (1957): 764–68; the citation here is on 766.

58. "Memorandum from the Secretary of State's Staff Assistant (Boster) to the Secretary of the Cabinet (Paterson)," Washington, September 12, 1958, in *Foreign Relations of the United States, 1958–1960, American Republics,* vol. 5 (Washington, D.C.: U.S. Government Printing Office, 1991), 246–48.

59. "Intervention of Roy Rubottom Jr.," *A Review of the Relations of U.S. and Other American Republics, Hearings before a Subcommittee on Intergovernmental Affairs of the Committee on Foreign Affairs, House of Representatives, 85 Congress July 31, 1958* (Washington, D.C.: U.S. Government Printing Office, 1958), 15, record group 287, NA.

60. "Statement of M. N. Hardesty, Acting Regional Director, Latin American Operations, Foreign Operations Administration," in *The Mutual Security Act of 1954, 83rd Congress, April, May, June 1954* (Washington, D.C.: U.S. Government Printing Office, 1954)," 371, record group 287, NA.

61. See Nicholas Cull, "The Man Who Invented Truth: The Tenure of Edward R. Murrow as Director of the United States Information Agency during the Kennedy Years," in Mitter and Major, *Across the Blocs,* 23–49; Rabe, *Eisenhower and Latin America,* 33.

62. "Statement of Dr. Hyde," in *The United States and International Health, Hearings before a Subcommittee of the Committee on Interstate and Foreign Commerce, House of Representatives, 84th Congress, February 8 and 9, 1956* (Washington, D.C.: U.S. Government Printing Office, 1956), 49, record group 287, NA.

63. Rubottom, "Communism in the Americas," 183.

64. Francis O. Wilcox, "The First Ten Years of the World Health Organization," *Department of State Bulletin* 38 (1958): 987–88, 989.

65. Williard L. Beaulac, "Technical Cooperation as an Instrument of Foreign Policy," *Department of State Bulletin* 35 (1955): 964–70. A similar perspective was supported by international health agencies.

66. Wilcox, "First Ten Years," 989. Years later, a newspaper editorial would relate

Notes to Pages 31–34

international health efforts with the U.S. foreign policy of "waging for peace"; "Health for Peace," *New York Times,* January 18, 1958.

67. On the ICA, see International Cooperation Administration, *Technical Cooperation Health* (1956, 1961). The ICA's malaria program became a malaria eradication branch in USAID. See Ronald Scheman, ed., *The Alliance for Progress: A Retrospective* (New York: Praeger, 1988).

68. The overlapping of these agencies rules out a simple chronological or functional review. "Survey on U.S. Aid since 1945," *Congressional Quarterly Almanac, 84th Congress, 2nd Session 1956* 12 (1956): 432–39. NA. The succession of three directors between 1955 and 1959 makes it difficult to establish the contribution of each. These directors were John Baker Hollister (July 1, 1955, to September 13, 1957), James H. Smith Jr. (October 8, 1957, to January 31, 1959), and James W. Riddleberger (March 9, 1959, to February 22, 1961). U.S. Department of State, *Principal Officers,* 42.

69. "Act of International Development," in *United States Statutes at Large, Containing the Laws and Concurrent Resolutions Enacted during the Second Session of the Eighty-First Congress of the USA 1950–1951 and Proclamation, Treaties, International Agreements, other Than Treaties and Reorganization Plans,* (Washington, D.C. U.S. Government Printing Office, 1952), vol. 64, part 1, 204, NA Library.

70. "Survey on U.S. Aid since 1945," *Congressional Quarterly Almanac, 84th Congress, 2nd Session 1956,* 12 (1956): 432–39 (the citation here is on 433), NA.

71. J. H. Smith, Jr., "The Mutual Security Program: A Fight for Peace," *Department of State Bulletin* 39 (1958): 380–84. "President Awaits Aid Chief Views," *New York Times,* May 5, 1955. "Survey on U.S. Aid since 1945," 439, NA.

72. "President Awaits Aid Chief's Views"; "New Aid Director Defends Program," *New York Times,* July 17, 1955; and "U.S. Agency Urges Global Aid Plan, ICA Survey Offers Program Providing for Preparation of Long-Range Goals," *New York Times,* September 11, 1955.

73. International Cooperation Administration, *Technical Cooperation in Health* (1956), 441.

74. Eugene P. Campbell, "The Role of the International Cooperation Administration in International Health," *Archives of Environmental Health* 1, no. 6 (1960): 502–11; the citation here is on 509.

75. International Cooperation Administration, *Technical Cooperation in Health* (1956), 7.

76. "Statement of Dr. Hyde," in *The United States and International Health, 84th Congress, February 8 and 9, 1956* (Washington, D.C.: U.S. Government Printing Office, 1956), 78, record group 287, NA.

77. Paul F. Russell, "Symposium Nation-wide Malaria Eradication Projects in the Americas, Introductory Remarks by the President," *Journal of the National Malaria Society* 10, no. 2 (1951): 98–99. The Symposium was held at the Thirty-Third Annual Meeting of the National Malaria Society, Savannah, November 8, 1951.

78. "Fifth International Congress on Malaria and Tropical Medicine," *Journal of Tropical Medicine and Hygiene* 56, no. 10 (1953): 225–42. The Sixth International Congress, which took place in 1958 in Lisbon, devoted an entire section to malaria eradication, reflecting "the optimism in many eminent malariologists." The meeting discussed successful examples of eradication such as Gabaldón's work reported in "Malaria Division," *Journal of Tropical Medicine and Hygiene* 61 (1958): 251.

79. Rockefeller Foundation, *Confidential Monthly Report for the Information of the Trustees, 1 November 1956,* RAC Reference Library.

80. Cited by Socrates Litsios, *The Tomorrow of Malaria* (Karori, N.Z.: Pacific Press, 1997) as a phrase used by Paul F. Russell in 1955, p 144.

81. Also participating in the meeting was the Venezuelan Arnoldo Gabaldón, head of the Malaria training center in Maracay. Organización Sanitaria Panamericana, *Actas de la Decimocuarta Conferencia Sanitaria Panamericana, Sexta Reunión del Comité Regional de la Organización Mundial de la Salud para las Américas, Santiago, Chile, 7–22 Octubre 1954, Documentos Oficiales N. 14* (Washington, D.C.: Oficina Sanitaria Panamericana, 1955), Resolution XLII, "Erradicación de la malaria en las Américas," 675. The document "Situación de la Lucha Antimalárica en el Continente Americano, V Informe presentado sobre lucha antimalárica, por el Dr. Carlos A. Alvarado, 5 Octubre 1954," was published as *Situación de la Lucha antimalárica en las Americas V Informe* (Washington, D.C.: Oficina Sanitaria Panamericana, 1956).

82. Mary Elizabeth Bedwell, "A Bio-Bibliography of Dr. Fred L. Soper (1893–), Director Emeritus of the Pan-American Sanitary Bureau" (master's thesis, Catholic University of America, 1963); Malcom Gladwell, "The Mosquito Killer: Millions of People Owe Their Lives to Fred Soper, Why Isn't He a Hero?" *New Yorker,* July 2, 2001, 42–51; Paul F. Russell, "Obituary: Fred Lowe Soper," *Transactions of the Royal Society of Tropical Medicine and Hygiene* 71, no. 3 (1977): 272–73; Socrates Litsios, "Rene J. Dubos and Fred L. Soper: Their Contrasting Views on Vector and Disease Eradication," *Perspectives in Biology and Medicine* 141, no. 1 (1997): 138–49. See also Fred L. Soper, "El concepto de la erradicación de las enfermedades transmisibles," *Boletín de la Oficina Sanitaria Panamericana* 42, no. 1 (1957): 1–5; "The Epidemiology of a Disappearing Disease: Malaria," *American Journal of Tropical Medicine and Hygiene* 8 (1960): 357–66; "Rehabilitation of the Eradication Concept in Prevention of Communicable Diseases," *Public Health Reports* 80 (1965): 855–69.

83. "Table I: United States Contributions to International Organizations from Fiscal Year 1956 Funds."

84. According to Pampana, malaria eradication did not require eradication of the *anopheline* species in a given area. See Emilio J. Pampana, "Changing Strategy in Malaria Control," *Bulletin of the World Health Organization* 11 (1954): 513–20. Some years later, he wrote a textbook on malaria eradication that was translated into Spanish: *A Textbook of Malaria Eradication* (London: Oxford University Press, 1963); and *Erradicación de la Malaria* (Mexico City: Limusa-Wiley, 1966).

85. According to Alvarado, eradication required "engineering virtuosity" like a "complex symphony . . . which cannot be played by ear," in "Speech by Dr. Carlos A. Alvarado, Director Division of Malaria Eradication, WHO, Geneva, at the Opening Session International Conference on Malaria Eradication, Addis Ababa, Ethiopia, 16–21 November 1959," box 14, folder correspondence (miscellaneous), A-Al. Fred L. Soper Papers, MC 359 (hereafter Soper Papers), NLM.

86. "E. Pampana: 40 Years against Malaria," *World Health* 13, no. 2 (1960): 26–29.

87. The interventions of Neghma, of Dr. Sánchez Vigil from Nicaragua, and of an unidentified representative of El Salvador appear in *Actas de la Decimocuarta Conferencia Sanitaria Panamericana,* Resolution XLII, "Erradicación de la malaria en las Américas," Organización Sanitaria Panamericana (Washington, D.C.: Oficina Sanitaria Panamericana, 1954), 367–68.

88. L. J. Bruce-Chwatt, "Man against Malaria: Conquest or Defeat," *Transactions of the Royal Society of Tropical Medicine and Hygiene* 73, no. 6 (1979): 605–17; the citation here is on 611.

89. Soper intervention in Organización Sanitaria Panamericana, *Actas de la Decimocuarta Conferencia Sanitaria Panamericana,* Resolution XLII, "Erradicación de la malaria en las Américas," 366, 675.

90. Intervention of Myron E. Wegman, in Industrial Council for Tropical Health, *Industry and Tropical Health: Proceedings of the Third Tropical Health Conference Sponsored by the Harvard School of Public Health.* (Boston: Harvard School of Public Health and International Council for Tropical Health, 1960), 42. Wegman was then secretary general of the PASB.

91. Soper to Nelson Rockefeller, February 9, 1955, folder Pan-American Sanitary Bureau, 1955, box 2, Louis Laval Williams Papers, MS C 169 (hereafter Williams Papers), NLM.

92. "Interview with Victor Soler-Sala by John Charnow," February 19, 1984, CF/RAI/USAA/DB01/HS/1996-0063, UNICEF Library, New York.

93. John Maclaurin, *The United Nations and Power Politics* (New York: Harper & Brothers, 1951), 235.

94. Maggie Black, *The Children and the Nations: The Story of UNICEF* (Sydney: UNICEF, 1986); and Virginia M. Gray, *Love Is Not Enough: Recollections of a Capitol Hill Lobbyist for UNICEF* (Washington, D.C.: Klinge Press, 1984). The size of donations was decided by governments—not determined by a UN scale. UNICEF, *Children of the Developing Countries: A Report by UNICEF* (Cleveland: World Publishing, 1963). "Oral History Interview to Carl M. Marcy, chief of staff, Foreign Relations Committee, 1955–73," National Archives, gpo.gov/lps12426/www.senate.gov/, 88. "UNICEF's New Goals," *New York Times,* October 10, 1955.

95. "Table I: United States Contributions to International Organizations from Fiscal Year 1956 Funds."

96. On Pate, see "Maurice Pate of UNICEF Dead, Helped World's Needy Children," *New York Times,* January 20, 1965; and John Charnow, *Maurice Pate: UNICEF Executive Director, 1947–1965* (Geneva: UNICEF, 1989).

97. *The Mutual Security Act of 1954, 83rd Congress, April, May, June 1954* (Washington, D.C.: U.S. Government Printing Office, 1954), 5, record group 287, NA.

98. "United Nations Children's Fund," in *U.S. Participation in the UN: Report by the President to the Congress for the Year 1955* (Washington, D.C.: U.S. Government Printing Office, 1955), 155.

99. Donald R. Hopkins, "Yaws in the Americas, 1950–1975," *Journal of Infectious Diseases* 4, no. 136 (1977): 548–54. Fed L. Soper, "YAWS: Its Eradication in the Americas," Washington, D.C., 1956, http://profiles.nlm.nih.gov/VV/B/B/D/H/.

100. "UN Fund to Spur War on Malaria," *New York Times,* March 6, 1955; "Paludismo: Problema mundial," *Chronicle of the World Health Organization* 9, no. 2 (1955): 35–104 (the citation here is on 50–51); UNICEF, "Policy on UNICEF Aid to Malaria Control and Eradication, Preliminary Draft, Microfiche, 1958 1/3 78.CF.0431," UNICEF Library; and Black, *The Children and the Nations,* 126.

101. The report of the director of the Pan-American Sanitary Bureau to the UNICEF Regional Board is cited as "Malaria Eradication in the Americas," E/ICEF/282, and appears as annex 2, "Excerpt from Report of the UNICEF Executive Board, March 1955

Session, WHO Malaria Eradication, Proposal by the Director General, 3 May 1955," 25–26, WHO Library.

102. "Recommendation of the Executive Director for an Allocation, Mexico, Malaria Eradication, 30 July 1957, E/ICEF/L.1099," UNICEF, Program Committee, Series Malaria Research Collection, box WHO7.0078, folder Mexico 1957–1958, WHO Archives.

103. "May 1–6, 1955," Paul F. Russell Diaries (hereafter Russell Diaries), RFA, record group 12.1, RAC.

104. "UN Fund to Spur War on Malaria"; "Paludismo," 50–51. Even in 1963, a report appraised UNICEF's allocations devoted to malaria for the "past few years" as the largest single item in its budget, sometimes counting for over one-third. UNICEF, *Children of the Developing Countries,* 32.

105. Louis L. Williams, "Malaria Eradication, 1955," box 2, folder: Reprints, Lectures, 1955–1957, Williams Papers, NLM.

106. "WHA8.30 Malaria Eradication," Eighth World Health Assembly, Mexico City, May 26, 1955; http://policy.who.int/cgi-bin/om_isapi.dll?infobase=WHA&softpage=Browse_Frame_Pg42.

107. "Octava Asamblea Mundial de la Salud," *Crónica de la Organización Mundial de la Salud* 9, no. 7 (1955): 217–23.

108. "Biographical Note Dr. M. G. Candau," WHO, August 27 1958, Historical Section, WHO Library.

109. "Dr. M. G. Candau and WHO," *British Medical Journal* 5864 (1973): 433. On WHO, see Javed Siddiqi, *World Health and World Politics: The World Health Organization and the UN System* (London: Hurst, 1995); Sung Lee, "WHO and the Developing World: The Contest for Ideology," in *Western Medicine as Contested Knowledge,* ed. Andrew Cunningham and Bridie Andrews (Manchester: Manchester University Press, 1997), 24–45; and Marcos Cueto, *El valor de la salud: Historia de la Organización Panamericana de la Salud* (Washington, D.C.: Organización Panamericana de la Salud, 2004).

110. In 1956, WHO received from the U.S. government $3,349,787, which represented 33.33 percent of its total assessments; "Table I: United States Contributions to International Organizations from Fiscal Year 1956 Funds." During the 1960s, the proportion amounted to 40 percent. In 1974, the U.S. contribution to most UN agencies was limited to 25 percent; Gray, *Love Is Not Enough,* 166.

111. "World Health Organization," in *U.S. Participation in the UN,* 137.

112. John Sibley, "UN Health Unit Marks a Decade," *New York Times,* April 6, 1958; "WHO to Get New Building," *New York Times,* December 6, 1960; "Marcolino Gomez Candau," *Revista de Malariologia e Doenças Tropicais* 34 (1982): 119–22; "In Memory of Dr. M. G. Candau," *WHO Chronicle* 37, no. 4 (1983): 144–47.

113. "Candau Intervention in Eight World Health Assembly, Mexico, D.F., 10–27 May 1955," in "Resolutions and Decisions, Plenary Meetings Verbatim Records, Committees, Minutes and Annexes," *Official Records of the WHO, No. 63* (WHO: Geneva, 1955), 65–66.

114. A prominent advocate of eradication explained the dilemma in the following terms: "The phenomenon of *Anopheles* tolerance to residual toxicants indicates that the choice is either for malaria eradication or indefinitely enduring a disease transmitted by increasingly resistant vectors. Paul F. Russell, "The Status of Malaria Today," in *Industry and Tropical Health,* 26.

115. In the second quotation, I used a phrase spoken by Candau in 1958. It is found in "Health Agency Hailed: Service of UN Unit Is Cited by Its Leader on Anniversary," *New York Times,* April 7, 1958.

116. Mentioned in "E. Pampana: 40 Years against Malaria," 29.

117. Biographical information on Russell is found in "Dr. Paul F. Russell, 89; Specialist on Malaria," *New York Times,* November 9, 1983; Paul F. Russell, "The World Wide Malaria Eradication," *Industrial Medicine and Surgery* 27, no. 8 (1958): 378–83; Andrew Spielman and Michael D'Antonio, *Mosquito: A Natural History of Our Most Persistent and Deadly Foe* (New York: Hyperion, 2001), 146; Paul F. Russell, "The United States and Malaria Debits and Credits," *Bulletin of the New York Academy of Medicine* 44, no. 6 (June 1968): 623–53; Russell, *Man's Mastery of Malaria* (Oxford: Oxford University Press 1955); Paul F. Russell Diaries, May 7–23, 1955, Mexico, Russell Diaries, RFA, record group 12.1, RAC. Rockefeller Foundation, "Confidential Monthly Report for the Information of the Trustees, No. 178, November 1, 1956," RAC Reference Library. For a study on Rockefeller interests on malaria, see Darwin H. Stapleton, "Lessons of History? Anti-Malaria Strategies of the International Health Board and the Rockefeller Foundation from the 1920s to the Era of DDT," *Public Health Reports* 119, no. 2 (2004): 206–15.

118. "Russell Intervention in Eight World Health Assembly, Mexico, D.F., 10–27 May 1955," in *Resolutions and Decisions, Plenary Meetings, Verbatim Records, Committees, Minutes and Annexes, Official Records of the WHO, No. 63* (WHO: Geneva, 1955), 198.

119. WHO, "Malaria Eradication, Proposal by the Director General, 3 May 1955," A8/P&B/10. WHO Library.

120. "Hurtado, Delegate for Cuba, Intervention in Eight World Health Assembly, Mexico, D.F., 10–27 May 1955," in *Resolutions and Decisions, Plenary Meetings, Verbatim Records, Committees, Minutes and Annexes, Official Records of the WHO, No. 63,* 200. According to the delegate from Ecuador—a country that was multiplying its malaria budget—an urgent situation certainly existed in the Americas. "Dr. Montalvan, Ecuador," in *Resolutions and Decisions, Plenary Meetings, Verbatim Records, Committees, Minutes and Annexes, Official Records of the WHO, No. 63,* 203.

121. "Dr. Pierre Noel, Haiti, and Dr. Duren, Belgium, Interventions in Eighth World Health Assembly, Mexico, D.F., 10–27 May 1955," in *Resolutions and Decisions, Plenary Meetings, Verbatim Records, Committees, Minutes and Annexes, Official Records of the WHO, No. 63,* 203.

122. Eric Pridie, Delegate, Great Britain and Northern Ireland, and Dr. Garcin, France, Dr. Duren, Belgium, Interventions in Eighth World Health Assembly, Mexico, D.F., 10–27 May 1955," in *Resolutions and Decisions, Plenary Meetings, Verbatim Records, Committees, Minutes and Annexes, Official Records of the WHO, No. 63,* 200, 201.

123. WHO, "Malaria Eradication, Proposal by the Director General, 3 May 1955," A8/P&B/10 WHO Library. 22.

124. "Dr. Duren, Belgium, Interventions in Eighth World Health Assembly," in *Resolutions and Decisions, Plenary Meetings, Verbatim Records, Committees, Minutes and Annexes, Official Records of the WHO, No. 63,* 201.

125. The argument was part of a growing notion to leave Africa aside from the campaign. "Dr. Togba, Liberia, Intervention in Eighth World Health Assembly," in *Resolutions and Decisions, Plenary Meetings, Verbatim Records, Committees, Minutes and Annexes, Official Records of the WHO, No. 63,* 201.

126. Bruce-Chwatt, "Man against Malaria," 606. Solitary voices criticized malaria eradication at WHO assemblies. For example, in the meeting held in Geneva in 1957, the Pakistani representative objected to the "urgency" of eradication and adamantly criticized the practice of blocking control programs because they were not converted into nationwide eradication programs. The intervention of the Pakistani representative, who appears with no name, is in *Ninth World Health Assembly, Geneva, May 8–25, 1956: Report of the Chairman of the U.S. Delegation (Excerpts),* American Foreign Policy, Current Document, 1956, Department of State Publication 6811 (Washington, D.C.: U.S. Government Printing Office, 1959), 254–65; the citation here is on 257.

127. M. Dobson, M. Malowany, and R. Snow, "Malaria Control in East Africa: The Kampala Conference and the Pare-Taveta Scheme—A Meeting of Common and High Ground," *Parassitologia* 42, nos. 1–2 (2000): 149–66.

128. "Intervention of Vargas-Mendez, Costa Rica Delegate," and Russell interventions, in *Resolutions and Decisions, Plenary Meetings, Verbatim Records, Committees, Minutes and Annexes, Official Records of the WHO, No. 63,* 200, 205.

129. WHO, "Appraisal: The Programme of the WHO for 1959–1964," 10.

130. "Dr. Williams, USA, Intervention," in *Resolutions and Decisions, Plenary Meetings, Verbatim Records, Committees, Minutes and Annexes, Official Records of the WHO, No. 63,* 201.

131. See Tudda, "Reenacting the Story of Tantalus."

132. The idea appears in UNICEF, "Malaria Eradication: A Report to the UNICEF Executive Board by the Director General of the WHO, 3 May 1961," microfilm E/ICEF/417, New York Public Library.

133. George Giglioli was an Italian doctor trained at London's School of Tropical Medicine. A biographical account appears in "The Demarara Doctor," by Donna J. Reynolds, *Perspectives: Pan-American Health Organization* 1, no. 2 (1996), http://www.paho.org/English/DPI/Number2_article1.htm. Some of his works considered instrumental for malaria eradication include Giglioli, "Eradication of *Anopheles Darlingi* from the Inhabited Areas of British Guiana by DDT Residual Spraying," *Journal of the National Malaria Society* 10, no. 2 (1951): 142–61; Giglioli, "Malaria Control in British Guiana," *Bulletin of the World Health Organization* 11, nos. 4–5 (1954): 849–53; and Giglioli, "Residual Effect of DDT in a Controlled Area of British Guiana tested by the Continued Release of *Anopheles Darlingi* and *Aedes Aegypti:* A Practical Guide for the Standardized Evaluation of Overall Residual Efficiency under Field Conditions," *Transactions of the Royal Society of Tropical Medicine and Hygiene* 48, no. 6 (1954): 506–21.

134. Mario Pinotti, "The Nation-wide Malaria Eradication Program in Brazil," *Journal of the National Malaria Society* 10, no. 2 (1951): 162–82; the citation here is on 170.

135. See Alfredo G. Kohn Loncarica and Abel L. Agüero, "Carlos Alberto Alvarado y los planes de salud rural: Las condiciones del éxito y del fracaso en técnica médica," *Saber y Tiempo* 4, no. 1 (1997): 489–96; and Ana Teresa Gutiérrez, *Tiempos de guerra y paz: Arnoldo Gabaldón y la investigación sobre malaria en Venezuela (1936–1990)* (Caracas: Cendes; 1998).

136. "México Abre Brecha en la lucha para erradicar ya el paludismo," *El Universal* (Mexico City), May 22, 1955.

137. Expert Committee on Malaria, WHO, *Athens, 20–28 June 1956: Sixth Report* (Athens: WHO, 1956), http://whqlibdoc.who.int/malaria/WHO_Mal_180.pdf. The origin of the committee could be traced to the origins of WHO. WHO, "Appraisal: The Programme of the WHO for 1959–1964."

138. WHO also standardized the use of terms for malaria. See Expert Committee on Malaria, WHO, *Malaria Terminology: Report of a Drafting Committee Appointed by WHO* (Geneva: WHO, 1953).

139. Expert Panel on Malaria, International Cooperation Administration, "Report and Recommendations on Malaria: A Summary," *American Journal of Public Health* 10 (1961): 451–502; the citation here is on 459.

140. Herbert M. Gilles and David A. Warrell, eds., *Bruce-Chwatt's Essential Malariology,* 3rd ed. (London: Arnold, 1993), 132.

141. Chloroquine was first synthesized by Bayer chemists in Germany in 1934, under the name Resochin. At the end of World War II, U.S. and British scientists renamed it Chloroquine and used it for military purposes. See David P. Earle Jr. and Robert W. Berliner, "Chloroquine," in *Fourth International Congress on Tropical Medicine and Malaria, Washington D.C., May 10–18, 1948* (Washington, D.C.: U.S. Government Printing Office, 1948), 57–58.

142. G. Robert Coatney (head, section on chemotherapy, Laboratory of Tropical Diseases, National Microbiological Institute), "Therapy and Chemoprophylaxis: The Present Status of Chloroquine, Pyrimethamine (Darapim) and Primaquine," reprinted from *Industry and Tropical Health,* box 7, Williams Papers, NLM. A manual reprinted several times and translated into Spanish was Pan-American Health Organization, *Manual for the Microscopic Diagnosis of Malaria (2nd Edition)* (Washington, D.C.: Pan-America Health Organization, 1963). The techniques were also based on work done at the National Institutes of Health, *Manual for the Microscopical Diagnosis of Malaria in Man, Bulletin No. 180* (Washington, D.C.: U.S. Public Health Service, 1942).

143. "Día Mundial de la Salud, 7 Abril 1956, bajo el lema 'Guerra a los insectos portadores de enfermedades,'" fondo Secretaría de Salubridad y Asistencia (hereafter SSA), sección: Secretaría Particular, caja 33, expediente 4 [1953–60], Archivo Histórico de la Secretaría de Salud (hereafter AHSS), Mexico City.

144. Paul F. Russell, "Diary, April 9–13, 1956," Russell Diaries, RFA, record group 12.1, RAC. The report is also described in Harry Cleaver, "Malaria en the Political Economy of Public Health," *International Journal of Health Services* 7, no. 4 (1977): 557–79; the citation here is on 571.

145. *Foreign Aid Activities of Other Free Nations, A Study Prepared at the Request of the Special Committee to Study Foreign Aid Programs, U.S. Senate by Stuart Rice Associates, Inc., May 1957* (Washington, D.C.: U.S. Government Printing Office, 1957).

146. Campbell remained in his position until 1961, when the ICA became part of USAID and he was transferred to India. During the period 1942–50, 163 malaria control projects were developed in fifteen Latin American countries with an expenditure of $9.5 million. "Finding Aid to the Eugene P. Campbell Papers, 1941–1986, MS C 467" (hereafter Campbell Papers), NLM.

147. "Statement of Dr. Hyde," in *The United States and International Health, Hearings before a Subcommittee of the Committee on Interstate and Foreign Commerce, House of Representatives, 84th Congress, February 8 and 9 1956* (Washington, D.C.: U.S. Government Printing Office, 1956).

148. Campbell, "Role of the International Cooperation Administration."

149. J. H. Smith, Jr., "The Mutual Security Program: A Fight for Peace," *Department of State Bulletin* 39 (1958): 380–84; the citation here is on 381. Smith was then director of the ICA.

150. "Oral History Interview with Henry Van Zile Hyde," Truman Presidential Library and Museum, http://www.trumanlibrary.org/oralhist/hydehvz1.htm.

151. "Entry for 13 December 1956," Journals, vol. 8, Campbell Papers, NLM; and "Entry 13 December 1956," box 12, folder "Diary, January–December 1956," Soper Papers, NLM.

152. Fred L. Soper. "International Health Work in the Americas, 3 May 1948," RFA, record group 1.2, series 114, box 111, folder 932, RAC.

153. "Entry 27 May 1954," box 12, folder "January–December 1954," Soper Papers, NLM.

154. "Entry 4 September 1956," Journals, vol. 8, Campbell Papers, NLM.

155. "Dr. Alvarado's Intervention, the Americas," in "Malaria Eradication Discussions, WHO, PASB and ICA Participating, 4 April 1958," Journals, vol. 9, Campbell Papers, NLM.

156. "Dr. Viwanathan's Intervention," in "Malaria Eradication Discussions."

157. G. Davidson "Studies on Insecticide Resistance in *Anopheline* Mosquitoes," *WHO Bulletin* 18 (1958): 579–621.

158. In 1961, a U.S. report explained: "Eradication requires continuous international cooperation." Expert Panel on Malaria, International Cooperation Administration, "Report and Recommendations on Malaria."

159. Russell intervention, in "United States Department of Health, Education and Welfare Public Health Service, Division of International Health, Minutes of Meeting for Discussion of Global Malaria Eradication, 3 June 1955," 2, box 63, folder "Malaria Miscellaneous Meetings, 1955–56," Soper Papers, NLM.

160. From Arnold Rivkin to John J. Hanlon, 18 June 1956 [U.S. Government Office Memorandum], box 18, folder Correspondence Malaria H-K, Soper Papers, NLM.

161. Division of International Health, Public Health Service, U.S. Department of Health, Education, and Welfare, "Minutes of Meeting for Discussion of Global Malaria Eradication, 3 June 1955," 4, box 63, folder "Malaria Miscellaneous Meetings, 1955–56," Soper Papers, NLM.

162. "Entry 4 September 1956," Journals, vol. 8, Campbell Papers, NLM.

163. The origin of the ICA can be traced to a new foreign aid proposals from Congress that merged military and economic programs with technical assistance in a new foreign aid agency, the Foreign Operations Administration. This agency, located in the Department of State, was transformed in 1954 into the International Cooperation Administration. See Organización Sanitaria Panamericana, *Actas de la Decimocuarta Conferencia Sanitaria Panamericana;* and Donald J. Pletsch, "Progress toward Malaria Eradication in the Americas with Special Reference to Mexico," *American Journal of Public Health* 48 (1958): 713–16.

164. By 1961, U.S. bilateral assistance had provided $8.5 million, or 94 percent, of the PASB's (then renamed the Pan-American Health Organization) Special Account. See "U.S. Contribution to Help Fight Malaria in American Republics," *Department of State Bulletin* 36 (1957): 56–66; and Milton Eisenhower, *The Wine Is Bitter: The United States and Latin America* (New York: Doubleday, 1963). The participation of Milton S. Eisenhower was significant. In 1955, he was president of Johns Hopkins University, where many of the leaders of eradication had been trained. In addition, from September 1956 to May 1957, he was the chairman of the Inter-American Committee, which submitted recommendations on public health that prioritized malaria eradication. His recommendations

appeared in Roy R. Rubottom, "The Significance of Latin America in the Free World," *Department of State Bulletin* 37 (1957): 923–29. See also "Inter-American Committee Completes Work," *Department of State Bulletin* 36 (1957): 1014–16; and International Cooperation Administration, *Technical Cooperation in Health* (1956), 459, 467.

165. "The Budget Battle," *New York Times* March 17, 1957; Bruce J. Schulman, *Lyndon B. Johnson and American Liberalism: A Brief Biography with Documents* (Boston: Bedford/St. Martins, 1995), 43.

166. "Oral History Interview to Carl M. Marcy," 7.

167. "Statement of the Public Health Service, Department of Health, Education and Welfare on Malaria Eradication," "Statement of the Assistant Secretary of Defense (Health and Medical) Department of Defense, on Malaria Eradication," and "Statement of Dr. Eugene P. Campbell, Acting Chief, Public Health Division, ICA," all in *Mutual Security Act of 1957, Hearings before the Committee on Foreign Affairs House of Representatives, 85th Congress, 1st Session on the Executive Branch Proposed Draft Bill to Amend the Mutual Security Act of 1954, June 21, 24, 25, 26 and 28, 1958, Part V* (Washington, D.C.: U.S. Government Printing Office, 1958).

168. Williams also participated in the antimalaria work of the Tennessee Valley Administration Project and in malaria surveys in India and China. See Louis L. Williams, "The Entomologist and the International Health Program," *Journal of Economic Entomology* 42, no. 4 (1949): 710–12; and "Autobiography, Medical Director Louis L. Williams Jr. U.S. Public Health Service," box 1, folder Biographical Data, Williams Papers, NLM. In 1957, he wrote: "I never had the feeling of being usefully successful until I changed my view from control of malaria to eradication of malaria and I recommend that you do likewise." Louis J. Williams to W. C. Frohne, January 5, 1957, box 1, folder Correspondence 1957–58, Williams Papers, NLM.

169. These ideas are presented in Chester Bowles, "Why Foreign Aid?" *Department of State Bulletin* 48 (1963): 777–84. An account on the criticism to foreign aid appears in "Is Foreign Aid Unpopular?" *New York Times,* July 6, 1958.

170. "Entry September 4 1956," Journals, vol. 8, Campbell Papers, NLM.

171. The information in this paragraph is from *Mutual Security Appropriation for 1958, Hearings before the Subcommittee of the Committee on Appropriations House of Representatives, 85th Congress, Subcommittee of Foreign Operations Appropriations* (Washington, DC.: U.S. Government Printing Office, 1957).

172. "Survey on U.S. Aid since 1945," 439

173. *Mutual Security Appropriation for 1958,* 983.

174. Williams intervention is narrated in "Entry for 4 June 1957," Journals, vol. 8, Campbell Papers, NLM. The decision also appears in "Global Malaria War," *World of Medicine, Medical Magazine* 1, no. 9 (1957): 325.

175. UNICEF, "Malaria Eradication: A Report to the UNICEF Executive Board."

176. The debate is in "Latin America: A Decade of Decision," by Robert C. Cook, *Population Bulletin* 17, no. 2 (1961): 17–38.

177. "Excerpts from a Statement by Charles L. Williams before the Senate Appropriations Committee, *Congressional Record,* Proceedings and Debates on the 85th Congress, First Session, Washington, D.C., Tuesday 27 August 1957, Vol. 103, No. 156," 14638, Journals, vol. 8, Campbell Papers, NLM.

178. Wilcox, "First Ten Years," 988.

179. Wilcox, "World Population," 862.

180. See J. M. Jones, *Does Overpopulation Mean Poverty? The Facts about Popula-*

tion Growth and Economic Development (with a foreword by Eugene R. Black, president of the World Bank) (Washington, D.C.: World Bank, 1962); Robin Barlow, "The Economic Effects of Malaria Eradication," *American Economic Review* 57, no. 2 (1968): 130–48; and R. Symonds and M. Carder, *The United Nations and the Population Question, 1945–1970* (New York: McGraw-Hill, 1973).

181. *Mutual Security Act of 1957, Hearings before the Committee on Foreign Affairs House of Representatives, 85th Congress, 1st Session on the Executive Branch Proposed Draft Bill to Amend the Mutual Security Act of 1954,* 1080. "El Costo de la Erradicación del Paludismo en las Américas," *Crónica de la OMS* 12, no. 1 (1958): 337–41; the citation here is on 340.

182. "La Enfermedad Más Cara del Mundo: Nueva estrategia antipalúdica," *Crónica de la OMS* 13, nos. 9–10 (1959): 355–62; the citation here is on 356.

183. In 1958, the subtitle of a WHO publication would define malaria as "the most expensive disease in the world." WHO, *Malaria Eradication: A Plea for Health* (Geneva: WHO, 1958), 7.

184. Expert Committee on Malaria, WHO, *Eight Report,* WHO Technical Report 205 (Geneva: WHO, 1961), 15.

185. Luís Vargas, "Consideraciones Generales sobre la Epidemiología de la Malaria Evanescente en México," *Gaceta Médica de México* 88 (1958): 613–33.

186. WHO, *Malaria Eradication,* 3.

187. WHO, "Appraisal: The Programme of the WHO for 1959–1964," 51. In an official publication of 1957, the figure was raised to more than $350 million a year.

188. "International Organizations: Aid to World Trade and Prosperity," *Department of State Bulletin* 37 (1957): 749–54; the citation here is on 752.

189. "Doom of Malaria by '67 Envisioned," *New York Times,* December 22, 1957.

190. "Malaria," *Journal of Tropical Medicine and Hygiene* (London) 61 (1958): 53–54.

191. "Malaria Eradication Would Cost Millions," *New York Times,* September 16, 1955; and "Interamerican Committee Completes Work," *Department of State Bulletin* 36 (1957): 1014–16 (the citation here is on 1016).

192. "Doom of Malaria by '67 Envisioned."

193. "Disease Curb Foreseen, End of Contagious Ailments Predicted by WHO Head," *New York Times,* May 16, 1958, 49.

194. "Statement by Eugene P. Campbell, M.D., Acting Chief, Public Health Division, International Cooperation Administration before the Senate Appropriations Committee, *Congressional Record,* 85th Congress, First Session, Washington, D.C., 27 August 1957, Vol. 103, No. 156," 14637, vol. 8, Journals, Campbell Papers, NLM.

195. Although the precise proportion devoted to insecticides and drugs in malaria eradication projects was presented as variable, its seems that these figures were significant everywhere. Carlos Alvarado, *Situación de la lucha antimalárica en el continente americano, IV informe presentado sobre la lucha antimalárica* (Washington, D.C. Oficina Sanitaria Panamericana, 1951), 33.

196. *Mutual Security Appropriations for 1959, Hearing before a Subcommittee on the Appropriations House of Representatives, 85th Congress, 2nd Session, Subcommittee on Foreign Operations Administrations* (Washington, D.C.: U.S. Government Printing Office, 1958), 1191.

197. "'Buy American'–and Foreign Aid," *New York Times,* October 26, 1959.

198. Donald Johnson and Roy Fritz, "Status Report on Malaria Eradication,"

Mosquito News 22, no. 2 (1962): 80–81. About 48 percent of the cost of malaria eradication operations in Latin America was spent on insecticides, spraying equipment, and transportation. WHO, "Appraisal: The Programme of the WHO for 1959–1964," 51.

199. National Institutes of Health, U.S. Department of Health and Human Services, *Malaria* (Washington, D.C. National Institute of Allergy and Infectious Diseases, 2002), 11.

200. Wallace Peters, *Chemotherapy and Drug Resistance in Malaria* (London: Academic Press, 1970), 10.

201. See Gary Gereffi, *The Pharmaceutical Industry and Dependency in the Third World* (Princeton, N.J.: Princeton University Press, 1983); Walsh McDermott, "Pharmaceuticals: Their Role in Developing Societies," *Science* 89 (1980): 240–45; and P. Temin, *Taking Your Medicine: Drug Regulation in the United States* (Cambridge, Mass.: Harvard University Press, 1980).

202. Jules Backman, *Chemicals in the National Economy* (Washington, D.C.: Manufacturing Chemists' Association, 1964); Alfred D. Chandler Jr., *Shaping the Industrial Century: The Remarkable Story of the Evolution of the Modern Chemical and Pharmaceutical Industries* (Cambridge, Mass.: Harvard University Press, 2005).

203. Douglas L. Murray, *Cultivating Crisis: The Human Cost of Pesticides in Latin America* (Austin: University of Texas Press, 1994), 15.

204. Davis Dyer and David B. Sicilia, *Labor of a Modern Hercules: The Evolution of a Chemical Company* (Boston: Harvard Business School Press, 1990), 347.

205. F. W. Knipe, "Nozzles of Insecticide Sprayers: Comments from the Point of View of Malaria Control," *Bulletin of the World Health Organization* 12, no. 3 (1955): 401–9.

206. Shell Oil Company, *Annual Report 1956* (New York: Shell Oil Company, 1956), 14. In 1957, the manager of the Chemical Sales Division of Shell Chemical celebrated its collaboration with the U.S. Public Health Service. "F. W. Hatch to Justin Andrews, 13 November 1957," and "Justin M. Andrews to Louis L. Williams, 18 November 1957," box 1, folder Correspondence 1957–1958, Williams Papers, NLM.

207. "Entry 12 June 1954," Journals, vol. 8, Campbell Papers, NLM. Kendall Beaton, *Enterprise in Oil: A History of Shell in the United States* (New York: Appleton-Century-Crofts, 1957), 681; Dan J. Forrestal, *Faith, Hope and $5,000: The Story of Monsanto—The Trials and Triumphs of the First 75 Years* (New York: Simon & Schuster, 1977).

208. "Doom of Malaria by '67 Envisioned."

209. "33,000,000 Pounds of DDT Shipped Overseas in Malaria Program," *Department of State Bulletin* 39 (1958): 290–91.

210. Johnson and Fritz, "Status Report on Malaria Eradication."

211. "Donald R. Johnson to Louis L. Williams, 8 July 1962," box 1, folder Correspondence 1963–67, Williams Papers, NLM. USAID was formed after an Act for International Development of 1961 that abolished the ICA and established a new agency to administer foreign economic and technical programs. Its director had the rank of an undersecretary within the Department of State. U.S. Department of State, *Principal Officers,* 42.

212. "Malaria," *Journal of Tropical Medicine and Hygiene.* During the 1960s, the proportion progressively declined to 40 percent and remained in that level until 1974, when the U.S. matching ratio of most UN agencies was limited to 25 percent. "Contri-

butions by the U.S. Governments to the General Resources of UNICEF, 1947–1979," in *Love Is Not Enough,* by Gray, 166; "Doom of Malaria by '67 Envisioned."

213. Campbell, "Role of the International Cooperation Administration," 507.

214. "World's Top Experts Convene Here in Campaign to Wipe Out Malaria, *Anopheles* Mosquito Racked Down," *Washington Post,* February 29, 1960. Donald Johnson, "Development of the Worldwide Eradication Program," *Mosquito News* 26, no. 2 (1966): 113–17; the citation here is on 114.

215. Alfonso Castrejón, *Algunas consideraciones sobre el paludismo que se observa en el Estado de Oaxaca* (Oaxaca: Tall. De Artes Graficas Julián S. Soto, 1923), 43. "Vuelven a los habitantes apáticos e indolentes, muchos vi que permanecieron acostados, cubriéndose la cara con las manos o con su sombrero durmiendo. El semblante de la mayoría acusa cansancio, indiferencia."

216. Organización Panamericana de la Salud, *La Malaria en las Américas: Bosquejo de la Batalla que libra el hemisferio para terminar con un viejo enemigo* (Washington, D.C. Oficina Sanitaria Panamericana, 1963).

217. "Mensaje a los habitantes del Estado de Guerrero," in *Costas de Guerrero: Boletín para el personal de la zona IX Sur* (Chilpancingo Guerrero, August 1967, no number), p. 2, fondo SSA, serie Comisión Nacional para la Erradicación del Paludismo (hereafter CNEP), sección Zona 9, caja 1 Expediente 2, AHSS. "Las cadenas del paludismo, es un ser cuyas iniciativas no adelantan y que desalentado por lo inutil de sus esfuerzos, se abandona a un cierto fatalismo [firme esta cita]."

218. "Intervention of Dr. Judd," in *Mutual Security Act of 1957, Hearings before the Committee on Foreign Affairs House of Representatives, 85th Congress, 1st Session on the Executive Branch Proposed Draft Bill to Amend the Mutual Security Act of 1954,* 1077.

219. "Doom of Malaria by '67 Envisioned."

220. According to Dulles, workers in communist countries "have become virtually slaves" (statement of Secretary Dulles made at the Tenth Inter-American Conference, March 11, 1954, Caracas). "Intervention of International communism in the Americas," *Department of State Bulletin* 30 (1954): 419–26, 421.

221. Rubottom, "Communism in the Americas," 182.

222. "Aiding Fight on Malaria: An Analysis of the Importance of U.S. Fiscal Help to Battle against the Disease," *New York Journal,* December 15, 1957, newspaper clipping, Journals, vol. 8, Campbell Papers, NLM.

223. "Malaria," *Journal of Tropical Medicine and Hygiene.* "United States Gives $7 Million to Malaria Eradication Campaign," *Department of State Bulletin* 37 (1957): 1000–3.

224. "Discurso pronunciado por el excelentísimo señor Joaquín Salazar, Embajador de la República Dominicana en los Estados Unidos de América 5 de abril de 1957, OSP," 2, fondo Secretaría de Salubridad y Asistencia, sección Sub SyA Subsecretaría, caja 42, expediente 3, años 1951–59, Nombre Oficina Sanitaria Panamericana, Archivo de la Secretaría de Salubridad, Mexico City.

225. UNICEF, "Policy on UNICEF Aid to Malaria Control and Eradication, Preliminary Draft," microfiche, 1958 1/3 78.CF.0431, UNICEF Library.

226. "Marcolino Candau to Miguel E. Bustamante, 1 October 1959," fondo Secretaria de Salubridad y Asistencia, sección CNEP, serie Dirección, caja 5, expediente 2, AHSS. The letter includes a table titled "Estado de la cuenta especial para la erradicación paludismo el 15 de Septiembre de 1959," which presents as the second most impor-

tant donor the Federal Republic of Germany, contributing $95,238, and the USSR, contributing $82,500. Candau's complaint appears also in "UN Agencies Urges Speed on Malaria," *New York Times,* April 7, 1960.

227. International Cooperation Administration, *Technical in Health* (1961), 459, 467.

228. Pampana, *Textbook of Malaria Eradication,* 475.

229. Campbell asked Soper to be part of the panel in a letter that discreetly stated the following: "As you know, we are running into many problems in the worldwide eradication program." "Campbell to Soper," no date, box 14, folder Campbell, Eugene, Soper Papers, NLM. Expert Panel on Malaria, International Cooperation Administration, "Report and Recommendations on Malaria."

230. International Cooperation Administration, "Report and Recommendations on Malaria," 486, 484.

231. UNICEF, *Children of the Developing Countries,* 32.

232. International Cooperation Administration, "Report and Recommendations on Malaria," 483.

233. Entry 21, April 1960, Journals, vol. 10, Campbell Papers, NLM. "Statement of Eugene Campbell, Director Office of Public Health, International Cooperation Administration, on Special Assistance Health Programs before the House Foreign Affairs Committee, *Congressional Record,* Appendix, March 9, 1960," newspaper clipping, Journals, vol. 10, Campbell Papers, NLM.

234. Comité de Expertos en Paludismo de la Agencia de Desarrollo Internacional, *El Paludismo, métodos para su erradicación* (Mexico City: Limusa-Wiley, 1963). In June 1960, the ICA was authorized to use $85 million for antimalaria campaigns around the globe and planned to request $38 million more for the following fiscal year. "World's Top Experts Convene," *Washington Post,* February 29, 1960.

235. L. J. Bruce-Chwatt, "Malaria Research and Eradication in the USSR: A Review of Soviet Achievements in the Field of Malariology," *Bulletin of the World Health Organization* 21 (1959): 737–72.

236. Campbell, "Role of the International Cooperation Administration," 505.

237. For example, see Servicio Nacional de Erradicación de la Malaria, Colombia, *Plan de erradicación de la malaria* (Bogotá: Servicio Nacional de Erradicacion de la Malaria, 1957).

238. O. K. Armstrong, "All Out Attack on Malaria," *Reader's Digest,* July 1958, 188–91; the citation here is on 188.

239. Murray Morgan, *Doctors to the World* (New York: Viking Press, 1958), cited in "The Days of the Mass Campaigns," by Glen Williams, *World Health Forum* 9 (1988): 7–23; the quotation here is on 16.

Chapter 3. National Decisions

1. "Comienza hoy la Campaña para la erradicación del paludismo," *El Universal* (Mexico City), September 7, 1956; "Es para bien de la patria la campaña contra el paludismo," *El Universal,* September 8, 1956; "Ruiz Cortines dará hoy la orden de marcha contra el paludismo," *Excelsior* (Mexico City), September 7, 1956; "Cada Mexicano es un Cruzado en la lucha contra el paludismo," *Excelsior,* September 8, 1956. These journals are kept at the Biblioteca Nacional, Mexico City. The headline of a newspaper an-

nounced the crusade: "Cada Mexicano es un Cruzado en la lucha contra el paludismo," *Excelsior,* September 8, 1956.

2. Murray Morgan, *Doctors to the World* (New York: Viking Press, 1958), 12.

3. The declaration of Pletsch is cited in "The Malaria Eradication Campaign in México, Report Submitted to the Program Committee on 25 October 1956 by Mr. R. Davee, Director, the Americas Regional Office, 30 October 1956," E/ICEF/329, United Nations Children's Fund, folder México 1955–56, box WHO 7.0078, series Malaria Research Collection, WHO Archives.

4. "A Big Day in Mexico," *New York Times,* September 8, 1956.

5. "Informe de la Situación Sanitaria que prevalece en la Actualidad y los recursos que se cuentan en el Estado de Oaxaca, 1978," fondo Poder Ejecutivo del Estado, sección Dirección General de Gobernación, serie Secretaría General del Despacho, expediente 281, Archivo General del Estado de Oaxaca, Oaxaca (hereafter AGEO).

6. "Recommendation of the Executive Director for an Apportionment, México Malaria Eradication, 10 August 1955, E/ICEF/L.809 UNICEF Programme Committee," folder Mexico 1955–56, box WHO 7.0078, series Malaria Research Collection, WHO Archives. J. Armas Domínguez, *Las Defunciones por Paludismo en la República Mexicana: Desde el punto de vista de su diagnóstico médico y su clasificación estadística* (Mexico City: Dirección General de Bioestadística, 1956), 2. The average malaria mortality for the country during the previous five years (1950–54) was 90 per 100,000 population, with a higher rate of 449 in Oaxaca, 321 in Tabasco, 308 in Chiapas, 200 in Puebla, and 177 in Veracruz. Malaria maintained third place among the main causes of death in the country starting in the 1930s; "Nombre Informe presidencial, Generalidades, 1961," fondo Secretaría de Salubridad y Asistencia (hereafter SSA), sección Sub-Secretaría de Salubridad, caja 2, expediente 4, 1960–61, Archivo Histórico de la Secretaría de Salud (hereafter AHSS).

7. J. Alvarez Amézquita, M. Bustamante, A. L. Picazos, and F. Fernández del Castillo, "Servicios médicos rurales cooperativos en la historia de la salubridad y de la asistencia en México," in *La Atención médico rural en México 1930–1980,* ed. Héctor Hernández Llamas (Mexico City: Instituto Mexicano del Seguro Social, 1984), 95–108 (the citation here is on 97). Michael C. Meyer and William H. Beezley, *The Oxford History of Mexico* (New York: Oxford University Press, 2000), 586.

8. "Mexico," in *The International Yearbook and Statesmen's Who's Who 1958,* ed. L. G. Pine (London: Burke's Peerage Limited, 1958), 415–20; the citation here is on 416.

9. This is equivalent to 2 billion pesos a year; "Recommendation of the Executive Director for an Apportionment." This figure also appears in "Facts and Figures Concerning the Economic Damage Caused by Malaria in Some Countries," July 1, 1957, WHO.

10. E.g.: José Alvarez Amézquita, "La obra de la revolución mexicana en el campo de la salud pública," *Salud Pública de México* 3 (1961): 9–14; and Luís Vargas, "Fundamentos evolutivos de la teoría del estado y sus alcances en la erradicación el paludismo en México," *Salud Pública de México* 2 (1960): 489–99.

11. Xavier de la Riva Rodríguez, "Salubridad y asistencia medico social," in *México, Cincuenta Años de Revolución, la Vida Social,* ed. Julio Duran Ochoa (Mexico City: Fondo de Cultura Económica, 1961); "Decreto que crea la Secretaría de Salubridad y Asistencia, 18 Octubre 1943," *Gaceta Médica de México* 73 (1943): 435–37; Ana Cecilia Rodríguez de Romo and Martha Eugenia Rodríguez, "Historia de la salud pública en México: Siglos XIX y XX," *História, Ciências, Saúde—Manguinhos* 5, no. 2 (1998):

293–310; and Fernando Lasso Echevarría, *Historia de los servicios de salud en el Estado de Guerrero* (Mexico City: N.p., 2003), 31.

12. Ignacio Avila Cisneros, "El Dr. Manuel Martínez Báez," *Revista de Investigaciones de Salud Pública* (Mexico City) 29, no. 3 (1969): 173–78.

13. Manuel Martínez Báez, *Obras,* ed. Adolfo Martínez Palomo (Mexico City: El Colegio Nacional, 1994); Raúl Arreola Cortés, *Manuel Martínez Báez: Científico y Humanista* (Morelia: Universidad Michoacana de San Nicolás de Hidalgo, 1994); Manuel Martínez Báez, *Manual de Parasitología Médica* (Mexico City: La Prensa Médica Mexicana, 1953).

14. The Plan Tripartito was signed on December 6, 1955. Manuel Martínez Báez, "Consecuencias sociales y económicas del paludismo de México," *Gaceta Médica de México* 87 (1957): 11–17.

15. "Morones Prieto, Ignacio," in *Mexican Political Biographies: 1935–1975,* by Roderic Camp (Tucson: University of Arizona Press, 1976), 226–27.

16. "Dr. Ignacio Morones Prieto, President of the Eight World Health Assembly," *Chronicle of the World Health Organization* 9, no. 6 (1955): 208.

17. See Michelle Dion, "The Political Origins of Social Security in Mexico during the Cárdenas and Avila Camacho Administrations," *Mexican Studies/Estudios Mexicanos* 21, no. 1 (2005): 59–95; and Gustavo Sánchez Vargas, *Orígenes y Evolución de la Seguridad Social en México* (Mexico City: Universidad Nacional Autonoma de Mexico, 1963).

18. John B. Ross, *The Economic System of Mexico* (Stanford, Calif.: California Institute of International Studies, 1971), 93.

19. Héctor Hernández Llamas, "Historia de la participación del estado en las instituciones de atención medica en México, 1935–1980," in *Vida y muerte del mexicano,* ed. Federico Ortiz Quesada (Mexico City: Folios Ediciones, 1982), vol. 2, 49–81; the citation here is on 75.

20. "Mexico: The Taming of a Revolution," in *Modern Latin America,* by Thomas E. Skidmore and Peter H. Smith (New York: Oxford University Press, 2001), 237–38.

21. Inter-American Affairs Office, *Mexico: Next Door Neighbor* (Washington, D.C.: U.S. Government Printing Office, 1943), 2.

22. Nils Gilman, *Mandarins of the Future: Modernization Theory in Cold War America* (Baltimore: Johns Hopkins University Press, 2003).

23. See Juan José Rodríguez Prats, *El poder presidencial: Adolfo Ruíz Cortines* (Mexico City: Miguel Angel Porrua, 1992); and José Luís Reyna and Raúl Trejo Delarbre, *De Adolfo Ruíz Cortines a Adolfo López Mateos: (1952–1964)* (Mexico City: Siglo Veintiuno, 1981).

24. Robert R. Miller, *Mexico: A History* (Norman: University of Oklahoma Press, 1985), 330.

25. Rodríguez Prats, *El poder presidencial.*

26. "Plan Tripartito de Operaciones para un Proyecto de Erradicación del Paludismo en México, 1955," fondo SSA, sección Comisión Nacional para la Erradicación del Paludismo 9 (hereafter CNEP), serie Dirección, caja 1, expediente 10. "Acuerdo entre el gobierno de los Estados Unidos Mexicanos y el Fondo de las Naciones Unidas para la Infancia, 1954," fondo SSA, sección CNEP, serie Dirección, caja 1, expediente 3, AHSS.

27. Mexico contribution for the years 1960 to 1962 was 500,000 per year; UNICEF, *Children of the Developing Countries: A Report by UNICEF* (Cleveland: World Pub-

lishing, 1963), 105. In 1961, Mexico annual contribution to the PASB was $245,340; "Puntos resolutivos del comité ejecutivo de la OPS en su 43 reunión," fondo SSA, sección SubSecretaría de Salubridad, caja 2, expediente Informe presidencial, generalidades, 1960–61.

28. Sarah Babb, *Managing Mexico: Economists from Nationalism to Neoliberalism* (Princeton, N.J.: Princeton University Press, 2001).

29. Ruíz Cortines, cited in Instituto Nacional Indigenista, *¿Que es el INI?* (Mexico City: INI, 1955), 9.

30. John B. Ross, *The Economic System of Mexico* (Stanford, Calif.: California Institute of International Studies, 1971), 3.

31. "Afirman que sistema ejidal no ha mejorado a nuestros campesinos," *Excelsior,* January 6, 1957. Also see U.S. Department of Commerce, *Investment in Mexico: Conditions and Outlook for United States Investors* (Washington, D.C. U.S. Government Printing Office, 1956), 26.

32. See Sergio de la Peña and Marcel Morales Ibarra, *Historia de la cuestión agraria mexicana: El agrarismo y la industrialización de México, 1940–1950* (Mexico City: Siglo XXI, 1990), vol. 6.

33. "México," in *Britannica Book of the Year 1958* (Chicago: Encyclopaedia Brittanica, 1958), 438.

34. "México," in *Britannica Book of the Year 1955* (Chicago: Encyclopaedia Brittanica, 1955), 503. R. J. Alexander, "Nature and Progress of Agrarian Reform in Latin America," *Journal of Economic History* 23, no. 4 (1963): 559–73; the citation here is on 567.

35. In WHO, "Facts and Figures Concerning the Economic Damage Caused by Malaria in Some Countries," July 1, 1957, fondo SSA, serie CNEP, sección Dirección, caja 1, expediente 7, AHSS.

36. See Cynthia Hewitt de Alcantara, *Modernizing Mexican Agriculture: Socioeconomic Implications of Technological Change, 1940–1970* (Geneva: United Nations Research Institute for Social Development, 1976); Deborah Fitzgerald, "Exporting American Agriculture: The Rockefeller Foundation in Mexico, 1943–1953," and Joseph Cooter, "The Rockefeller Foundation's Mexican Agricultural Project: A Cross-Cultural Encounter, 1943–1949," both in *Missionaries of Science: The Rockefeller Foundation and Latin America* (Bloomington: Indiana University Press, 1994), ed. Marcos Cueto, 72–96 and 97–125, respectively.

37. "Summary of Agricultural Fellowships and Scholarship Program 1957," RFA, record group 1.2, series 100E, box 45, folder 339, Rockefeller Archive Center (hereafter RAC). "The Rockefeller Foundation, Current fellowship program, 1951–1956," RFA, record group 1.2, series 100E, box 45, folder 335, 17, RAC.

38. "Robert A. Lambert to Raymond B. Fodsick, Subject Visit to México, March 14, 1941," RFA, record group 1.1, series 223, box 13, folder 95; "Report of Fellowships for Travel and Training Grants 1955–1958," RFA, record group 1.2, series 100E, box 45, folder 345; and "Latin American Awards, Fellows, Scholars, Trainee Awards 1917–1960, 3 March 1960" (the total was 1,430), RFA, R.G. 1.2, series 300, box 2, folder 8, RAC.

39. Jesús Alanis, "Homenaje a Arturo Rosenblueth," *Acta Physiologica Lationoamericana Americana* 21, no. 1 (1971):1–7.

40. Mildred Garret, "The United States–Mexico Border Public Health Association," *Nursing Outlook* 7, no. 5 (May 1959): 295–97; and Humberto Romero Alvarez, *Health*

without Boundaries: Notes for the History of the United States–Mexico Border Public Health Association, on the Celebration of its 30 Years of Active Life, 1943–1973 (Mexico City: United States–Mexico Border Public Health Association, 1975).

41. "Table 110: Twin City Populations, 1900–1980," in *United States–Mexico Border Statistics, since 1900,* ed. David E. Lorey (Los Angeles: UCLA Latin American Center Publications, 1990), 33. The other twin-city populations with significant populations (over 5,000 in the 1950) were Matamoros and Brownsville; Reynosa and McAllen (located in Tamaulipas and Texas respectively); Nuevo Laredo, Tamaulipas, and Laredo, Texas; Piedras Negras, Coahuila, and Eagle Pass, Texas; Nogales, Sonora, and Nogales, Arizona; Mexicalli, Baja California, and Calexico, California; and Tijuana, Baja California, and San Diego. During the mid–twentieth century, the population of Ciudad Juarez grew significantly from 39,669 in 1930 to 122,566 in 1950. "Table 112: Ciudad Juarez Population, 1850–1974," in *United States–Mexico Border Statistics,* ed. Lorey, 34.

42. "United States–Mexico Border Public Health Association," *Public Health Reports* 73, no. 12 (1958): 1133–40.

43. Joseph E. Potter, "Population and Development in Mexico since 1940: An interpretation," *Population and Development Review* 12, no. 1 (1986): 47–75; the citation here is on 61.

44. A sign of PRI dominance was the fact that President Ruíz Cortines had won the 1953 election (for the 1953–58 period) with more than 74 percent of the total vote. Michael C. Meyer and William L. Sherman, *The Course of Mexican History* (New York: Oxford University Press, 1979), 596–651.

45. See Peter H. Smith, *Talons of the Eagle: Dynamics of U.S.–Latin American Relations* (New York: Oxford University Press, 1996).

46. "Mexico," in *International Yearbook,* ed. Pine, 416.

47. Stepen A. Nibblo, "Allied Policy towards Axis Interests in Mexico during World War II," *Mexican Studies/Estudios Mexicanos* 17, no. 2 (2001): 351–73.

48. Herbert L. Matthews, "Anti-U.S. feeling in Mexico Easing," *New York Times,* April 7, 1957.

49. Sidney Gruson, "Pro-U.S. Feeling Grows in Mexico," *New York Times,* September 1, 1954.

50. Walter M. Daniels, *Latin America in the Cold War* (New York: H. W. Wilson, 1952), 57.

51. "Mexico Installs a New President," *New York Times,* December 2, 1958.

52. Ana María Carrillo, "Miguel Bustamante," in *Ciencia y tecnología en México en el siglo XX: Biografías de personajes ilustres,* ed. Secretaría de Educación Pública (Mexico City: Academia Mexicana de Ciencias, 2003), vol. 3, 143–59; and Anne-Emanuelle Birn, "Miguel Enrique Bustamante (1898–1986)," in *Doctors, Nurses and Medical Practitioners: A Biographical Source Book,* ed. Lois N. Magner (Westport, Conn.: Greenwood Press, 1977), 30–36.

53. Frank Brandenburg, *The Making of Modern Mexico* (Englewood Cliffs, N.J.: Prentice-Hall, 1964), 115.

54. "Ceremony at Mexican Border Marks Settlement of Chamizal Dispute," *Department of State Bulletin* 51 (1964): 545–52; "President Johnson and President López Mateos of Mexico Hold Talks in California," *Department of State Bulletin* 50 (1964): 396–403.

55. Remarks by Secretary Rusk, "The United States and Mexico: Partners in a Common Task," *Department of State Bulletin* 46 (1962): 919–21. According to Aguayo, the

U.S. government accepted Mexico as it was because once the pros and cons had been taken into account, the status quo was favorable to U.S. interests. Sergio Aguayo, *Myths and [Mis]perceptions: Changing U.S. Elite Visions of Mexico* (San Diego: Center for U.S.-Mexican Studies at the University of California, 1998), 46.

56. "Mexico Now Seeks Goodwill of U.S., Ruíz Cortines Quietly Orders Shift in Policy to Silence Talk of 'Anti-Yankeeism,'" *New York Times,* June 4, 1954.

57. Sidney Gruson, "Prestige of Reds Wanes in Mexico," *New York Times,* October 17, 1954.

58. Roy R. Rubottom Jr. (assistant secretary of state for inter-American affairs), "Communism in the Americas," *Department of State Bulletin* 38 (1958): 180–85; the citation here is on 181.

59. U.S. Department of State, "National Intelligence Estimate: The Outlook for Mexico, Washington, D.C., August 13, 1957, NIE 81-57," in *Foreign Relations of the United States, 1955–1957: American Republics, Multilateral, Mexico, Caribbean,* ed. John P. Glennon (Washington, D.C.: U.S. Government Printing Office, 1987), 684–85

60. "Diary Entry 20 July 1954," folder "January–December 1954," box 12, Fred L. Soper Papers (hereafter Soper Papers), National Library of Medicine, Bethesda, Md. (hereafter NLM).

61. "Mikoyan in Mexico Defends Red Policy," *New York Times,* November 28, 1959.

62. Max J. Smedley, "Mexican–United States Relations and the Cold War, 1945–1954" (Ph.D. thesis, University of Southern California, 1981).

63. Stepen R. Niblo, *War, Diplomacy and Development: The United States and Mexico, 1938–1954* (Wilmington, Del.: Scholarly Resources, 1995).

64. *Health and Sanitation, Cooperative Program in Mexico: Agreement between the United States of America and Mexico, Effected by Exchange of Notes Signed at Mexico, September 20 and November 23, 1950, Entered into Force January 22, 1951; Operative Retroactively from June 30, 1950* (Washington, D.C.: U.S. Department of State, 1951), NLM.

65. Mentioned in "Airgram from Foreign Operations Administration, 31 March 1954," R.G. 469, entry 1948–55, box 14, folder "Mexico," National Archives, Maryland.

66. Miguel E. Bustamante, "Hechos sobresalientes en la historia de la Secretaría de Salubridad y Asistencia," *Salud Pública de México* 25, no. 5 (1983): 465–82; Secretaría de Salubridad y Asistencia, *Memoria, 1947–1950* (Mexico City: Secretaría de Salubridad y Asistencia, 1951), 8.

67. *Oaxaca, 1ª Convención Regional Para la Campaña Nacional contra el Paludismo 21–27 Marzo 1938* (Oaxaca: N.p., 1938), Fundación Cultural Bustamante, Vasconcelos, Oaxaca.

68. "Programa General de Labores mencionado en Joaquín Astorga a Ignacio Morones Prieto, 18 Abril 1947," fondo SSA, sección Subsecretaría de Salubridad y Asistencia, caja 15, expediente 4, AHSS.

69. Dirección General de la Campaña Nacional contra el Paludismo, Secretaría de Salubridad y Asistencia, México, *Trabajos realizados en la Zona Norte de Petróleos Mexicanos* (Mexico City: Secretaría de Salubridad y Asistencia, 1949).

70. Bustamante, "Hechos sobresalientes," 472. A. W. A. Brown, *Insecticide Resistance in Arthropods* (Geneva: World Health Organization, 1958), 123.

71. See table, "Resumen de los trabajos de rociado residual con DDT en México hasta 1951," in *II Congreso Nacional de Paludismo: Programa de sesiones, convocado por la Secretaría de Salubridad y Asistencia de los Estados Unidos Mexicanos en la*

ciudad de México durante los días 12, 13 y 14 de abril, 1951, ed. Secretaría de Salubridad y Asistencia (Mexico City: Secretaría de Salubridad y Asistencia, 1952), 189–200.

72. J. B. Gahan and G. C. Payne, "Control of *Anopheles Pseudopunctipennis* in Mexico with DDT Residual Sprays Applied in Buildings," *American Journal of Hygiene* 45 (1947): 123–32; and Wilburg C. Downs, "Actividades de la Oficina de Especialización Sanitaria," *Medicina, Revista Mexicana* 31, no. 629 (1951): 213–14. This was part of a broader effort by the Rockefeller Foundation to test DDT as a means of controlling malaria.

73. In the towns of Temixco and Acatlipa, the number of malaria cases for the period 1939–44, before spraying, was averaged 258. In contrast, after intense spraying with DDT, from the mid-1940s to 1949, the annual average was 82. See Wilburg Downs, Heliodoro Celis, and James B. Gahan, "Control of *Anopheles Pseudopunctipennis* in Mexico with DDT Residual Sprays Applied in Buildings, Part III: Malariological Observations after Five Years of Annual Spraying," *American Journal of Hygiene* 52, no. 3 (1950): 348–52 (the citation here is on 349).

74. E. Bordas y W. G. Downs, "Ecología de *Anopheles aztecus* en la region de Xochimilco," *Revista del Instituto de Salubridad y Enfermedades Tropicales* 11 (1951): 48–56.

75. W. G. Downs, E. Bordas, and A. Enriquez Chávez, "El control del paludismo en la región de Xochimilco, D.F.," *Revista del Instituto de Salubridad y Enfermedades Tropicales* 11, nos. 1–3 (1950): 99–103; the citation here is on 103.

76. Enrique Beltrán and Luís Vargas, "El Paludismo en el Distrito Federal: Características de una cepa de *Plasmodium vivax* aislada en Xochimilco," *Revista del Instituto de Salubridad y Enfermedades Tropicales* 9, no. 1 (1948): 21–26.

77. "Si el porvenir de la Patria, como en muchas ocasiones se ha dicho, esta en manos del campesino, el porvenir del campesino esta en manos de los maestros y médicos rurales." "Notes on Malaria Control in México, no author, November 1940, restricted," folder Mexico 1947–49, box WHO 7.0078, WHO Archives. "Manuel Márquez Escobedo to Felipe García Sánchez, 6 February 1956," fondo SSA, sección CNEP, serie Dirección, caja 2, expediente 1, AHSS. "Carta de Antonio J. Bermúdez a Ignacio Morones Prieto julio 18, 1956," fondo SSA, sección CNEP, serie Dirección, caja 2, expediente 1, AHSS. "Proyecto de Convenio de Coordinación entre la Comisión del Papaloapán y la Comisión Nacional para la Erradicación del Paludismo en México, 1956," fondo SSA, sección CNEP, serie Dirección, caja 2, expediente 5, AHSS. Secretaría de Salubridad y Asistencia, *Memoria, 1947–1950* (Mexico City: Secretaría de Salubridad y Asistencia, 1950). Departamento de Salubridad Pública, "Ley que declara de utilidad pública la Campaña contra el Paludismo y que crea la Comisión de Saneamiento Antimalárico, Lázaro Cárdenas, Agosto 29, 1938," fondo SSA, sección Secretaría Particular, caja 232, expediente 1, AHSS.

78. "José I .Cano a Subsecretario de Salubridad y Asistencia, 2 March 1948," fondo SSA, sección Subsecretaría de Salubridad y Asistencia, caja 27, expediente 3, AHSS. "Julián Garza Tijerina to Subsecretario de Salubridad, 'Relativo a la Desintectización de braceros que se internen en los EEUU 27 de julio 1948,' Horacio Terán to Rafael Gamboa, 9 September 1949," fondo SSA, sección Subsecretaría de Salubridad y Asistencia, caja 27, expediente 3, AHSS.

79. Antonio Loaeza, *Breve resumen de los estudios acera del paludismo en los Estados Unidos Mexicanos* (Mexico City: Tipográfica de la Viuda, 1911); Alfonso G. Alarcón, *La sobrealimentación en los niños de pecho: El paludismo en la primera infancia*

(Tampico: Imp. Nacional, 1921); Alfonso G. Alarcón, *Estudios clínicos y terapéuticos acerca del paludismo infantil* (Mexico City: Nipos, 1938); Enrique Beltrán and Eduardo Aguirre Pequeño, *Lecciones de paludología* (Monterrey: Universidad de Nuevo León, 1948); Felipe McGregor Giacinti, *Mosquitos y Paludismo* (Mexico City: Oficina Central del Servicio de Puertos y Fronteras, 1940); Ignacio Alcaraz Rivera, *El paludismo en Mochicahui, Sinaloa* (Mexico City: Facultad de Medicina, 1950).

80. Manuel Martínez Báez, "El Instituto de Salubridad y Enfermedades Tropicales," *Anales de la Sociedad Mexicana de Historia de la Ciencia y de la Tecnología* 1 (1969): 143–62; Manuel González Rivera, "Diez años de trabajo en el Instituto de Salubridad y Enfermedades Tropicales," *Revista del Instituto de Salubridad y Enfermedades Tropicales* 10, no. 1 (1949): 3–16.

81. See "Campaña Nacional contra el Paludismo," in *Memoria, 1947–1950,* ed. Secretaría de Salubridad y Asistencia, 117–45.

82. Galo Soberón y Parra, "La importancia de los estados de resistencia orgánica en las campañas antipalúdicas," in *II Congreso Nacional de Paludismo,* ed. Secretaría de Salubridad y Asistencia, 19.

83. "Observaciones que hace la Sección Técnica dependiente de la Campaña Nacional contra el Paludismo y de Profilaxis de la Fiebre Amarilla al Trabajo del Dr. Carlos Calero titulado la Campaña contra el Paludismo en el Puerto de Veracruz, 1952, sin firma," 10, fondo SSA, sección Subsecretaría de Salubridad y Asistencia, caja 19, expediente 3, AHSS.

84. Dirección General de la Campaña contra el Paludismo, Secretaría de Salubridad y Asistencia, "Labores desarrolladas en el periodo comprendido del 1 de diciembre de 1946 al 31 de agosto de 1947," fondo SSA, sección Subsecretaría de Salubridad y Asistencia, caja 19, expediente 3, AHSS.

85. "Informe de la Situación Sanitaria que prevalece en la actualidad y los recursos que se cuentan en el Estado de Oaxaca, 1978." 33, fondo Poder Ejecutivo del Estado, sección Dirección General de Gobernación, serie Secretaria General del Despacho, expediente 281, AGEO.

86. "Mi padre . . . estaba convencido de que una medida aislada [DDT] no sería efectiva y que era necesario reforzarla con una campaña antilarvaria y la detección y el tratamiento de enfermos portadores. No obstante, la presión política para realizar la campaña de erradicación era abrumadora. . . . Para tranquilizar su conciencia enviaría una carta a la Academia Nacional de Medicina en la que dejaría constancia de sus reservas al respecto, la cual se conservaría cerrada hasta después de su muerte." Guillermo Soberón Acevedo, "Remembranzas de mi padre," in *Galo Soberón y Parra, 1896–1956* (Mexico City: Fundación Mexicana para la Salud 1998), 12–21; the citation here is on 18 [however, the letter was never found].

87. "Octava Asamblea Mundial de la Salud," *Crónica de la Organización Mundial de la Salud* 9, no. 7 (1955): 217–23.

88. "Socios honorarios," in *Directorio de la Academia Nacional de Medicina de México, Cuerpo Consultivo del Gobierno Federal* (Mexico: N.p., 1962), 10.

89. Carlos Calero—cited in "México escogido para el mas colosal ensayo antipalúdico," *Excelsior,* May 10, 1955, 12—said it was "una lucha de cuyos resultados dependerá el bienestar de nuestra patria y el provenir inmediato de la campaña mundial."

90. During the mid-1950s, twenty-five species of malaria mosquitoes were identified in Mexico. Of these, the main *Anopheles* were *A. pseudopunctipennis pseudopunctipennis* and *A. albimanus. Plasmodium vivax* was the most common of the three versions

of malaria that exist in the Western Hemisphere (88 percent of all malaria cases); Manuel E. Pesquiera, "Programa de Erradicación del Paludismo en México," *Boletín de la Oficina Sanitaria Panamericana* 42, no. 6 (1957): 537–47. A document that explains the campaign is kept at the WHO Library: "Malaria Eradication, Mexico," in *The Work of WHO 1956* (Geneva: WHO, 1957), 60–63. Historical studies of malaria work in Mexico include Domingo G. Cervantes, *Breve Reseña de la Lucha Antipalúdica en México* (Mexico City: Secretaría de Salubridad y Asistencia, 1979); A.-E. Birn, "Eradication, Control or Neither? Hookworm versus Malaria Strategies and Rockefeller Public Health in México," *Parassitologia* 40, nos. 1–2 (1998): 137–47; and Héctor Gómez-Dantes and Anne-Emanuelle Birn, "Malaria and Social Movements in México: The Last 60 Years," *Parassitologia* 42, nos. 1–2 (2000): 69–85.

91. "El Arzobispo Primado Bendice la Campaña para la Erradicación del Paludismo," *Boletín Zona VI CNEP Año 1 No. 3 Ciudad Valles San Luís Potosí,* August 15, 1956, 1, fondo SSA, sección CNEP, serie Zona VI, caja 1, expediente 2, AHSS.

92. "Nuestra entidad, paulatinamente deja de ser víctima del terrible paludismo," *El Imparcial* (Oaxaca) 23 (October 1958), 1, Hemeroteca Municipal Oaxaca, Oaxaca.

93. "Anti-Malaria Campaign, México Seeks to Eliminate Disease in Next Five Years," *New York Times,* December 7, 1955, 10. "World Health Talk Opened in Mexico," *New York Times,* May 12, 1955, 7. On Padilla Nervo, see "Notas Biográficas Luís Padilla Nervo," *Testimonios de 40 años de Presencia de Mexico en las Naciones Unidas* (Mexico City: Secretaría de Relaciones Exteriores, 1985). Padilla Nervo was Mexico's representative to the UN, again, between 1958 and 1963.

94. UNICEF, *Children of the Developing Countries,* 32.

95. In 1963, the amounts donated by UNICEF to other Mexican programs included $185,000 to Salud Materno-Infantil y Saneamiento del Medio Ambiente and $393,000 to Adiestramiento de Personal Rural de Salud. "Informe preparado por el Secretario de Salubridad y Asistencia, February 1963" and "Informes de labores rendidos por el Departamento General de Epidemiología," fondo SSA, sección Subsecretaría de Salubridad y Asistencia, caja 35, expediente 2, AHSS. Also see Expert Panel on Malaria, International Cooperation Administration, "Report and Recommendations on Malaria: A Summary," *American Journal of Public Health* 10, no. 4 (1961): 451–502.

96. "Donald J. Pletsch y Luís Vargas, 'Daños económicos causados por la malaria, 8 August 1957,'" in "Informes elaborados por el Dr. Donald J. Pletsch en relación con el programa para la erradicación del paludismo en México, 1956," fondo SSA, sección CNEP, serie Dirección, caja 1, expediente 7, AHSS.

97. "Recommendation of the Executive Director for an Allocation, Mexico, Malaria Eradication, 28 February 1957, E/ICEF/L.1005, UNICEF, Program Committee," folder Mexico 1955–56, box WHO 7.0078, series Malaria Research Collection, WHO Archives. "Recommendations of the Executive Director for an Allocation México, Malaria Eradication, E/ICEF/L.1099, UNICEF, Program Committee," folder Mexico 1955–56, box WHO 7.0078, series Malaria Research Collection, WHO Archives.

98. "A Lottery That Helped to Build a Nation," *WLA Magazine,* March 2005, 20–21; http://www.world-lotteries.org/documents/magazine/wla16/wla16_mexico.pdf.

99. Ignacio Morones Prieto, "Informe presentado ante la VI Reunión de Directores de los Servicios Nacionales," V Región de Directores de los Servicios Nacionales de Erradicación de la Malaria de Centro América, México y Panamá, San José, Costa Rica, 24–29 de Junio 1957, Informe Final," 25–26 (the citation here is on 26), fondo SSA, sección CNEP, serie Dirección, caja 2, expediente 15, AHSS.

100. "Más y mejores mexicanos, Campaña Nacional de Erradicación del Paludismo, 1955," 8, fondo SSA, sección CNEP, serie Dirección, caja 1, expediente 6, AHSS.

101. "Entry January 1956, Geneva," folder January–December 1956, box 12, Soper Papers, NLM.

102. "Decreto presidencial que declara de interés público y de beneficio social la campaña para erradicar el paludismo," *Diario Oficial, órgano del gobierno constitucional de los Estados Unidos Mexicanos* (Mexico City) 212, no. 41 (December 17, 1955), fondo SSA, sección CNEP, serie Dirección, caja 1, expediente 5, AHSS; and José Alvarez Amézquita, Miguel Bustamante, Antonio López Picazos, and Francisco Fernández del Castillo, *Historia de la Salubridad y de la Asistencia de México* (Mexico City: Secretaría de Salubridad y Asistencia, 1960), vol. 2, 593.

103. "Convenio de Relaciones de Trabajo entre la CNEP y los Asesores Internacionales," October 30, 1956, fondo SSA, sección CNEP, serie Dirección, caja 2, expediente 2, AHSS.

104. U.S. foreign policy supported Taiwan over continental China starting in the late 1940s. In 1955, President Harry Truman and the U.S. Congress established an American commitment to defend Formosa (later known as Taiwan) as a matter of national security. See Robert Accinelli, *Crisis and Commitment: United States Policy toward Taiwan, 1950–1955* (Chapel Hill: University of North Carolina Press, 1996).

105. David A. Dame, "Donald James Pletsch: Six Decades of International Commitment," *Journal of the American Mosquito Control Association* 21, no. 3 (2005): 331–36. In the mid-1960s, Pletsch joined the U.S. Agency for International Development and worked in Ethiopia and Central America as a malariologist.

106. "Informe de inspección de la Zona VIII, Puebla, 22 Mayo 1956, José Roffe to Donald J. Pletsch, OPS," fondo SSA, sección CNEP, serie Dirección, caja 1, expediente 7, AHSS.

107. Cervantes, *Breve Reseña*, 49.

108. "Report on a Visit to México, the United States and England by Julian de Zulueta, Medical Entomologist, Malaria Section WHO [restricted], 1957 (Pampana)," folder Mexico 1957–58, series Malaria Research Collection, box WHO 7.0078, WHO Archives.

109. Ignacio Chávez, *México en la cultura médica* (Mexico City: FCE, 1947 [1987]), 120.

110. "Diary Entry, January 1956, Geneva," folder January–December 1956, box 12, Soper Papers, NLM.

111. "Dirección de salubridad en el D.F.," in *Memoria, 1947–1950,* ed. Secretaría de Salubridad y Asistencia, 11.

112. Milton I. Roemer, *Medical Care in Latin America* (Washington, D.C.: Organization of American States, 1963), 120.

113. Morgan, *Doctors,* 9.

114. "Un ingeniero sanitario ingresa a la Academia Nacional de Medicina," in *Campeche, ciudad del Carmen: Historia, paludismo, inundaciones, petróleo,* by Antonio Uribe González (Campeche: N.p., 1992), 287.

115. Vargas worked under the direction of the parasytologist Carlos C. Hoffman, who trained a number of young researchers. See Sergio Ibáñez Bernal, "Daniel Luís Vargas García Alonso," in *Una institución académica mexicana y dieciséis investigadores distinguidos,* ed. José Luís Valdespino Gómez, Aurora del Rio Zolezzi, Alejandro Escobar Gutiérrez, and José Luís Mora Galindo (Mexico City: Secretaría de Salud, 1994),

127–30; Luís Vargas and Amado Martínez Palacios, *Anofelinos Mexicanos: Taxonomía y Distribución* (Mexico City: Secretaría de Salubridad y Asistencia, 1950), 9; and Luís Vargas and A. Martínez Palacios, "Distribución de los Anofelinos mexicanos," *Revista del Instituto de Salubridad y Enfermedades Tropicales* 15, no. 2 (1955): 81–123.

116. Luís Vargas, "Problemas de identificación de vectores del paludismo y su biología, en las principales zonas endémicas de México," *Boletín de Sanidad Militar* (Mexico City) 9 (1951): 435–39; the citation here is 436.

117. Luís Vargas, "Malaria along the Mexico–United Sates Border," *Bulletin of the World Health Organization* 2, no. 4 (1950): 611–20.

118. Paul F. Russell, *Paludismo: Compendio de principios básicos,* was originally published in English in 1952. Some years later, another important work on malaria eradication was published in Mexico: Emilio Pampana, *Erradicación de la Malaria* (Mexico City: Limusa-Wiley, 1966).

119. Luís Vargas and Martínez Palacios, *Estudio taxonómico de los mosquitos anofelicos de México* (Mexico City: Secretaría de Salubridad y Asistencia, 1950); and Paul F. Russell, Lloyd E. Roszenboom, and Alan Stone, *Keys to the Anopheline Mosquitoes of the World, with Notes On Their Identification, Distribution, Biology, and Relation to Malaria* (Philadelphia: American Entomological Society, 1943).

120. "Entry March 1 1956," folder January–December 1956, box 12, Soper Papers, NLM.

121. Cervantes, *Breve Reseña,* 49.

122. Humberto Romero Álvarez, *La Campaña Nacional para la Erradicación del paludismo: Su importancia para la salud pública* (Mexico City: Talleres Gráficos de la Nación, 1973), 20.

123. "Secretaría de la Defensa y la CNEP," *Boletín Zona VI CNEP, Año 1 No. 3 Ciudad Valles San Luís Potosí,* August 15, 1956, 1, fondo SSA, sección CNEP, serie Zona VI, caja 1, expediente 2, AHSS; and "The Malaria Eradication Campaign in México, Report Submitted to the Program Committee on 25 October 1956 by Mr. R. Davee."

124. "¿Quién comanda la Quinta Zona de la CNEP?" *Sol de Oaxaca,* January 1957, newspaper clipping, fondo SSA, sección CNEP, serie Zona V, caja 1, expediente 2, AHSS.

125. Luís Vargas, "Realizaciones del Programa de Erradicación," *Salud Pública de México* 7 (1965): 737–40.

126. Morgan, *Doctors,* 15.

127. "Decreto presidencial que declara de interés público y de beneficio social la campaña para erradicar el paludismo"; and "Informe narrativo y numérico de las actividades más importantes desarrolladas durante el año comprendido del 1 de septiembre de 1956 al 31 de agosto de 1957," fondo SSA, sección Subsecretaría de Salubridad y Asistencia, caja 80, expediente 1, AHSS.

128. *Memoria de la Secretaría de Salubridad y Asistencia Pública, Sexenio 1952–1958* (Mexico City: Secretaría de Salubridad y Asistencia Pública, 1959), 351.

129. "Noticias para la Publicación, Organización Panamericana de la Salud, 25 Septiembre 1956," fondo SSA, sección Subsecretaría de Salubridad y Asistencia, caja 42, expediente 3, AHSS.

130. "Report on a Visit to Mexico, the United States and England by Julian de Zulueta."

131. Márquez Escobedo, "La erradicación del paludismo en México," AHSS; and "Recommendation of the Executive Director for an Apportionment."

132. Program Committee, UNICEF, "Recommendation of the Executive Director for an Allocation, Mexico, Malaria Eradication, 28 February 1957, E/ICEF/L.1005," folder Mexico 1955–56, series Malaria Research Collection, box WHO 7.0078, WHO Archives.

133. E.g.: "Francisco Mújica Bahena to Presidente de la República, Acapulco, 23 December 1956," Archivo Ruíz Cortines, vol. 423, expediente 424/23, AGN México; and "Armín Monte de Honor to Adolfo Ruíz Cortines, 14 September 1955," Archivo Ruíz Cortines, vol. 423, expediente 424/23, AGN México.

134. See Marcos Cueto, "Sanitation from Above: Yellow Fever and Foreign Intervention in Perú, 1919–1922," *Hispanic American Historical Review* 72, no. 1 (1992): 1–22.

135. The Pan-American Health Organization was against the use of drugs because it did not consider them fully effective, but eventually, starting in 1957, it supported the use of drugs. See WHO Expert Committee on Malaria, *Sixth Report* (Geneva: World Health Organization, 1957). See also Humberto Romero Álvarez, "Comisión Nacional para la Erradicación del Paludismo," *Salud Pública de México* 6 (1964): 1123–52; Luís Vargas, G. Román y Carillo, and A. Almaraz y Ugalde, "Organization and Evaluation of the Malaria Eradication Campaign in Mexico during the First Year of Complete Coverage," *Bulletin of the World Health Organization* 19, no. 4 (1958): 621–35.

136. José Alvarez Amézqita, "Programa de Erradicación del Paludismo en México: Informe de actividades año de 1958, preparado para la VII Reunión de Directores de los Servicios Nacionales de Erradicación el Paludismo en México, Centro América y Panamá, celebrada en Panamá 13–17 abril 1969," fondo SSA, sección CNEP, serie Dirección, caja 44, expediente 7, AHSS.

137. Escobedo, "La Erradicación del Paludismo en México."

138. "Campana Antimosquito en el Istmo, Oaxaca," *El Imparcial* (Oaxaca), September 27, 1958.

139. This was announced in Department of Public Information, United Nations, Press Release, "Malaria Eradication Campaign in Mexico Begins with Aid of WHO and UNICEF, 31 January 1957," ICEF/636, UNICEF Archives.

140. On Chile, see M. Ulloa, "Malaria Eradication in Chile," *Parasitology Today* 5, no. 2 (1989): 31.

141. Vargas, "Realizaciones."

142. The draft was "Plan Tripartito de Operaciones para un Proyecto de Erradicación del Paludismo en México, 1954," fondo SSA, sección CNEP, serie Dirección, caja 1, expediente 3. The information of this paragraph comes from "Datos principales del desarrollo del programa de erradicación del paludismo en México, 1958," fondo SSA, sección Subsecretaría de Asistencia, caja 80, expediente 1, AHSS.

143. Vargas, "Realizaciones," 739.

144. J. Fernández de Castro, "El paludismo en México y la lucha para su control," *A cien años del descubrimiento de Ross: El paludismo en México,* ed. Jesús Kumate and Adolfo Martínez Palomo (Mexico City: Colegio Nacional, 1998), 227–35; the citation here is on 231.

145. Escobedo, "La Erradicación del paludismo en México."

146. "Notable abatimiento de la mortalidad por malaria fue logrado en el Año de 1959," *El Dictamen, Diario Independiente* (Veracruz), June 4, 1960; "Positivos frutos arroja la Campaña para la Erradicación del Paludismo," *El Sol de Puebla* (Puebla), June 19, 1960; "Rociado de casas se suspenderá," Tampico, July 26, 1960; "El paludismo fue

erradicado de la entidad," *El Mundo* (Tamaulipas), July 27, 1960; "La Campaña de Erradicación del Paludismo ha sido todo un éxito," *El Diario de ciudad Victoria* (Ciudad
Victoria), Tamps. 28 Julio 1960 [Zone VII]; "El paludismo ya no existe en el estado
de Durango," *El Diario de Culiacán* (Culiacán Sinaloa), September 1, 1960; "Ahorro
de 600 millones de pesos al vencer al paludismo," *El Dictamen* (Veracruz), January 18,
1961. These are all newspaper clippings in fondo SSA, sección CNEP, serie Dirección,
caja 5, expediente 8, AHSS.

147. Aimee Wilcox, *Manual for the Microscopical Diagnosis of Malaria in Man*
(Washington, D.C.: U.S. Government Printing Office, 1950 [1942]); also see G. Román
y Carrillo, "El paludismo en México," *Gaceta Médica de México* 110, no. 6 (1975):
401–10, Manuel B. Márquez Escobedo to Enrique Palafox Muñoz [jefe de la Zona II,
Tabasco, Villahermosa], 4 February 1956, fondo SSA, sección CNEP, serie Zona II, caja
1, expediente 3, AHSS.

148. José Álvarez Amézquita, "¿Hay defunciones por paludismo en México?" *Salud
Pública de México* 5 (1963): 748–49; the citation here is on 748.

149. "Población urbana y rural del país por entidades federativas 1960 y 1965," in
Anuario estadístico compendiado de los Estados Unidos Mexicanos, 1968, ed. Dirección General de Estadística, México (Mexico City: Dirección General de Estadística,
1969), 18. See also Gabriel Calderon Arias, "La malaria se localiza en dos entidades,"
Novedades de Acapulco, April 2, 1974, newspaper clipping, fondo SSA, sección CNEP,
serie Zona IX, caja 2, expediente 9, AHSS. The localities mentioned in this article were
Oaxaca and Guerrero.

150. "Tratamiento Intensivo Antipalúdico," *Novedades de Acapulco,* January 13,
1973, newspaper clipping, fondo SSA, sección CNEP, serie Zona IX, caja 2, expediente
9, AHSS. The localities mentioned in this article were Oaxaca and Guerrero.

151. "Guillermo E. Samame to Soper, 2 June 1958," folder Correspondence-Malaria,
L-S, box 18, Soper Papers, NLM.

152. "Prórroga del Plan Tripartito de Operaciones para un Proyecto de Erradicación
del Paludismo en México, 31 Agosto 1961," fondo SSA, sección CNEP, serie Dirección,
caja 44, expediente 15, AHSS.

153. "Editorial," *Boletín CNEP, Zona IX, Enero 1961* [no number, no day], 1, fondo
SSA, sección CNEP, serie Zona IX, caja 1, expediente 2, AHSS.

154. "Plan de Distribución en las Zonas del Material Educativo entregado a la CNEP
por la Dirección de Educación Higiénica de la SSA," August 11, 1960, fondo SSA, sección CNEP, serie Dirección, caja 2, expediente 24, AHSS.

155. Poder Ejecutivo Federal, México, *Acción educativa del gobierno federal del 1
de Septiembre de 1954 al 31 de Agosto de 1955* (Mexico City: Secretaría de Educación
Pública, 1955), 74–79.

156. *Memorias del Instituto Nacional Indigenista,* vol. 6, ed. Alfonso Caso, Silvio
Zavala, José Miranda, Moisés Gonzáles Navarro, Gonzalo Aguirre Beltrán, and Ricardo
Pozas (Mexico City: Instituto Nacional Indigenista, 1954), 248.

157. Manuel Gonzáles Rivera, *Las enfermedades transmisibles en el medio agrario:
Cartilla para uso de los maestros rurales por el Dr.* (Mexico City: Secretaría de Salubridad y Asistencia, 1946), 7.

158. Dirección General de Higiene Escolar y Servicios Médicos, Secretaría de Educación Pública, *Manual de técnicas y procedimientos, zonas médico escolares* (Mexico City: Secretaría de Educación Pública, 1958) and Idem., *Higiene Escolar Mexicana*
(Mexico City: Secretaría de Educación Pública, 1959).

159. "Convenio celebrado entre la Secretaría de Educación Pública y la de Salubridad y Asistencia para coordinar actividades en el Distrito Federal y en otras entidades del país, en la Campaña Nacional para la Erradicación del Paludismo en México," February 3, 1956, in *Legislación y Reglamentación, 1921–1958,* ed. Secretaría de Educación Pública (Mexico City: Secretaría de Educación Pública, 1958), 113–17.

160. "Convenio celebrado entre la Secretaría de Educación Pública y la de Salubridad y Asistencia."

161. "Enrique Escobedo Valdez to Manuel Márquez Escobedo, 19 January 1956," fondo SSA, sección CNEP, serie Dirección, caja 2, expediente 24, AHSS.

162. The illustration and poster appear in *Magisterio Nacional y Paludismo,* by Dirección General de Higiene Escolar y Servicios Médicos (Mexico City: Secretaría de Educación Pública, 1957), 9, 13.

163. "Enrique Escobedo Valdez to Manuel Márquez Escobedo, 19 January 1956."

164. "El Magisterio en la Campaña," 5, *Boletín Zona VI CNEP Año 1 No 2 Ciudad Valles San Luís Potosí,* May 15, 1956, 4, fondo SSA, sección CNEP, serie Zona VI, caja 1, expediente 2, AHSS.

165. "Profesor Antonio M. García [Cuicatlan, Oaxaca] a Ignacio Morones Prieto, 5 September 1956," fondo SSA, sección CNEP, serie Zona V, caja 1, expediente 1, AHSS.

166. Manuel E. Pesqueira, "A Year of Antimalarial Activities, April 1957," in folder Mexico 1957–58, box WHO 7.0078, series Malaria Research Collection, WHO Archives.

167. "Mario Moreno 'Cantinflas' en la guerra antipalúdica," *Boletín de la Comisión Nacional para la Erradicación del Paludismo, Zona VI, Ciudad valles San Luís Potosí, Año 2. No. 6-7,* July 1, 1957, series Malaria Research Collection, folder Mexico 1955–56, box WHO 7.0078, WHO Archives.

168. In 1960, officers of CNEP's educational program explained the important role played by audiovisual materials. F. Villaseñor, "Los medios audiovisuales en la enseñanza," *Salud Pública de México* 2 (1960): 77–80; and J. Chargoy Martínez, "La cinematografía y la educación higiénica," *Salud Pública de México* 2 (1960): 81–84.

169. Pablo González Casanova, *La Democracia en México* (Mexico City: Era, 1967), 90.

170. "Radio," in *Encyclopaedia of Mexico, History, Society and Culture,* ed. Michael S. Werner (London: Fitzroy Dearborn, 1997), vol 2, 1218–26; the citation here is on 1221.

171. Jorge Ayala Blanco, *La aventura del cine mexicano en la epoca de oro y después* (Mexico City: Grijalbo, 1993).

172. Rafael Manrique Paz, *Informe médico-sanitario del pueblo de Chicomuselo, Chiapas y breves consideraciones sobre el paludismo,* Thesis, examen profesional de médico cirujano, Facultad de Medicina (Mexico City: Tipográfica Ortega, 1955).

173. "La opinión del día: Campaña moderna," *Rumbo Nuevo,* July 11, 1956, Villahermosa, Tabasco, fondo SSA, sección CNEP, serie Zona II, caja 1, expediente 6, AHSS.

174. "Donald J. Pletsch to Manuel B. Márquez Escobedo, 3 September 1956," fondo SSA, sección CNEP, Serie Dirección, caja 2, expediente 24, AHSS.

175. This is in the pamphlet *Yo soy patriota: Colaboro en la guerra al paludismo,* 2 [no date, but it appears at the beginning of the campaign], fondo SSA, sección CNEP, serie Zona I, caja 1, expediente 1, AHSS.

176. These posters are kept at fondo SSA, sección CNEP, serie Dirección, caja 8, expediente 4, AHSS.

177. "¡A la guerra! A sumarnos todos en la gran movilización de ciudadanos de

extremo a extremo de la Patria para combatir al enemigo que siega vidas, que siembra desolación y muerte," in *Yo soy patriota.*

178. "México esta en guerra, el enemigo es el paludismo," *Rumbo Nuevo* (Villahermosa, Tabasco), July 10, 1956, newspaper clipping, fondo SSA, sección CNEP, serie Zona II, caja 1, expediente 6, AHSS.

179. *Boletín Zona VI CNEP: Año 1 No. 2 Ciudad Valles San Luís Potosí,* May 15, 1956, fondo SSA, sección CNEP, serie Zona VI, caja 1, expediente 2, AHSS.

180. Edmund Russell, *War and Nature: Fighting Humans and Insects with Chemicals from World War I to Silent Spring* (Cambridge: Cambridge University Press, 2001).

181. Lini de Vries, *The People of the Mountains: Health Education among Indian Communities in Oaxaca, Mexico* (Cuernavaca: Centro Intercultural de Documentacion, 1969), 55.

182. Alicja Ianska, "The Mexican Indian: Image and Identity," *Journal of Interamerican Studies* 6, no. 4 (1964): 529–36.

183. Alan Knight, "Peasant into Patriots: Thoughts on the Making of the Mexican Nation," *Mexican Studies/Estudios Mexicanos* 10, no. 1 (1994): 135–61.

184. See Scott Cook and Jong-Taick Joo, "Ethnicity and Economy in Rural Mexico: A Critique of the Indigenista Approach," *Latin American Research Review* 30, no. 2 (1995): 33–59.

185. In "Memoria del CNEP," *Boletín del CNEP* 11, no. 4 (1958): 3–55.

186. "La Mujer mexicana ante la Campaña para la Erradicación del Paludismo por Rebeca Fernández Gonzáles," *Boletín Zona VI CNEP Año 1 No. 2 Ciudad Valles San Luís Potosí,* May 15, 1956, 4, fondo SSA, sección CNEP, serie Zona VI, caja 1, expediente 2, AHSS.

187. "Dueño de su destino y por tanto un hombre superado: Más y mejores mexicanos—Campaña Nacional de Erradicación del Paludismo, 1955," 1, 2, fondo SSA, sección CNEP, serie Dirección, caja 1, expediente 6, AHSS.

188. Luís Vargas, "Consideraciones generales sobre la epidemiología de la malaria evanescente en México," *Gaceta Médica de México* 88, no. 9 (1958): 613–33.

189. "En la lucha por erradicar el paludismo deben participar todos los Mexicanos como un solo hombre. Únase a nosotros: su colaboración ilustrada y eficaz significara la salvación de muchos compatriotas, quizás la de usted mismo y la de los suyos." Dirección General de Higiene Escolar y Servicios Médicos, *Magisterio Nacional y Paludismo* (Mexico City: Secretaría de Educación Pública, 1957), 28.

190. "¡Guerra al paludismo! Oiga: Notas del Director," Marzo 18, 1957, *La Voz del Sureste,* newspaper clipping, fondo SSA, sección CNEP, serie Zona II, caja 1, expediente 6, AHSS. "Dirije a su parcela, llena de ilusiones, pensando que ese día podrá sembrar o podrá cosechar. Al poco rato sus ilusiones mueren, el paludismo lo vence, las calenturas lo postran y busca una sombra para refugiarse. Ahí bajo un árbol delira y cuando le pasa el furor de la fiebre, regresa a su hogar, triste y agotado. Mientras tanto las tierras exuberantes quedan en el peor de los abandonos . . . en las escuelas los niños no pueden asimilar la enseñanza del maestro, el pupitre lo utilizan como dormitorio. . . . El comerciante, el profesionista, todo sufren viendo pasar los años sin poder gozar de salud. Con mucha razón se comenta: MIENTRAS EL NORTE TRABAJA EL SURESTE DUERME. Es verdad duerme y mucho, no porque el pueblo sea flojo, no, duerme porque la enfermedad obliga a dormir. . . . Hoy ha llegado el día de la salvación. Acabando con el paludismo el Sureste despertara de su letargo. Veremos hombres fuertes, dispuestos a cultivar sus tierras. Veremos mujeres y niños alegres, llenos de satisfacción y deseosos de cooperar

para lograr un México grande. Al pueblo le corresponde ayudar para que la campaña antipalúdica triunfe, no se les pide dinero, porque la campaña es completamente gratuita, ni tampoco se les exige trabajo, únicamente se les pide colaboración, fe y entusiasmo. Estimado lector pensemos todos en el futuro de nuestros hijos y de nuestra patria. Acabar con el paludismo es nuestra meta."

191. José Alvarez Amézqita (secretario de salubridad y asistencia), "Programa de Erradicación del Paludismo en México: Informe de actividades Año e 1958, preparado para la VII Reunión de Directores de los Servicios Nacionales de Erradicación el Paludismo en México, Centro América y Panamá, celebrada en Panamá 13–17 abril 1969," fondo SSA, sección CNEP, serie Dirección, caja 44, expediente 7, AHSS.

192. "Manuel B. Márquez Escobedo to Carlos Rus Ávila, Jefe de la Zona II de la CNEP, 31 August 1959," fondo SSA, sección CNEP, serie Zona II, caja 1, expediente 3, AHSS.

193. According to Pesquiera, the malaria mortality rate for Chiapas was 308.3 per 100,000 inhabitants. Pesquiera, "Programa de Erradicación," 541.

194. In *La Cotorra,* October 1960 [no day, no folder], fondo SSA, sección Subsecretaría de Asistencia, expediente 3, caja 84, AHSS.

195. "Editorial: El Rociador—pilar y gigante en el programa de erradicación del paludismo," *Boletín Mensual, para el Personal de la Zona II,* September 1960 [no day], fondo SSA, sección Subsecretaría de Asistencia, expediente 3, caja 84, AHSS.

196. José Romero Alzate (schoolteacher in Matatan, Rosario, Sinaloa), "Página poética, el paludismo mata," *El Humaya Órgano de Información para el Personal del CNEP Zona VIII Año IV, Culiacán,* February 1960, 4, fondo SSA, sección CNEP, serie Zona I, caja 1, expediente 3, AHSS.

197. "Editorial: Por que se hizo campaña," *La Cotorra, Periódico al Servicio del Personal CNEP, Zona VIII,* September 1960 [no day], fondo SSA, sección Subsecretaría de Asistencia, expediente 3, caja 84, AHSS.

198. Fernando Camara, "Contemporary Mexican Indian Cultures: The Problems of Integration," in *Indian Mexico: Past and Present—Symposium Papers, 1965,* ed. Betty Bell (Los Angeles: University of California, Los Angeles, 1967), 100–9; the citation here is on 104.

199. "Mountains, Rivers and Mayas of Chiapas," *New York Times,* May 9, 1954.

200. *El Tarasco; Boletín para el Personal CNEP Zona X* (Morelia, Michoacán), fondo SSA, sección Subsecretaría de Asistencia, caja 84, expediente 3, Años 1949–55, AHSS. ("¡Muera, muera el paludismo!/¡y viva la patria mía!")

201. This word means "secret" but is also used to refer to hell.

202. This is a popular name for death.

203. ¡Que bonito es el rociado / con DDT o Dieldrin; / Millones de mexicanos, / de las palúdicas zonas, / se salvaron del Arcano / de donde viene "la pelona . . ." ¡Guerra a toda esclavitud! / ¡Y viva la democracia! By Antonio Bautista y López, "Poesía y corrido del paludismo," Animas, Oaxaca, September 29, 1960, Producción Artística y Literaria, vol. 1273, expediente 33275, AGN México.

204. "Lid Moderna," 4, *El Huasteco Boletín Zonal CNEP Zona VI Ciudad Valles San Luís Potosí VI Julio 1961* [no day], fondo SSA, sección CNEP, serie Zona VI, caja 1, expediente 2, AHSS. "No será, sin embargo el acero El que empuñe el moderno adalid; / Hoy será un científico apero, / El que de la victoria en la lid. / Hoy la lucha feroz se ha iniciado / Por combate de un bicho falaz / El zancudo que ha propalado / La malaria mortal y tenaz."

205. "Himno al paludismo: Canto de Fe, por E. Méndez Pérez, Auxiliar Honorario de Educación Higiénica," Oaxaca, Oaxaca, September 17, 1960, fondo SSA, sección CNEP, serie Zona V, caja 1, expediente 3, AHSS.

206. Claudio Lommintz, *Death and the Idea of Mexico* (New York: Zone Books, 2005), 421.

207. In *El Transmisor: Órgano de información para el personal CNEP Zona VII* (Tamaulipas, Nuevo León, Coahuila) [no date, no folder], fondo SSA, sección Subsecretaría de Asistencia, caja 84, expediente 3. Spanish version: "La muerte muy indignada / de ver a todos contentos / 'me los llevo, me los llevo'/ gritaba con aspavientos // Me los llevo a todos junto / antes que se venga un sismo / me están quitando la chamba / todos los del Paludismo // La calaca se impresiona / y se tiro al abismo / al visitar esta Zona y no encontrar Paludismo."

208. "Una carta de amor de un malariólogo, anónimo," *Publicación Mensual al Servicio del Personal de la Zona VIII H. Puebla de Zaragoza,* February 1960 [no day], 3, fondo SSA, sección CNEP, serie Zona I, caja 1, expediente 3, AHSS.

209. According to Pampana, the idea of voluntary collaborators was born in Mexico and was later extended to the rest of the world. Emilio J. Pampana, *A Textbook of Malaria Eradication* (London: Oxford University Press, 1963), 409.

210. "Leobardo S. Jiménez [director of a school] to Manuel Márquez Escobedo, 7 Marzo 1956," fondo SSA, sección CNEP, serie Zona V, caja 1, expediente 1, AHSS.

211. Manuel Márquez Escobedo and Ignacio Gómez Mendoza, "Evaluation, Techniques and Surveillance in Malaria Eradication Programs in México," May 17, 1960 [presented to Expert Committee on Malaria], series Malaria Research Collection, folder Mexico 1958, box WHO 7.0078, WHO Archives.

212. In *Boletín Mensual, para el Personal, Zona II,* September 1960 [no day], fondo SSA, sección Subsecretaría de Asistencia, expediente 3, caja 84, AHSS.

213. The information on AHEH is from Ignacio Morones Prieto, Manuel Márquez, and Luís Vargas, "La erradicación del paludismo en México," paper presented to the VI Congreso de Medicina Tropical y Paludismo, Lisbon, September 15–18, 1958, fondo SSA, sección Secretaría Particular, caja 18, expediente 2, AHSS; and Guillermo Suárez Torres, *La Campaña Nacional para la Erradicación del Paludismo y su importancia para la salud pública* (Mexico City: Secretaría de Salubridad y Asistencia, 1973), 85.

214. On Cime, "El notificante, ciudadano ejemplar, ¿Quién es Olegario Cime?" *El Informador, Boletín CNEP Zona I Mérida, Yucatán,* May 1962 [no day], fondo SSA, sección Subsecretaría de Asistencia, serie CNEP, caja 93, expediente 1, AHSS.

Chapter 4. Local Responses

1. "Supervisión Efectuada a la Sección de Relaciones Públicas de Zona I, Septiembre 1961," fondo Secretaría de Salubridad y Asistencia (hereafter SSA), sección Comisión Nacional para la Erradicación del Paludismo (hereafter CNEP), serie Zona II, expediente 6, Archivo Histórico de la Secretaría de Salud (hereafter AHSS), Mexico City. Although the zones usually appeared in official publications in Arabic numbers, I will use roman numbers.

2. Ricardo Zebada Ochoa (chief of Zone IX), "Supervisión a la Sección de Relaciones Publicas, Zona IX, 18-4-1962," 2, fondo SSA, serie CNEP, sección Zona IX, caja 2, expediente 2, AHSS.

3. Luís Vargas, "Consideraciones generales sobre la epidemiología de la malaria evanescente de México," *Gaceta Médica de México* 88, no. 9 (1958): 613–33; the citation here is on 613.

4. "Armín Monte de Honor to Adolfo Ruíz Cortines, 14 September 1955," Archivo Ruíz Cortines, vol. 423, expediente 424/23, Archivo General de la Nación (hereafter AGN), Mexico City.

5. "Soper to Morones Prieto, 16 March 1956," fondo SSA, sección CNEP, serie Dirección, caja 2, expediente 17, AHSS. "The Malaria Eradication Campaign in Mexico, Report Submitted to the Program Committee on 25 October 1956 by Mr. R. Davee, Director, the Americas Regional Office, E/ICEF/329, United Nations Children's Fund," series Malaria Research Collection, folder Mexico 1955–56, box WHO7.0078, WHO Archives.

6. "1957 Annual Report Dieldrin Study Project, AMRO 105, Mexico, Compiled by Travis E. McNeel," folder "Dieldrin Project," box 9, Louis Laval Williams Papers (hereafter Williams Papers), National Library of Medicine, Bethesda, Md. (hereafter NLM).

7. "1957 Annual Report Dieldrin Study Project, AMRO 105, Mexico, Compiled by Travis E Mcneel," folder "Dieldrin Project," 54–55, box 9, Williams Papers, NLM.

8. Ibid., 118.

9. Ibid., 87.

10. "Manuel Márquez Escobedo to Jefe de la Zona I, 24 January 1957," fondo SSA, sección CNEP, serie Zona I, caja 1, expediente 2, AHSS. "Márquez Escobedo to Dávila, 19 October 1956," fondo SSA, sección CNEP, serie Zona IV, caja 1, expediente 2, AHSS.

11. By the late 1950s, the institute had linguists working in Bolivia, Brazil, Ecuador, Guatemala, Mexico, Peru, the Philippines, and the United States; "Información cronológica de las actividades planeadas y desarrolladas por el departamento de información, publicidad y educación higiénica de la CNEP, 1956," fondo SSA, sección CNEP, serie Dirección, caja 3, expediente 7, AHSS. Also see David Stoll, *Fishers of Men or Founders of Empire? The Wycliffe Bible Translators in Latin America* (London: Zed Press, 1982). Summer Institute of Linguistics, *Veinticinco años del Instituto Lingüístico de Verano en México, 1935–1960* (Mexico City: Summer Institute of Linguistics, 1960).

12. Manuel E. Pesqueira (undersecretary of health), "A Year of Antimalarial Activities, April 1957," series Malaria Research Collection, box WHO 7.0078, folder Mexico 1957–58, WHO Archives.

13. A letter suggests that these four measures were the main goal of the educational program; "Professor Carmen M. Hernández Guzmán to Carlos Ruz Avila (Jefe de la Zona II Villahermosa, Tabasco), 11 May 1962," fondo SSA, sección CNEP, serie Zona II, expediente 6, AHSS.

14. "Intervención del Dr. Carlos Alvarado," in "V Región de Directores de los Servicios Nacionales de Erradicación de la Malaria de Centro América, México y Panamá, San José, Costa Rica, 24–29 de Junio 1957, Informe Final, Mimeo," 25–26, fondo SSA, sección CNEP, serie Dirección, caja 2, expediente 15, AHSS.

15. "Mario Aguilar Sierra [chief of Zone XII] to CNEP, México, D.F., 2 January 1959," fondo SSA, sección CNEP, serie Zona XII, caja 1, expediente 4, AHSS.

16. "Sección de Epidemiología," a leaflet, fondo Secretaría de Salubridad y Asistencia, sección CNEP, serie Zona I, caja 1, expediente 3, AHSS.

17. Domingo Cervantes González, "Informe de la visita de orientación epidemiológica efectuada en la Zona IV, Chiapas, 6 al 20 de Agosto 1962," 10, fondo SSA, serie CNEP, sección. Zona IV, caja 1, expediente 8, AHSS.

18. Gordon Novell, Paul F. Russell, and N. H. Swellengrebel, *Malaria Terminology: Report of a Drafting Committee Appointed by the World Health Organization* (Geneva: World Health Organization, 1953).

19. These names were "amarillas, calenturas pega, calenturas, calentura con frío, calentura entre cuerpo y carne, ceel, costeado chahuiste, espantado, fiebre con fríos, fiebre del bazo, fiebre de la costa, fiebre remitente, fiebres barranqueñas, fríos costeños, fríos criollos, fríos y calenturas intermitentes, jacaltamal, latido con bazo, los fríos, maduro por los fríos, mal de espanto, miseria fisiológica por paludismo, morrongo, tenahuiste, tener bazo, tiricia, toahusite, tenahuistle." Luís Vargas, "Realizaciones del programa de erradicación," *Salud Pública de México* 7 (1965): 737–40; the quotaton here is on 739.

20. In 1970, in the states of Chiapas, Guerrero, and Oaxaca, the percentages of medical certificates were, respectively, 37.5, 39.8, and 23.3. José Luís Bobadilla, "La mortalidad en Mexico," in *Vida y muerte del mexicano I,* by Federico Quedasa (Mexico City: Folios Ediciones, 1982), 15–42; the citation here is on 38.

21. "Alfonso Caso, Director de Instituto Indigenista to Ignacio Morones Prieto, 9 February 1956," and response in "Ignacio Gómez Mendoza to Manuel Márquez Escobedo 22 February 1956," fondo SSA, sección CNEP, serie Dirección, caja 3, expediente 1, AHSS.

22. See Anne Doremus, "Indigenism, Mestizaje and National Identity in Mexico during the 1940s and 1950s," *Mexican Studies/Estudios Mexicanos* 17, no. 2 (2001): 375–402.

23. Henri Favre, *Cambio y Continuidad entre los Mayas de México* (Mexico City: Siglo XXI, 1972); and Jaime Tomas Page Pliego, *Política sanitaria dirigida a los pueblos indígenas de México y Chiapas 1857–1995* (Mexico City: Universidad Nacional Autonoma de México, 2002), 28 Agustín Romano Delgado, *Historia Evaluativa del Centro Coordinador Indigenista Tzeltal-Tzotzil,* vols. 1 and II (Mexico City: Instituto Nacional Indigenista, 2002).

24. Julio de la Fuente, "El Centro Coordinador Tzeltal-Tzotzil," *América Indígena* 13, no. 1 (1953): 55–64; Gonzalo Aguirre Beltrán, ed., *El Indigenismo en Acción: XXV Aniversario del Centro Coordinador Indigenista Tzeltal-Tzotzil, Chiapas* (Mexico City: Instituto Nacional Indigenista, 1976); Carlos Inchaustegui Díaz, Instituto Nacional Indigenista, "Informe sobre la Zona Triqui," fondo SSA, sección CNEP, serie Zona VIII, caja 2, expediente 1, AHSS. For a theoretical approach to analyzing midwives in México, see Verónica Sieglin, *Modernización y Devastación de la Cultura Tradicional Campesina* (Mexico City: Plaza y Valdez, 2004).

25. "Cambiar el concepto de la causa de enfermedad en las comunidades indígenas. Generalmente creen estas que la enfermedad no son el resultado de un proceso natural, sino que obedecen a causas mágicas. . . . Ese concepto mágico . . . es el principal motivo de que no se tomen las precauciones higiénicas y que los indígenas. . . . No tengan fe en la medicina científica." Instituto Nacional Indigenista, *¿Que es el INI?* (Mexico City: INI, 1955), 51.

26. Gonzalo Aguirre Beltrán, ed., *El Indigenismo en Acción: XXV Aniversario del Centro Coordinador Indigenista Tzeltal-Tzotzil, Chiapas* (Mexico City: Instituto Nacional Indigenista, 1976), 216.

27. Poder Ejecutivo Federal, Government of Mexico, *Acción Educativa del Gobierno Federal del 1 de Septiembre de 1954 al 31 de Agosto de 1955* (Mexico City: Secretaría de Educación Pública, 1955), 88.

28. Cited in Marion Wilhelm, "Hidden by Centuries: Mexican Indian Community Strides from Shadow," *Christian Science Monitor,* December 14, 1953, 3.

29. See Alan Knight, "Racism, Revolution and *Indigenismo:* México, 1910–1940," in *The Idea of Race in Latin America,* ed. Richard Graham (Austin: University of Texas Press, 1990), 71–113.

30. Luís Vargas and A. Almaraz Ugalde, "Evaluación epidemiológica de la erradicación del paludismo en 1959, tercer año de cobertura integral," *Salud Pública de México* 5 (1963): 257–69; the citation here is on 258.

31. Vargas, "Realizaciones del programa de erradicación," 740. Socioeconomic factors not studied in this chapter—e.g., urbanization and literacy—encouraged the Western medicalization of rural Mexico. Western medicine "penetration" followed prior efforts; see Ana María Kapeluz-Poppi, "Rural Health and State Construction in Post-Revolutionary Mexico: The Nicolaita Project for Rural Medical Services," *The Americas* 58, no. 2 (2001): 261–83; Anne-Emanuelle Birn, "A Revolution in Rural Health? The Struggle over Local Health Units in Mexico, 1928–1940," *Journal of the History of Medicine and Allied Sciences* 53, no. 1 (1998): 43–76; and Anne-Emanuelle Birn, "Wa(i)ves of Influence: Rockefeller Public Health in Mexico, 1920–50," *Studies in the History and Philosophy of Biological and Biomedical Sciences* 31, no. 3 (2000): 381–95.

32. An example of a less antagonistic perspective on indigenous medicine appeared in the most important periodical publication of CNEP. A field officer who worked in San Cristobal de las Casas, located in the center of the state of Chiapas, wrote an article that attempted to find a link between indigenous beliefs and the antimalaria campaign, revealing an appreciation of native healing: "Very often health workers criticize the Indians because their practices seem strange and unreasonable. However, when analyzed, these apparently strange beliefs are based on logic, and are part of a systematic, albeit different, way of seeing the world. [It is necessary] to be more tolerant and even to make some concessions to the traditional ways of healing malaria based on beverages, prayers and *temazcal* [therapeutic steambaths] . . . so campaign services will be accepted. These concessions are made, of course, trying not to hurt the prestige and effectiveness of our own prescriptions." "Medicina y Cultura," *El Chamula,* August 1961, fondo SSA, sección Subsecretaría de Salubridad y Asistencia, caja 84, expediente 3, AHSS.

33. Elsie Clews Parsons, "Curanderos in Oaxaca, Mexico," *Scientific Monthly* 32, no. 1 (1931): 60–68.

34. C. Sergio Escobar, "La erradicación del paludismo: Producto del esfuerzo conjunto nacional," *Salud Pública de México* 5 (1963): 727–31; the citation here is on 729.

35. This information appears in a pamphlet in fondo SSA, sección Secretaría Particular, caja 55, expediente 1, AHSS.

36. José Alvarez Amézqita (secretario de salubridad y asistencia, presidente del Consejo Directivo del CNEP), "Programa de erradicación del paludismo en México: Informe de actividades, 1958, VII Reunión de Directores de los Servicios Nacionales de Erradicación el Paludismo en México, Centro América y Panamá, celebrada en Panamá 13–17 Abril 1969," fondo SSA, sección CNEP, serie Dirección, caja 44, expediente 7, AHSS.

37. Juan Valdez, "El trabajo educativo todo lo vence" [Misión Cultural No. 29, Poblado de Mochitlán, Costas de Guerrero], *Boletín de Información para el personal de la Zona IX Sur,* Chipalcingo, Guerrero, November 1966, 5, fondo SSA, sección CNEP, serie Zona IX, caja 1, expediente 2, AHSS.

38. Carlos Ponce Escobar, "Solamente esfuerzo y voluntad," *Boletín del Personal del CNEP Zona II* Febrero 1960 [no number, no year], 3, fondo SSA, sección CNEP, serie Zona I, caja 1, expediente 3, AHSS.

39. The term "medical anthropology" was not widely used in American universities until 1962. Transcript of "George M. Foster: An Anthropologist in the Twentieth Century—Theory and Practice at UC Berkeley, the Smithsonian in Mexico and with the World Health Organization," interviews conducted by Susanne Riess in 1998 and 1999, Regional Oral History Office, BAN MSS 2001/116, Bancroft Library, University of California, Berkeley. A Society for Applied Anthropology was established in the early 1940s.

40. George M. Foster, *Applied Anthropology* (Boston: Little, Brown, 1969).

41. An American anthropologist who preceded Foster was Robert Redfield; see Redfield, *A Village That Chose Progress: Chan Kom Revisited* (Chicago: University of Chicago Press, 1950). Also see Gonzalo Aguirre Beltrán, *Programas de Salud en la Situación Intercultural* (Mexico City: Instituto Indigenista Interamericano, 1955).

42. George M. Foster, "Relationship between Theoretical and Applied Anthropology: A Public Health Program Analysis," *Human Organization* 11, no. 3 (1952): 5–16.

43. George M. Foster, "The Institute of Social Anthropology of the Smithsonian Institution, 1943–1952," *Anuario Indigenista* 27 (1967): 173–92.

44. George M. Foster, "Use of Anthropological Methods and Data in Planning and Operation," *Public Health Reports* 69, no. 9 (1953): 841–57; the citation here is on 342.

45. George M. Foster, "Bureaucratic Aspects of International Health Agencies," *Social Science and Medicine* 25 (1987): 1039–48.

46. Transcript of "George M. Foster: An Anthropologist in the Twentieth Century."

47. On Kelly, see Yólotl González, ed., *Homenaje a Isabel Kelly* (Mexico City: Instituto Nacional de Antropología e Historia, 1989); and "Isabel Kelly (1906–1982)," http://morgan.iia.unam.mx/usr/Actualidades/11/texto11/necrologia.html; Isabel Kelly, "El adiestramiento de parteras en México desde el punto de vista antropológico," *América Indígena* 15, no. 2 (1955): 109–17; and Isabel Kelly, *Folk Practices in North Mexico, Birth Customs, Folklore, Medicine and Spiritualism in the Laguna Zone* (Austin: University of Texas Press, 1965). A small collection of papers is kept at the Bancroft Library, University of California, Berkeley. Her first letter sent from Mexico is dated April 27, 1948, folder "Isabel Kelly, 1948–56," box 81, collection CU-23, Berkeley Department of Anthropology, Bancroft Library, University of California, Berkeley (hereafter Kelly Papers, BDA, BL).

48. "Isabel Kelly to Mary Anne Whipple, 16 May 1948," folder "Isabel Kelly, 1948–56," Kelly Papers, BDA, BL.

49. Ibid.

50. Ibid.

51. "Isabel Kelly to O. Lundberg, Controller Regents of the University of California, 18 January 1951," folder "Isabel Kelly, 1948–56," Kelly Papers, BDA, BL.

52. "Isabel Kelly to C. Crittenden [Secretary of Berkeley's Department of Anthropology], 19 February 1951," folder "Isabel Kelly, 1948–56," Kelly Papers, BDA, BL.

53. "Isabel Kelly to T. D. McCown 23 October 1951," folder "Isabel Kelly, 1948–56," Kelly Papers, BDA, BL.

54. "T. D. McCown to Robert G. Sproul, 17 October 1951," folder "Isabel Kelly, 1948–56," Kelly Papers, BDA, BL.

55. Isabel Kelly, "Preliminary Report on the Laguna Housing Project, Ejido El

Cuije, near Torreón, Cohauila," Institute of Inter-American Affairs, Mexico City, 1953. Kelly and García Manzanedo, "Santiago Tuxtla, Veracruz: Cultura y salud," Institute of Inter-American Affairs, Mexico City, 1956.

56. "Reglamento de Exámenes y Títulos Profesionales," *Periódico Oficial Organo Constitucional del Estado Libre y Soberano de Oaxaca,* May 13, 1944, 182–85.

57. See Cynthia Hewitt de Alcántara, *Anthropological Perspectives on Rural Mexico* (London: Routledge & Kegan Paul, 1984).

58. Héctor García Manzanedo and Isabel Kelly, "Comentarios al proyecto de Campaña para la Erradicación del Paludismo en México, 1955," fondo SSA, sección Subsecretaría de Salubridad y Asistencia, caja 49, expediente 6, AHSS. A copy of the report is kept at the NLM.

59. The national malaria mortality rate per year (for the period 1949–53) was 89.9 per 100,000 inhabitants; in Oaxaca, it was 449.2. Manuel E. Pesquiera, "Programa de erradicación del paludismo en México," *Boletín de la Oficina Sanitaria Panamericana* 42, no. 6 (1957): 537–47; the citation here is on 541.

60. "Informes e investigaciones," fondo SSA, sección Subsecretaría de Salubridad y Asistencia, caja 49, expediente 6, AHSS.

61. See Miguel León Portilla, "Panorama de la Población Indígena de México," *América Indígena* 19 (1959): 43–68; the citation here is on 45.

62. See Portilla, "Panorama de la población indígena"; and Miguel León Portilla, "México," *Indianist Yearbook* (Mexico City) 22 (1962): 65–82. This journal was published a Spanish and English edition by the Inter-American Indian Institute, based in Mexico City.

63. Emilio J. Pampama, *A Textbook of Malaria Eradication* (London: Oxford University Press, 1963), 365.

64. The malaria mortality rate for Chiapas was 308.3 per 100,000 inhabitants. Pesquiera, "Programa de erradicación," 541.

65. García Manzanedo and Kelly, "Comentarios al proyecto de Campaña."

66. See Jean P. Egbert, "Experiences in Mexico," *Nursing Outlook* (1964): 38–42. Previous efforts to articulate medical services in rural areas could be traced to the 1940s.

67. See Hernán García, Antonio Sierra, and Gilberto Balám, *Wind in the Blood: Maya Healing and Chinese Medicine* (Berkeley, Calif.: North Atlantic Books, 1999).

68. According to the *Diccionario enciclopédico de la medicina tradicional mexicana* (Mexico: Instituto Nacional Indigenista, 1994), published a few years ago, there are around nine types of fever in rural Mexico (fiebre blanca, fiebre de leche, fiebre de lombrices, fiebre de parto, fiebre escamosa, fiebre intestinal, fiebre pasada, fiebre roja, fiebre de la casa), 426–27.

69. Julio de la Fuente, "Creencias indígenas sobre la onchocercosis, el paludismo y otras enfermedades," *América Indígena* (México) 1, no. 1 (1941): 43–46; Claudia Madsen, *A Study in Mexican Folk Medicine* (New Orleáns: Middle American Research Institute, Tulane University, 1965), 124; Murray Morgan, *Doctors to the World* (New York: Viking Press, 1958), 21.

70. Fuente, "Creencias indígenas," 46; and *Oaxaca, 1ª Convención Regional Para la Campaña Nacional contra el Paludismo 21–27 Marzo 1938* (Oaxaca: N.p., 1938), 13, Fundación Cultural Bustamante Vasconcelos, Oaxaca.

71. "Antonio J Bermúdez [director general, Petróleos Mexicanos], 18 July 1956 to Ignacio Morones Prieto," fondo SSA, sección CNEP, serie Dirección, caja 2, expediente 1, AHSS.

72. As late as 1968, two articles in the *Bulletin* for Guerrero mention that fear: "Importancia de muestras de sangre" and "El Temor y la salud," *Costas de Guerrero, Boletín para el personal de la Zona IX Sur CNEP Chipalcingo, Guerrero* 1968 [no month], fondo SSA, serie CNEP, sección Zona IX, caja 1, expediente 2, AHSS, 2, 6; also see "Humberto Romero Álvarez, director general de enseñanza y obras públicas, to Noe Camacho Camacho [jefe de la Zona IV de CNEP, Tuxtla Gutiérrez, Chiapas], 24 January 1962," fondo SSA, sección CNEP, serie Dirección, expediente 1, AHSS. A similar conception of blood as intrinsic and nonregenerative existed in Guatemala; see Bruce Barret, "Identity, Ideology and Inequality, Methodologies in Medical Anthropology, Guatemala 1950–1955," *Social Science and Medicine* 44, no. 5 (1997): 579–87.

73. On the history of blood, see Douglas Star, *Blood and Epic History of Medicine and Commerce* (New York: Knopf, 1998); and John M. Ingham, "Human Sacrifices at Tenochitlan," *Comparative Studies in Society and History* 16 (1984): 379–400.

74. See "Sangre," in *Diccionario enciclopédico de la medicina tradicional mexicana,* 735–38; the citation here is on 737.

75. *El Señor José E Larumbe, descubridor de la causa eficiente de la ceguera onchocercosica: la microfilaria de los tejidos oculares,* (México: N.p., 1960), 8, biblioteca, Archivo General del Estado de Oaxaca, Oaxaca (hereafter AGEO).

76. See George M. Foster, "Medical Anthropology and International Health Planning," *Medical Anthropology Newsletter* 7, no. 3 (1976): 12–18 (the citation here is on 14); and Richard Adams, "A Nutritional Research Program in Guatemala," in *Health, Culture and Community,* ed. B. D. Paul (New York: Russell Sage Foundation, 1955), 435–58.

77. See Foster, "Use of Anthropological Methods."

78. "Editorial, A Vaccine against Malaria," *Boletín Indigenista* 14, no. 4 (1954): 231.

79. René Vargas Lozano, "Dirección de servicios médicos rurales cooperativos," *Salud Pública de México* 6, no. 6 (1964): 967–78; and Héctor Hernández Llamas, ed., *La Atención Médica Rural en México, 1930–1980* (Mexico City: Instituto Mexicano del Seguro Social, 1984). On medical pluralism, see Horacio Fabrega Jr. and Daniel Silver, *Illness and Shamanistic Curing in Zinacatan* (Stanford, Calif.: Stanford University Press, 1973); and Michael B. Whiteford, "Homeopathic Medicine in the City of Oaxaca, Mexico: Patients' Perspectives and Observations," *Medical Anthropology Quarterly* 13, no. 1 (1999): 69–78.

80. Ricardo Martell Ramírez, "La cultura trique," *Boletín de la Sociedad Oaxaqueña de Salud Pública* 7, no. 1 (1972): 11–18; the citation here is on 12. This paper was presented to a meeting of the Oaxaca Public Health Society.

81. "Partida de la Doctora Isabel Kelly," *Boletín Indigenista* (Mexico City) 17, no. 4 (1957): 294.

82. In a document kept at WHO and signed by C. J. Foll titled "Mexican Malaria Program (CNEP) 16 November–15 December 1962," series Malaria Research Collection, folder México 1961–63, box WHO 7.0079, WHO Archives.

83. World Health Organization, *World Directory of Medical Schools* (Geneva: World Health Organization, 1957), 178.

84. In Spanish: *Servicio social del pasante de medicina.* Inter-American Affairs Office, *Mexico: Next Door Neighbor* (Washington, D.C.: U.S. Government Printing Office, 1943), 17.

85. World Health Organization, *World Directory of Medical Schools* (Geneva: World Health Organization, 1957), 178.

86. Luís Cañedo, "Rural Health Care in Mexico," *Science* 185, no. 4157 (September 27, 1967): 1131–37.

87. José L. Villalobos Revilla, *Informe médico de la población de Jalpa, Zacatecas, Indice de Ross: Tratamiento de la ulcera gastroduodenal por la uroenterona (Kutrol)— tesis para sustentar examen profesional de médico cirujano y partero* (Mexico City: Universidad Nacional Autonoma de México, 1954), 10. It was published as a pamphlet and is kept at the Biblioteca Nacional de México.

88. Villalobos's comments appear in "Síntesis del trabajo realizado durante los años 1956–1959 en la región de Juchipila, Estado de Zacatecas, relacionado con la campaña de erradicación del paludismo," Fondo SSA, sección Secretaría Particular, caja 51, expediente 1, AHSS.

89. Luís Vargas, "Aspectos Socioeconómicos de las zonas rurales mexicanas en relación con la erradicación del paludismo," *Revista del Instituto de Salubridad y Enfermedades Tropicales* 18, nos. 3–4 (1958): 145–86; the citation here is on 160.

90. Secretaría de Industria y Comercio, "Viviendas urbanas y rurales en el país por entidades federativas, según el número de cuartos, 1960," in *Anuario Estadístico Compendiado de los Estados Unidos Mexicanos, 1968* (Mexico City: Dirección General de Estadística, 1969), 58.

91. Villalobos, "Síntesis del trabajo realizado," AHSS.

92. This is mentioned in "Gregorio Espinosa Cruz [malariólogo Espinosa Cruz] a Ricardo Zebadua Ochoa [jefe de la Zona IX] 27 June 1962," fondo SSA, sección CNEP, serie Zona IX, caja 2, expediente 1, AHSS.

93. M. A. Bravo-Becherelle and Luís Mazotti, "Distribución Geográfica de la Mortalidad por picadura de alacrán en México," *Revista del Instituto de Salubridad y Enfermedades Tropicales* 21, nos. 3–4 (1961): 129–40. See also M. A. Mazzotti and M. A. Bravo-Becherelle, "Escorpionismo en la República Mexicana," *Revista del Instituto de Salubridad y Enfermedades Tropicales* 21, nos. 1 and 2 (1961): 3–19.

94. Luís Vargas, "El tamaño de la localidad como factor epidemiológico en malariología," *Revista del Instituto de Salubridad y Enfermedades Tropicales* 20, no. 1 (1960): 193–211; the citation here is on 207. Luís Vargas and Arturo Alamaraz Ugalde, "La erradicación del paludismo en México durante el segundo año de cobertura integral," *Revista del Instituto de Salubridad y Enfermedades Tropicales* 20, no. 3 (1960): 193–221; the citation here is on 205. Today Dieldrin's use has ceased all over the world; see U.S. Environmental Protection Agency, *Health Effects Support Document for Aldrin/Dieldrin* (Washington, D.C.: U.S. Environmental Protection Agency, 2003).

95. According to a poem signed by "El Rociador," the sprayers were called "*matagatos*"; in Juan Angel Rabanales, Tuxtla Gutiérrez, September 1966, 5. Its new name is *Publicación Mensual Zona IV, CNEP*, September 1966. Tuxtla Gutiérrez, Chiapas, fondo SSA, sección CNEP, serie Zona IV, caja 1, expediente 3, AHSS. See also "Definiciones: DDT, una agüita que según las gentes que desconocen nuestros trabajos es muy práctica para acabar con los gatos y pollos de los vecinos," in *El Humaya, órgano de información para el personal del CNEP Zona VIII Año 4, Culiacán,* February 1960, 5, fondo SSA, sección CNEP, serie Zona I, caja 1, expediente 3, AHSS.

96. "May 29–31, 1955 meeting with Gabaldón," RFA, record group 12.1, Russell Diaries, RAC.

97. "F. J. Ramos Calcaneo to Presidente de la República [he worked at the Compañía Nacional de Seguros Sobre la Vida, Huixtla, Chiapas]." The letter is kept in "Oficina de

Quejas, Presidencia de la República, 20 Abril 1960," Archivo López Mateos, vol. 388, expediente 423/11, AGN.

98. "Celia Orozco y Laura Díaz de Orozco to Presidente de la República, 18 June 1960," Archivo López Mateos, vol. 388, expediente 423/9, AGN.

99. "Fernando Infazón Villalobos to Villalobos, 4 April 1960," Archivo Lopez Mateos, vol. 387, expediente 423/1, AGN. José Eutasio Almazan Nieto, the local authority of Pueblo Verde, San Luís Potosí, sent a telegram to Mexico's president March 1, 1957, Archivo Ruíz Cortinez, vol. 423, expediente 424/23, AGN.

100. "En Tecpan, los mosquitos se rien del DDT" [Tecpan de Galeana, Guerrero, *Excelsior,* February 12, 1957], newspaper clipping, fondo SSA, serie CNEP, serie Zona IX, caja 1, expediente 3, AHSS. According to the article, the same null effect was occurring in other localities of the state.

101. Villalobos, "Resultado de la Campaña Nacional para la Erradicación del Paludismo (CNEP) en la República Mexicana: Estudio y Conclusiones, 1957–1958," *El Heraldo de Aguascalientes,* October 4, 1958, fondo SSA, sección Secretaría Particular, caja 51, expediente 1, AHSS.

102. "Letter of Antonio Obispo de Zacatecas to José Villalobos, 19 November 1959." The note at the end of the letter written by Villalobos states: "México. D.F. 14 March 1960," fondo SSA, sección Secretaría Particular, caja 51, expediente 1, AHSS. However, this second letter is not kept in the archives.

103. See David Arnold, *Colonizing the Body: State, Medicine and Epidemic Disease in Nineteenth-Century India* (Berkeley: University of California Press, 1993); and L. White, *Speaking with Vampires: Rumor and History in Colonial Africa* (Berkeley: University of California Press, 2000).

104. Villalobos's references cite without major details: *Bulletin of the New York Academy of Medicine* 33 (1957): 397; *American Journal of Clinical Pathology* 27 (1957): 6; *Selecciones de Reader's Digest* (April 1959), 82 (September 1959): 139. The first article was probably Mark H. Adams, "The Nature of Viruses," 397–404; the second article may have been Harland Manchester, "The New Age of Atomic Crops," *Reader's Digest,* November 1959, 135–40. With regard to *Reader's Digest* as an imperialistic cultural tool, see Ariel Dorfman, "Salvación y sabiduría del hombre común: La teología de *Selecciones del Reader's Digest,"* in *Imperialismo y medios masivos de comunicación* [no author] (Lima: N.p., 1973), vol. 2, 5–38.

105. Rachel Carson, *Silent Spring* (Boston: Houghton Mifflin, 1962); Lewis Herber, *Our Synthetic Environment* (New York: Alfred A. Knopf, 1962). Latin American and Mexican critics of DDT and pesticides appeared some years later, around the early 1970s, see A. E. Olszyna-Marzys, "Residuos de plaguicidas clorados en la leche humana en Guatemala," *Boletín de la Oficina Sanitaria Panamericana* 74, no. 2 (1973): 93–107; Saúl Franco Agudelo, "El saldo rojo de los insecticidas en América Latina, a propósito de su utilización contra la malaria," *Revista Centroamericana de Ciencias de la Salud* 7, no. 20 (1981): 35–53; and Iván Restrepo, *Naturaleza muerta, los plaguicidas en México* (Mexico City: Oceano, 1988).

106. "José Villalobos Telegram to Frank J. Von Zuben, México D.F, 6 April 1960," fondo SSA, sección Secretaría Particular, caja 33, expediente 4, AHSS.

107. "Guillermo Suárez Torres to José Jiménez Cantú [Secretaría de Salubridad y Asistencia], 23 Jan. 1971 [Asunto: Relacionado con el documento del Dr. José Villalobos Revilla, México]," fondo SSA, sección Secretaría Particular, caja 51, expediente 1, AHSS.

108. In 1974, Villalobos attempted to reach the Health Secretariat and sent work complaining about contamination produced by insecticides. He reported a session of medical doctors that discussed his ideas in a new workplace, the General Hospital in Mexico City. José Villalobos, "Síndrome por organoclorados y su tratamiento (informe preliminar), 1974" [he signs as Médico Externo del Hospital General], fondo SSA, sección Subsecretaría de Salubridad y Asistencia, caja 127, expediente 1, AHSS.

109. Pesqueira, "Programa de erradicación," 541.

110. "Pablo Díaz Hernández to Juan Canales Cirilo, 23 August 1959," fondo SSA, sección CNEP, serie Zona VIII, caja 1, expediente 6, AHSS; and "Carta de Marcial Matías Velasco, Jefe de Brigada Sector 6, Oaxaca," August 20, 1959, fondo SSA, sección CNEP, serie Zona VIII, caja 1, expediente 6, AHSS. "Ya vienen estos desgraciados chincheros'; 'váyanse mucho a la chingada con sus porquerías, mi casa no dejo que se rocíe'; 'mi casa no la rocían, primero la quemo que dejar que me echan mas chinches."

111. Pablo González Casanova, *La democracia en México* (Mexico City: Era, 1967), 42.

112. "Pablo Díaz Hernández to Juan Canales Cirilo, 23 August 1959," fondo SSA, sección CNEP, serie Zona VIII, caja 1, expediente 6, AHSS. "Carta de Marcial Matías Velasco," August 20, 1959, fondo SSA, sección CNEP, serie Zona VIII, caja 1, expediente 6, AHSS. "Lo que ustedes quieren es únicamente chingar al pueblo, como siempre lo ha hecho el gobierno."

113. "Acta de la Reunión Acata Quiotepec, 22 Agosto 1959," fondo SSA, sección CNEP, serie Zona VIII, caja 1, expediente 6, AHSS. "Pablo Díaz Hernández to Juan Canales Cirilo [jefe de la Zona V CNEP], 23 Agosto de 1959," fondo SSA, sección CNEP, serie Zona VIII, caja 1, expediente 6, AHSS.

114. "Aviso al Público, por Acuerdo Presidencial su casa será rociada con insecticidas," The leaflet was attached to a letter from Filemón Ramírez [Zona IX] to CNEP, October 5, 1966, requesting over 85,000 copies of this material; fondo SSA, serie CNEP, caja 2, expediente 6, AHSS.

115. "Filemón Ramírez Huanosto to CNEP, 28 November 1972," fondo SSA, serie CNEP, sección Zona IX, caja 2, expediente 6, AHSS.

116. Ernesto Guzmán Clark, "Participación de las Autoridades Municipales en la solución de problemas de salud pública," *Boletín de la Sociedad Oaxaqueña de Salud Pública* 6, no. 3 (1971): 36–40.

117. "Brigada antipalúdica atacada en Oaxaca, 18 March 1957," no page, fondo SSA, sección CNEP, serie Zona V, caja. 1, expediente 2, AHSS.

118. "Editorial," *Boletín CNEP, Zona IX,* January 1961, 2, fondo SSA, serie CNEP, sección Zona IX, caja 1, expediente 2, AHSS.

119. These are mentioned in "Informe de la situación sanitaria que prevalece en la actualidad y los recursos que se cuentan en el Estado de Oaxaca, 1978," 46, fondo Poder Ejecutivo del Estado, sección Dirección General de Gobernación, serie Secretaría General del Despacho, expediente 281, AGEO.

120. "Zona V de la CNEP, Plan de Acción para la resolución del problema originado en la localidad de Mazatlán Villa de Flores, Oaxaca, con motivo de la agresión sufrida por el Jefe de Brigada de Rociado Bernardino Rodríguez, 23 February 1963," fondo SSA, sección CNEP, serie Zona VIII, caja 1, expediente 6, AHSS. A similar complaint is in "Presidente Municipal Alfonso Mota López 2 October 1959 to CNEP, Zona V," fondo SSA, sección CNEP, serie Zona VIII, caja 1, expediente 6, AHSS. "Testimonio de Manuel Cruz Ton," no date, in Pliego, *Política sanitaria dirigida,* 53; "En Tecpan,

los Mosquitos se Ríen del DDT," *El Excelsior,* February 12, 1957, newspaper clipping, fondo SSA, sección CNEP, serie Zona IX, caja 1, expediente 3, AHSS. "El rociado de insecticidas que la brigada antipalúdica hizo resulto poco menos que nulo, por la mala calidad del producto, que no ha tenido efecto en los mosquitos. . . . Lo mismo ha sucedido en las localidades de Tenexpa y Tetitlan."

121. Lini de Vries, *The People of the Mountains: Health Education among Indian Communities in Oaxaca, Mexico,* Cuaderno No 42 (Cuernavaca: Centro Intercultural de Documentación, 1969).

122. Pampama, *Textbook of Malaria Eradication,* 365.

123. "Márquez Escobedo to Antonio E. Izaguirre, 3 January 1959," fondo SSA, serie CNEP, sección Zona IV, caja 1, expediente 6, AHSS.

124. "¿Aumenta el Rociado los chinches?" *Boletín Zonal Mensual del CNEP Zona II No 8, Año 2,* February 1960, 2, fondo SSA, sección CNEP, serie Zona I, caja 1, expediente 3, AHSS. "Acta, San Juan de Coyula, Municipio de Cuicatlán, 10 January 1960," fondo SSA, sección CNEP, serie Zona VIII, caja 1, expediente 6, AHSS.

125. "Carlos Ruz Dávila [jefe de Zona II] to CNEP [no name], 22 March 1960," fondo SSA, sección CNEP, serie Zona II, caja 1, expediente 6, AHSS.

126. Paul R. Ehrlich, *The Population Bomb* (New York: Ballantine Books, 1971), 31.

127. Luís Vargas, "Anteproyecto para un programa de la CNEP de combate contra los chinches, 25 octubre 1962," fondo SSA, sección CNEP, serie Dirección, caja 8, expediente 1, AHSS; Vargas, "La interpretación epidemiológica del paludismo, con énfasis en campañas de erradicación," *Revista Venezolana de Sanidad y Asistencia Social* 28, no. 4 (1963): 339–509 (the citation here is on 341).

128. As early as 1958, WHO's biologist in the Division of Environmental Sanitation acknowledged that resistance to DDT and Dieldrin was a significant problem; see Anthony William A. Brown, *Insecticide Resistance in Arthropods* (Geneva: WHO, 1958).

129. A. Martínez-Palacios and J. De Zulueta, "Ethological Changes in *Anopheles Pseudopuntipennis* in Mexico after prolonged use of DDT," May 12, 1964, WHO/Mal/449, WHO Library, Geneva; Luís Vargas, "Las casas y la transmisión del paludismo," *Boletín Epidemiológico* (Mexico City), 20 (1956): 160–66.

130. R. W. Babione, "Special Technical Problems in Malaria Eradication in Latin America, 6 February 1964," World Health Organization, http://whqlibdoc.who.int/malaria/WHO_Mal_430.pdf.

131. See Douglas L. Murray, *Cultivating Crisis: The Human Cost of Pesticides in Latin America* (Austin: University of Texas Press, 1994), 18.

132. Murray, *Cultivating Crisis;* and David Bull, *Growing Problem: Pesticides and the Third World* (Oxford: Oxfam and Third World Publications, 1982).

133. The problem was addressed in a public health meeting of both countries that took place in May 1960. See "Report of Noé Camacho Camacho May 7, 1960 a Secretaría de Salubridad," fondo SSA, sección CNEP, serie Zona IV, caja 2, expediente 3, AHSS; and "Asociación Mexicano Guatemalteca de Salud Pública: Primera reunión anual, 13–14 enero 1961, Chiapas," fondo SSA, sección CNEP, serie Zona IV, caja 2, expediente 3, AHSS. On migration, see Servicios Coordinados de Salud Pública de Campeche, "Consideraciones sobre factores humanos para la erradicación del paludismo," *Salud Pública de México* 8, no. 3 (1966): 379–82; Mansell R. Prothero, "Malaria in Latin America: Environmental and Human Factors," *Bulletin of Latin American Research* 14, no. 3 (1995): 357–65; and Rafael Moreno Valle and Guillermo Suarez Torres,

"Evolución del paludismo en la frontera mexicano-guatemalteca en 1964 y Plan de Acción para 1965," *Salud Pública de México* 7, no. 1 (1963): 33–38.

134. David C. Halperin Frisch and Homero De León Montenegro, *México-Guatemala, Salud en la Frontera Guatemala-México* (San Cristóbal de las Casas: El Colegio de la Frontera Sur, 1996).

135. Lafe R. Edmunds (Malaria Eradication Branch, Pan-American Health Organization), "Observations on the Biology of *Anopheles Pseudopuntipennis Pseudopuntipennis* and *Theobald* and Its Relationship to the Transmission of Malaria in Mexico," 1966, unofficial draft, folder Mexico 1966, box WHO 7.0079, WHO Archives, 10.

136. J. De Zulueta and C. Garret-Jones, "An Investigation of the Persistence of *Malaria* Transmission in Mexico," *American Journal of Tropical Medicine and Higiene* 14, no. 1 (1965): 63–77; and Vargas, "El tamaño de la localidad como factor epidemiológico en malariologia."

137. "Enmienda no. 1 al Plan Tripartita de operaciones para un proyecto de erradicación de la malaria en México, 18 March 1959," fondo SSA, sección CNEP, serie Dirección, caja 1, expediente 10, AHSS.

138. Guillermo Suárez Torres, "Incremento de la lucha antipalúdica en el Estado de Oaxaca," *Boletín de la Sociedad Oaxaqueña de Salud Pública* 5, no. 1 (1970): 22.

139. This is stated by Ignacio Gómez Mendoza, director of epidemiology, CNEP, in "WHO/MAL/527.65 1965," folder 1965, box WHO 7.0079, WHO Archives.

140. "G. G. Gramiccia, Chief, ME/EA, Report on a Visit to America (8 August–2 September 1966)," folder Mexico 1966, box WHO 7.0079, WHO Archives. Also see Rafael Moreno Valle and Guillermo Suárez Torres, "La erradicación del paludismo en México, Informe de Actividades en 1964," *Salud Pública de México* 8, no. 1 (1966): 83–97.

141. "Tabla 2: Número de localidades clasificadas según su población: número de notificantes existentes y número de notificantes productivos, evaluación epidemiológica Enero 1957–Junio 1960," fondo SSA, sección CNEP, serie Dirección, caja 44, expediente 8, AHSS. "Editorial: El Informador" *Boletín CNEP Zona I, Mérida Yucatán,* February 1961, fondo SSA, sección CNEP, serie Zona I, caja 1, expediente 3, AHSS. The problem of insufficient facilities was mentioned before: "Horwitz to Robert L. Davee, 24 October 1960, Programme for Malaria Eradication in Mexico. Project Files," folder Mexico 200, box WHO10/4, WHO Archives.

142. "CNEP para autoridades de Pochutla, Oaxaca, 1962," and "Circular de Vicario General Guillermo Álvarez Varela a señores párrocos de Pochutla, 31 Octubre 1960," series Malaria Research Collection, folder México 1961–63, box WHO 7.0079, WHO Archives. Morgan, *Doctors to the World,* 16. M. Cahn and E. Levy, "The Tolerance to Large Weekly Doses of Primaquine and Amodiaquine In Primaquine-Sensitive and Non-Sensitive Subjects," *American Journal of Tropical Medicine and Hygiene* 11 (1962): 605–6.

143. In Martín Baranda López, "Pochutla, Oaxaca 18 Octubre 1962," Malaria Research Collection, folder México 1961–63, box WHO 7.0079, WHO Archives.

144. The draft of a 1966 report by an officer in charge of the PASB malaria program explained some of these factors: Lafe R. Edmunds, "Observations on the Biology of *Anopheles Pseudopuntipennis Pseudopuntipennis* and Its Relationship to the Transmission of Malaria in Mexico," 1966, unofficial draft, 10, Malaria Research Collection, folder Mexico 1966, box WHO 7.0079, WHO Archives.

145. For a discussion, see "Rural Health Services in Latin America," *WHO Chronicle* 22, no. 6 (1968): 249–53.

146. See Luís Vargas, "Notas sobre la transfusión sanguínea y el paludismo inducido en México," *Salud Pública de México* 14 (1972): 353–63; and L. J. Bruce-Chwatt, "Transfusion Malaria," *Bulletin of the World Health Organization* 50 (1970): 337–46.

147. Rolando Medina Aguilar, *El Banco de Sangre, Organización, Funcionamiento, Legislación* (Mexico City: Prensa Médica Mexicana, 1963), 125.

148. "Enmienda No. II al Plan Tripartito de Operaciones para un proyecto de erradicación del paludismo de México, 7 February 1963," signed by Mexican Government, UNICEF, and PAHO, fondo SSA, serie CNEP, serie Dirección, caja 1, expediente 10, AHSS.

149. "Informe preparado por el secretario de salubridad y asistencia, Febrero 1963," fondo SSA, sección Subsecretaría de Salubridad y Asistencia, caja 35, expediente 2, AHSS.

150. "Horowitz to Candau, 4 August 1964, and Horwitz to Candau, 4 August 1964," in "Programme for Malaria Eradication in Mexico: Project Files," folder Mexico 200, box WHO 10/4, WHO Archives.

151. "Malaria Eradication in 1966," *WHO Chronicle* 21, no. 9 (1967): 373–88; the citation here is on 375.

152. Glen Williams, "WHO: The Days of the Mass Campaigns," *World Health Forum* 9 (1988): 7–23; the citation here is on 16.

153. The new policy appears in *Informe de los Seminarios sobre la Misión de los Servicios Generales de Salud en la Erradicación de la Malaria, Pocos de Caldas, Brasil, 26 de junio-4 de julio de 1964/Cuernavaca, México 4-13 Marzo, 1965,* Pan-American Health Organization (Washington, D.C.: Pan-American Health Organization, 1965); and World Health Organization, *Twenty-Second World Health Assembly, Boston, Massachusetts, 8–25 July 1969, Part II, Plenary Meetings, Committees, Summary Records and Reports* (Geneva: World Health Organization, 1969).

154. "WHA22.39 Re-examination of the Global Strategy of Malaria Eradication," Twenty-Second World Health Assembly, Boston, July 24; http://policy.who.int/cgi-bin/om_isapi.dll?infobase=WHA&softpage=Browse_Frame_Pg42.

155. "Filemón Ramírez Huanosto [jfe Zona IX] to CNEP, 26 October 1966," fondo SSA, sección CNEP, serie Zona IX, expediente 7, AHSS.

156. Kenneth Newell, "Selective Primary Health Care: The Counter Revolution," *Social Science and Medicine* 26, no. 9 (1988): 903–6; the citation here is on 903.

157. "Malaria Campaign to Be Reappraised," *New York Times,* March 16, 1969.

158. "Interventions of Dr. Vargas Mendez from Costa Rica, Dr. N'Diaye from Senegal and Dr. Ferreira from Brazil, In *Twenty-Second World Health Assembly,* ed. World Health Organization, 239, 233.

159. "Intervention of Dr. Vargas Mendez from Costa Rica and Dr. N'Diaye from Senegal," in *Twenty-Second World Health Assembly,* ed. World Health Organization, 239, 243.

160. See Williams, "WHO," 17.

161. Guillermo Suárez Torres, "El Programa de Erradicación del paludismo, plan de seis años," *Salud Pública de México* 12, no. 6 (1970): 751–73.

162. J. W. Tuthill, "Malathion Poisoning," *New England Journal of Medicine* 258, no. 20 (1958):1018–19.

163. Thomas R. Dunlap, *DDT, Scientists, Citizens, and Public Policy* (Princeton, N.J.: Princeton University Press, 1981), *Pesticides in South America and México* (New York: Frost and Sullivan, 1981); and Jesús Gracia Fadrique, ed., *Estado y fertilizantes, 1760–1985* (Mexico City: Universidad Nacional Autonoma de México / FCE, 1988) (on DDT

environmental problems in México, see 613–42). L. López Carrillo, L. Torres-Arreola, L. Torres-Sánchez, F. Espinosa-Torres, C. Jiménez, Mariano Cebrian, S. Waliszeski, and O. Saldate, "Is DDT Use a Public Health Problem in Mexico?" *Environmental Health Perspectives* 104, no. 6 (1996): 584–87.

164. "Filemón Ramírez Huanosto [Zona IX] to CNEP, 17 April 1970," fondo SSA, sección CNEP, serie Zona IX, caja 2, expediente 6, AHSS.

165. "Plan de Seis Años para la Erradicación del Paludismo Residual en México," Mexico City, January 1965, fondo SSA, sección CNEP, serie Dirección, caja 8, expediente 1, AHSS. "Guillermo Suárez Torres to Héctor Acuña Monteverde, 26 April 1973," fondo SSA, sección CNEP, serie Dirección, caja 1, expediente 10, AHSS.

166. Maggie Black, *The Children and the Nations: The Story of UNICEF* (Sydney: UNICEF, 1986), 129, 131. In 1969, UNICEF estimated that his worldwide eradication investment, since 1955, came to $100 million. "Intervention of Dr. Bowles from UNICEF," in *Twenty-Second World Health Assembly*, ed. World Health Organization, 232. See also Socrates Litsios, "Criticism of WHO's Revised Malaria Eradication Strategy," *Parassitologia* 42 (2000): 167–72.

167. Joseph M. Jones, *Does Overpopulation Mean Poverty? The Facts about Population Growth and Economic Development*, foreword by Eugene R. Black, president of the World Bank (Washington, D.C.: Center for International Economic Growth, 1962), 7. See also R. Barlow, "The Economic Effects of Malaria Eradication," *American Economic Review* 57, no. 2 (1968): 130–48; and R. Symonds and M. Carder, *The United Nations and the Population Question, 1945–1970* (New York: McGraw-Hill, 1973).

168. Jones, *Does Overpopulation Mean Poverty?* includes comparisons of annual population growth by region; see 17 and the table on 32.

169. An indication that overpopulation was a growing concern in the United States is a 1962 newspaper article that underscored population growth in Mexico: James Reston, "Mexico City: Love Is the Problem, Birth Rate More Vexing than Death Rate South of the Border," *New York Times,* December 10, 1962, 8.

170. Ehrlich, *Population Bomb,* 31.

171. L. E. Rozeboom, "DDT: The Life Saving Poison," *Johns Hopkins Magazine* 22 (Spring 1971): 29–32. Cited by Mohyeddin A. Farid, "The Malaria Programme: Euphoria to Anarchy," *World Health Forum* 1 (1980): 8–33 (the citation here is on 16).

172. Donald T. Critchlow, "Birth Control, Population Control and Family Planning: an Overview," *Journal of Health Policy* 7, no. 1 (1995): 1–21; and John Sharpless, "World Population Growth, Family Planning and American Foreign Policy," *Journal of Policy History* 7, no. 1 (1995): 72–102.

173. Center for Policy Studies of the Population Council, "Population Brief: Latin America," *Population and Development Review* 6, no. 1 (1980): 126–52; the citation here is on 127, 142.

174. R. J. Alexander, "Nature and Progress of Agrarian Reform in Latin America," *Journal of Economic History* 23, no. 4 (1963): 559–73; the citation here is on 567.

175. "Table 100: State Population, Urban and Rural, 1900–1980," in *United States–Mexico Border Statistics since 1900,* ed. David E. Lorey (Los Angeles: UCLA Latin American Center Publications, 1990), 8.

176. Frank Brandenburg, *The Making of Modern Mexico* (Englewood Cliffs, N.J.: Prentice-Hall, 1964), 236.

177. Richard Symonds and Michael Carder, *The United Nations and the Population Question, 1945–1970* (New York: McGraw-Hill, 1973).

178. Donald Pletsh, "Malaria Control and Economics," *Science,* 149, no. 3687 (August 27, 1965): 926.

179. *United Nations Fund for Population Activities: An Agenda for People—The UNFPA through Three Decades,* ed. Nafis Sadik (New York: New York University Press, 2002).

180. Arnoldo Gabaldón, "Influencia del Rociamiento Intradomiciliario con DDT sobre las tasas específicas de mortalidad general en Venezuela," *Boletín de la Oficina Sanitaria Panamericana* 40, no. 35: (1956): 93–106.

181. An example of a medical publication that sustains that perspective is Miguel García Cruz, "Los Problemas Demográfico de México," *Suplemento de Medicina* (1964): 9–14.

182. Carson, *Silent Spring.* See James Whorton, *Before Silent Spring: Pesticides and Public Health in Pre-DDT America* (Princeton, N.J.: Princeton University Press, 1974).

183. Tom J. Cade, Jeffrey L. Lincer, Clayton M. White, David G. Roseneau, and L. G. Swartz, "DDE Residues and Eggshell Changes in Alaskan Falcons and Hawks," *Science* 172, no. 3986 (1971): 955–57; W. Bowerman, J. Giesy, D. Best, and V. Kramer, "A Review of Factors Affecting Productivity of Bald Eagles in the Great Lakes Region: Implications for Recovery," *Environmental Health Perspectives* 103, supplement 4 (1995): 51–59; J. Grier, "Ban of DDT and Subsequent Recovery of Reproduction in Bald Eagles," *Science* 218, no. 4578 (1982): 1232–35.

184. "DDT Dilemma: Poor Countries Insist Pesticide Is Essential Despite Its Dangers," *Wall Street Journal,* February 14, 1970.

185. Alfred Friendly, "Wide Curb on DDT Opposed in FAO," *New York Times,* November 29, 1969.

186. "Interventions of Dr. Sambasivan, Director, Division of Malaria Eradication and Dr. N'Diaye from Senegal," in *Twenty-Second World Health Assembly,* ed. World Health Organization, 243, 245.

187. Philip Handler, "The Federal Government and the Scientific Community," *Science* 171, no. 3967 (1971): 144–51; the citation here is on 148.

188. United Nations Environment Program, *The United Nations Environment Program: A Brief Introduction* (Nairobi: United Nations Environment Program, 1975).

189. "Organización Panamericana de la Salud, Departamento de Erradicación de la Malaria para la reunión de los jefes de Zona; El Uso del DDT y su repercusión sobre el hombre y el ambiente, Julio 1970," fondo SSA, sección CNEP, serie Dirección, caja 8, expediente 4, AHSS. Donald R. Johnson, "Recent Developments in Mosquito-Borne Diseases: Malaria," *Mosquito News* 33, no. 3 (1973): 341–48; the citation here is on 345.

190. The phrase "circle of poison" was used by environmentalist after the publication of David Weir and Mark Schapiro, *Circle of Poison: Pesticides in a Hungry World* (San Francisco: Institute for Food and Development Policy, 1981). Angus Wright, *The Death of Ramón González: The Modern Agricultural Dilemma* (Austin: University of Texas Press, 1997), demonstrated the extension of the problem to Mexico.

191. Andres J. Yoder, "Lessons from Stockholm: Evaluating the Global Convention on Persistent Organic Pollutants," *Indiana Journal of Global Legal Studies* 10, no. 2 (2003): 113–56; the citation here is on 116.

192. According to an article, WHO recognized in the early 1980s 14,000 cases per year of fatal poisoning and some 750,000 cases of nonfatal consequences, produced by pesticides; see Angus Wright, "Rethinking the Circle of Poison: The Politics of Pesticide Poisoning among Mexican Farm Workers," *Latin American Perspectives* 13, no. 4 (1986): 26–59.

193. Rachel L. Carson, *Primavera silenciosa* (Barcelona: Luis de Caralt, 1964).

194. Humberto Romero Alvarez, "Contaminación ambiental y salud," in *La Evolución de la Medicina en México durante las últimas cuatro décadas,* ed. Ramon de la Fuente (Mexico City: El Colegio Nacional, 1984).

195. Another example of a low-tone opposition was Leonard J. Bruce-Chwatt, "Man against Malaria: Conquest or Defeat," *Transactions of the Royal Society of Tropical Medicine* 73, no. 6 (1979): 605–16.

196. E.g., see Arnoldo Gabaldón, "Global Malaria Eradication: Changes of Strategy and Future Outlook," *American Journal of Tropical Medicine and Higiene* 18, no. 5 (1969): 641–56; and Gabaldón, "Problemas actuales del control y erradicación de la malaria en América Latina," *Boletín de la Dirección de Malariología y Saneamiento Ambiental* 28, nos. 1–2 (1988): 1–12. Another distinguished malariologist in Latin America, G. Giglioli, died in 1975.

197. Leonard J. Bruce-Chwatt, "Malaria Eradication at the Crossroads," *Bulletin of the New York Academy of Medicine* 45, no. 10 (1969): 999–1012; the citation here is on 1009.

198. Farid, "Malaria Programme," 18.

199. USAID supported antimalaria activities in Haiti. According to a study done by the U.S. General Accounting Office in 1980, the total amount donated by USAID to Latin American malaria projects between 1950 and 1980 was $96,632 million; see Alexandrina Schuler, *Malaria: Meeting the Global Challenge* (Boston: Oelgeschlager, Gunn & Hain, 1985), 18–19.

200. J. Mayone Stycos, "Population Control in Latin America," *World Politics* 20, no. 1 (1967): 66–82; the citation here is on 78–79.

201. "Epitaph for Global Malaria Eradication?" *The Lancet,* July 5, 1975, 15–16; William C. Reeves, "Can the War to Contain Infectious Disease Be Lost?" *American Journal of Tropical Medicine and Hygiene* 21, no. 3 (1972): 251–59.

202. Cited by L. J. Bruce-Chwatt, "Need for New Weapons," *World Health Forum* 1 (1980): 23–24; the citation is on 24.

203. Newell, "Selective Primary Health Care," 903.

204. "Guillermo Suárez Torres to Carmen Gómez Sigler, 21 July 1965," fondo SSA, sección CNEP, caja 1, expediente 4, AHSS.

205. Lázaro Vargas, "Importancia de la Coordinación en Salud Pública y sus Perspectivas," *Boletín de la Sociedad Oaxaqueña de Salud Pública* 5, no. 2 (1970): 28–31, 29, 31.

206. "Travel Report Summary by Jacques Hamon, Visit to the III Meeting of the Directors of the National Services for the Eradication of Malaria in the Americas, 2 April 1979," folder Mexico 1979–93, box WHO 7.0081, WHO Archives; and Guillermo Suárez Torres, "Resumen de la Revisión de la Estrategia para la Campaña para la Erradicar el Paludismo en México, Mayo 1972," folder Mexico 1972, box WHO 7.0080, WHO Archives.

207. Robert A. Packenham, *The Dependency Movement: Scholarship and Politics in Development Studies* (Cambridge, Mass.: Harvard Univ. Press, 1992).

208. Dean C. Tipps, "Modernization Theory and the Comparative Study of Societies: A Critical Perspective," *Comparative Studies in Society and History* 15, no. 2 (1973): 199–226.

209. Rodolfo Stavenhagen, *El campesinado y las estrategias del desarrollo rural* (Mexico City: Colegio de México, 1977).

210. See Guillermo Bonfil Batalla, *México Profundo: Una Civilización Negada* (Mexico City: Secretaría de Educación Pública, 1987); and María del Consuelo Ros Romero, *La imagen del Indio en el discurso del Instituto Nacional Indigenista* (Mexico City: Centro de Investigaciones y Estudios Superiores en Antropología Social, Secretaría de Educación Pública, 1992).

211. Jerome Levinson and Juan de Onis, *The Alliance That Lost Its Way: A Critical Report on the Alliance for Progress* (Chicago: Quadrangle Books, 1970).

212. Bruce J. Schulman, *Lyndon B. Johnson and American Liberalism: A Brief Biography with Documents* (New York: St. Martin's Press, 1995); Maurice Isserman and Michael Kazin, *America Divided: The Civil War of the 1960s* (New York: Oxford University Press, 2004).

213. Wallace Peters, *Chemotherapy and Drug Resistance in Malaria* (London: Academic Press, 1970), 14.

214. Ibid.

215. Johnson, "Recent Developments," 341; Nate Haseltine, "Resistant Malaria Hits U.S. Forces in Vietnam," *Washington Post,* August 3, 1965. Today, Artesimin is considered one of the most important antimalaria drugs.

216. I. Guerrero, B. Weniger, and M. Schultz, "Transfusion Malaria in the United States, 1972–1981," *Annals of Internal Medicine* 99, no. 2 (1983): 221–26; and Mary Mungai, Gary Tegtmeier, Mary Chamberland, and Monica Parise, "Transfusion-Transmitted Malaria in the United States from 1963 through 1999," *New England Journal of Medicine* 26, no. 344 (2001): 1973–78.

217. Humberto Romero Alvarez, "Comisión Nacional para la Erradicación del Paludismo," *Salud Pública de México* 6, no. 6 (1964): 1123–52 (the citation here is on 1151); and later Miguel E. Bustamante, "La Lucha antipalúdica en el mundo y en México," *Gaceta Médica de México* 110, no. 6 (1975): 389–91.

218. *La Salud en Oaxaca, su evolución hacia el siglo XXI 1998–2004* (Oaxaca: Servicios de salud de Oaxaca, 2004), 115.

219. "Información sucinta sobre los factores administrativos que originaron el deterioro de la Campaña contra el Paludismo en México, 1983," fondo SSA, sección Secretaría Particular, caja 249, expediente 2, AHSS. See also Joseph S. Tulchin, "The United States and Latin America in the 1960s," *Journal of Interamerican Studies and World Affairs* 30, no. 1 (1988): 1–36. See C. Manfredi, "Can the Resurgence of Malaria Be Partially Attributed to Structural Adjustment Programmes?" *Parassitologia* 41 (1999): 389–90. The feelings of uncertainty in CNEP positions and demands that malaria eradication continued indefinitely appears in a number of letters, poems, and *Bulletin* articles during the 1960s. Fernando Lasso Echevarría, *Historia de los servicios de salud en el estado de guerrero* (Mexico City: N.p., 2003), 41, Wellcome Library; "Editorial: Nuestro futuro en paludismo," 2, *El Chamula, Boletín CNEP,* Zona IV Año V Num. 6, June 1961, fondo SSA, sección CNEP, serie Zona IV, caja 1, expediente 3, AHSS. "Jorge Ordóñez Utrilla de Tierra Blanca, Veracruz to Presidente de la República, 2 February 1961," Adolfo López Mateos, vol. 938, expediente, 703.2/423, AGN.

220. Arnoldo Gabaldón, "Difficulties Confronting Malaria Eradication," *American Journal of Tropical Medicine and Hygiene* 21, no. 5 (1972): 634–39; the citation here is on 638.

221. "Información sucinta sobre los factores administrativos que originaron el deterioro de la Campaña contra el Paludismo en México, 1983."

222. "Grant-in-Aid to el Colegio de Mexico toward the Cost of a Latin American

Regional Conference on Population, December 1 1969," RFA. R.G. 1.2, series 323, box 63, folder 487, RAC.

223. These policies were continued by President Lopez Portillo (1976–82), who established a specialized Mexican agency to promote changes in what was considered a "prolific" population's reproductive behavior. Joseph E. Potter, "Population and Development in Mexico since 1940: An Interpretation," *Population and Development Review* 12, no. 1 (1986): 47–75.

224. Thomas E. Skidmore and Peter H. Smith, *Modern Latin America* (New York: Oxford University Press, 2001), 242–46; and Donald K. Freebairn, "Agricultural Interactions between Mexico and the United States," *Journal of Interamerican Studies* 25, no. 3 (1983): 275–98; the citation here is on 277.

225. "Juan José Bremer, Private Secretary of the Presidency, to Dr. Jorge Jiménez Cantú, March 22, 1974," copy of a letter directed to the president of the republic on February 18, 1974, in which he asks "for a more profound study of the malaria problem." The letter is signed by Laureano Solano, Gonzalo M. Torres, and Lusio Herrera Gomes Cosolapa, Oaxaca, fondo SSA, sección Secretaría Particular, caja 249, expediente 2, AHSS.

Spanish versión: "Nada mas un derroche de dinero para la nación mejicana y perder el tiempo útil y por la otra sentimos mucho que nuestra nación la aigan engañado que con este polbo se acabaría el paludismo . . . ni los mismos doctores se dan cuenta lo que es el paludismo. el paludismo tiene varios orígenes

1. mala alimentación

2. esta trabajando y se va a bañar o le llovió el cielo . . .

3. cuando toma mucha agua antes de comer . . .

4. cuando el paciente tiene frió y después le entra la calentura. . . .

desde que ese polbo yego todos los campesinos están perdiendo. Todos los poyos y gallinas y cochinos y asta uno que otro perro y gato . . . las brigadas vienen . . . no les importa rociar en el agua o en la comida ¿es justo? Y si ay un enfermo de grabeda no les importa le rosian . . . nos amenasan si nos oponemos, nos meten a cárcel. ¿Eso esta bien? No señor presidente debe usted de quitar todas las brigadas y salbaremos nuestra nación y nosotros los Mexicanos le agradeceremos que supo usted ver por sus hijos."

226. In 1971, a Special Technical Committee of the Health Secretariat began a thorough examination of CNEP's work but confirmed the decision to eradicate the disease. "Consejo Técnico de la Campaña Nacional para la Erradicación del Paludismo, Acta de las Sesiones, 1971, México DF," fondo SSA, serie Dirección, caja 55, expediente 1, AHSS. It was formed by malaria eradication advocates: Miguel E. Bustamante, Márquez Escobedo, Manuel Martínez Báez, Guillermo Romas y Carrillo, and Luís Vargas. A report of its activities appears in Humberto Romero Alvarez, "Estrategia y tácticas de la erradicación," *Gacéta Médica de México* 110, no. 6 (1975): 410–19.

227. Ibid., 417.

228. G. Gramicia "Health Education in Malaria Control, Why Has It Failed?" *World Health Forum* 2, no. 3 (1981): 385–89. Some authors criticized health authorities for concentrating on malaria instead of other devastating illnesses in southern Mexico; e.g., see Rosendo Pérez García, *La Sierra Juárez: Apuntes sobre arqueología, orografía, hidrografía, historia, estadística, economía, sociología, lingüística, biología, etc. de los pueblos del distrito de Ixtlán de Juárez* (Mexico City: Gráfica Cervantina, 1956), 245–48.

229. "Francisco Linares Carbajal [schoolteacher in Jayacatlan] to Jefe de Servicios Coordinados de Salubridad y Asistencia Publica en el Estado, Oaxaca, 9 March 1957,"

fondo Poder Ejecutivo del Estado, sección Dirección General de Gobernación, serie Secretaría General del Despacho Expediente 539, AGEO.

230. World Health Organization, *Malaria Control as Part of Primary Health Care: Report of WHO Study Group,* Technical Report 712 (Geneva: World Health Organization, 1984). On the history of primary health care, see Marcos Cueto, "The Origins of Primary Health Care and Selective Primary Care," *American Journal of Public Health* 94, no. 11 (2004): 1864–74. A valuable effort to implement these perspectives is described in Manuel Sánchez Rosado, "Horizontalización de la lucha contra el paludismo en México," *Boletín de la Oficina Sanitaria Panamericana* 106, no. 2 (1959): 163–67.

231. This information appears in Schuler, *Malaria: Meeting the Global Challenge,* 26.

Chapter 5. Conclusions: The Return of Malaria and the Culture of Survival

1. For the first figure, see Jesús Kumate, "Las enfermedades infecciosas en México," in *Vida y muerte del mexicano,* ed. Federico Ortiz Quesada (Mexico City: Folios Ediciones, 1982), vol. 1, 53.

2. Secretaria de Salud del Estado de Oaxaca, "Información epidemiológica de morbilidad, Estado de Oaxaca, 1988," table 12, Biblioteca, Archivo General del Estado de Oaxaca, Oaxaca (hereafter AGEO).

3. Secretaria de Salud del Estado de Oaxaca, "Información epidemiológica," tables 7, 9, 12.

4. Philip Musgrove, "The Impact of the Economic Crisis on Health and Health Care in Latin America and the Caribbean," *WHO Chronicle* 40, no. 40 (1986): 152–57; Asa Cristina Laurell, "Crisis, Neoliberal Health Policy, and Political Processes in Mexico," *International Journal of Health Services* 21, no. 3 (1991): 457–70.

5. Leonel Espinoza Guzmán, "Situación actual y perspectivas de las instituciones formadoras de recursos humanos para la salud," Oaxaca, May 29, 1986, 2. This paper appears as part of a bound volume titled *Situación actual y perspectivas de la salud en el Estado de Oaxaca* (Oaxaca, 1986), found in the Biblioteca, AGEO.

6. Juan Javier Montesinos Camarillo, "Medicina tradicional," Oaxaca, n.p., 1986. This paper appears as part of the bound volume titled *Situación actual y perspectivas de la salud en el Estado de Oaxaca.*

7. "Situación de la Malaria en las Américas," *Boletín Epidemiológico de la Organización Panamericana de la Salud* 17, no. 4 (1996): 1–3.

8. "Malaria, Mexico," http://www.cdc.gov/malaria/control_prevention/mexico .htm.

9. See http://irptc.unep.ch/pops/indxhtms/manexp11.html and http://www.idrc.ca/ reports/read_article_english.cfm?article_num=1094.

10. Medical Entomology Research and Training Unit, "Guatemala," http://www .cdc.gov/malaria/cdcactivities/guatemala.htm.

11. David Bull, *Growing Problem: Pesticides and the Third World* (Oxford and Birmingham: Oxfam and Third World Publications, 1982), 43.

12. Andres J. Yoder, "Lessons from Stockholm: Evaluating the Global Convention on Persistent Organic Pollutants," *Indiana Journal of Global Legal Studies* 10, no. 2 (2003): 113–56.

13. An example of a work that advocates a return to DDT spraying in Latin Amer-

ica is D. R. Roberts, S. Magin, and J. Mouchet, "DDT House Spraying and Re-emerging Malaria," *The Lancet* 356, no. 9226 (2000): 330–32.

14. Reed Karaim, "Not So Fast with the DDT: Rachel Carson's Warnings Still Apply," *American Scholar* 74, no. 3 (2005): 53–59.

15. C. Rehwagen, "WHO Recommends DDT to Control Malaria," *British Medical Journal* 333, no. 7569 (2006): 622.

16. World Health Organization, *Implementation of the Global Malaria Control Strategy: Report of a WHO Study Group on the Implementation of the Global Plan of Action for Malaria Control 1993–2000* (Geneva: World Health Organization, 1993); World Health Organization, *The Work of WHO 1992–1993: Biannual Report of the Director General to the World Health Assembly and to the United Nations* (Geneva: World Health Organization, 1994).

17. Global Partnership to Roll Back Malaria, *Roll Back Malaria Country Strategies & Resource Requirements* (Geneva: World Health Organization, 2001); D. Nabarro and K. Mendis, "Roll Back Malaria Is Unarguably Both Necessary and Possible," *Bulletin of the World Health Organization* 78, nos. 1–2 (2000): 1454–55. For a discussion, see "Rolling Back Malaria: Action or Rhetoric?" *Bulletin of the World Health Organization* 78, nos. 1–2 (2000): 1450–54.

18. R. S. Desowit, "The Malaria Vaccine: Seventy Years of the Great Immune Hope," *Parassitologia* 42 (2000): 173–82.

19. P. E. Duffy and T. K. Mutabingwa, "Artemisinin Combination Therapies," *The Lancet* 367, no 9528 (2006): 2037–39.

20. Robert Walgate, "Global Fund for AIDS, TB and Malaria Opens Shop," *Bulletin of the World Health Organization* 80, no. 3 (2002): 259–59. See also Global Fund to Fight Aids, Tuberculosis, and Malaria, *The Framework Document of the Global Fund,* at http://www.theglobalfund.org/en/files/publicdoc/Framework_uk.pdf.

21. Elizabeth A. Casman and Hadi Dowlatabadi, eds., *Contextual Determinants of Malaria* (Washington, D.C.: Resources for the Future, 2002).

22. U.S. Government Accountability Office, "Global Health: The Global Fund to Fight AIDS, TB and Malaria Is Responding to Challenges but Needs Better Information and Documentation for Performance-Based Funding," report to Congressional Committees, U.S. Government Accountability Office, Washington, June 2005, 6.

23. Pan-American Health Organization, 26th Pan-American Sanitary Conference, 54th Session of the Regional Committee, "Status Report on Malaria Programs in the Americas (Based on 2001 Data)," document PAHO/HCP/M217/02, Pan-American Health Organization, Washington, September 23–27, 2002.

24. U.S. House of Representatives, *HIV/AIDS, TB, and Malaria: Combating a Global Pandemic—Hearing before the Subcommittee on Health of the Committee on Energy and Commerce, House of Representatives, 108th Congress, First Session, 20 March 2003* (Washington, D.C.: U.S. Government Printing Office, 2003), 1.

25. Uriel Kitron, "Malaria, Agriculture and Development: Lessons from Past Campaigns," *International Journal of Health Services* 17, no. 2 (1987): 295–326.

26. Marguerite Owen, *The Tennessee Valley Authority* (New York: Praeger, 1973).

27. Geoffrey M. Jeffery, "Malaria Control in the Twentieth Century," *American Journal of Tropical Medicine and Hygiene* 25, no. 3 (1976): 361–71.

Bibliography

Archives and Libraries
Mexico

Archivo General del Estado de Oaxaca, Oaxaca, Mexico
    Biblioteca del Archivo General del Estado de Oaxaca
    Fondo Poder Ejecutivo del Estado, Sección Dirección General de Gobernación,
        Serie Secretaria General del Despacho
Archivo General de la Nación, Mexico City
    Archivo López Mateos
    Archivo Ruíz Cortines
Archivo Histórico de la Secretaría de Salud, Mexico City
    Fondo Secretaría de Salubridad y Asistencia
        Sección: Comisión Nacional para la Erradicación del Paludismo
        Sección: Secretaría de Salubridad y Asistencia
        Sección: Secretaría Particular
        Sección: Subsecretaría de Salubridad y Asistencia
        Sección: Subsecretaría de Salubridad
Biblioteca Municipal de Oaxaca, Oaxaca, Mexico
Biblioteca Nacional, Mexico City

United States

Bancroft Library, University of California, Berkeley
    Isabel Kelly, 1948–56, Collection CU-23, Berkeley Department of Anthropology
    "George M. Foster: An Anthropologist in the Twentieth Century," Regional Oral
        History Office, BAN MSS 2001/116
Pan-American Health Organization Library, Washington
Rockefeller Archive Center, New York City
    Rockefeller Foundation Archives
        Record Group 1.1, Series 223
        Record Group 1.2, Series 100E, 114, 300, 323
        Record Group 12.1, Paul F. Russell Diaries

Stanford University Library, Stanford, California
Truman Presidential Library and Museum, Independence, Missouri
UNICEF Library, New York City
U.S. National Archives, College Park, Maryland, Records Groups 59, 469, 287
U.S. National Library of Medicine, Bethesda, Maryland
    Eugene Campbell Papers, 1941–86, MS C 467
    Fred L. Soper Papers, 1919–75, MS C 3590
    Louis Laval Williams Papers, 1921–70, MS C 169

Switzerland

Malaria Research Collection, World Health Organization Archives, Geneva

Newspapers
Mexico

El Diario de Ciudad Victoria, Ciudad Victoria
El Diario de Culiacán, Culiacán, Sinaloa
El Dictamen, Diario Independiente, Veracruz
Excelsior, Mexico City
El Imparcial, Oaxaca
El Mundo, Tamaulipas
Periódico Oficial, Órgano Constitucional del Estado Libre y Soberano de Oaxaca,
    Oaxaca
El Sol de Puebla, Puebla
El Universal, Mexico City
Rumbo Nuevo, Villahermosa, Tabasco

United States

Christian Science Monitor, Boston
New York Times, New York City
Wall Street Journal, New York City
Washington Post, Washington

Articles and Books

Aandahl, Frederick, ed. *Foreign Relations of the United States, 1951: The United Nations, the Western Hemisphere.* Washington, D.C.: U.S. Government Printing Office, 1979.
Abel, Christopher. "External Philanthropy and Domestic Change in Colombian Health Care: The Role of the Rockefeller Foundation, ca. 1920–1950." *Hispanic American Historical Review* 75, no. 3 (1995): 339–76.
———. *Health, Hygiene and, Sanitation in Latin America c. 1870 to c. 1950.* London: Institute of Latin American Studies, 1996.
Academia Nacional de Medicina de México. *Directorio de la Academia Nacional de*

Medicina de México, Cuerpo Consultivo del Gobierno Federal. Mexico City: Academia Nacional de Medicina de México, 1962.

Accinelli, Robert. *Crisis and Commitment: United States Policy toward Taiwan, 1950–1955.* Chapel Hill: University of North Carolina Press, 1996.

Adams, Richard. "A Nutritional Research Program in Guatemala." In *Health, Culture and Community,* ed. Benjamin D. Paul. New York: Rusell Sage Foundation, 1955.

Aguayo, Sergio. *Myths and [Mis]perceptions: Changing U.S. Elite Visions of Mexico.* San Diego: Center for U.S.-Mexican Studies at the University of California, 1998.

Agudelo, Saúl Franco. "El Saldo Rojo de los insecticidas en América Latina, a propósito de su utilización contra la malaria." *Revista Centroamericana de Ciencias de la Salud* 7, no. 20 (1981): 35–53.

Aguirre Beltrán, Gonzalo. *Obra antropológica IV: Formas de gobierno indígena.* Mexico City: Fondo de Cultura Económica, 1992.

———. *Programas de salud en la situación intercultural.* México: Instituto Indigenista Interamericano, 1955.

Aguirre Beltrán, Gonzalo, ed. *El indigenismo en acción: XXV aniversario del Centro Coordinador Indigenista Tzeltal-Tzotzil, Chiapas.* Mexico City: Instituto Nacional Indigenista, 1976.

Alanis, Jesus. "Homenaje a Arturo Rosenblueth." *Acta Physiologica Lationoamericana Americana* 21, no. 1 (1971): 1–7.

Alarcón, Alfonso G. *Estudios clínicos y terapéuticos acerca del paludismo infantil.* Mexico City: Nipos, 1938.

———. *La sobrealimentación en los niños de peche: El paludismo en la primera infancia.* Tampico: Imp. Nacional, 1921.

Alcaraz Rivera, Ignacio. *El paludismo en Mochicahui, Sinaloa.* Mexico City: Facultad de Medicina, 1950.

Alexander, Robert J. *Communism in Latin America.* New Brunswick, N.J.: Rutgers University Press, 1957.

———. "Nature and Progress of Agrarian Reform in Latin America." *Journal of Economic History* 23, no. 4 (1963): 559–73.

"Alianza para el Progreso, address by President Kennedy, 13 March 1961, Washington, D.C." *Department of State Bulletin* 44 (1961): 471–74.

Almeida, Marta de. "Combates sanitários e embates científicos: Emílio Ribas e a febre amarela em São Paulo." *História, Ciências, Saúde—Manguinhos* 6, no. 3 (2000): 577–607.

Alvarado, Carlos. *Situación de la lucha antimalárica en el continente americano: IV informe presentado sobre la lucha antimalárica.* Washington, D.C.: Oficina Sanitaria Panamericana, 1951.

Álvarez Amézquita, José. "¿Hay defunciones por paludismo en México?" *Salud Pública de México* 5 (1963): 748–49.

———. "La obra de la Revolución Mexicana en el campo de la Salud Pública." *Salud Pública de México* 3 (1961): 9–14.

Álvarez Amézquita, J., M. Bustamante, A. López Picazos, and F. Fernández del Castillo. *Historia de la Salubridad y de la Asistencia de México.* Mexico City: Secretaría de Salubridad y Asistencia, 1960.

———. "Servicios médicos rurales cooperativos en la historia de la Salubridad y de la Asistencia en México." In *La atención médico rural en México 1930–1980,* ed. Héctor Hernández Llamas. Mexico City: Instituto Mexicano del Seguro Social, 1984.

Anderson, Warwick. "Postcolonial Histories of Medicine." In *Locating Medical History: The Stories and Their Meanings,* ed. Frank Huisman and John Harley Warner. Baltimore: Johns Hopkins University Press, 2004.

Armas Domínguez, J. *Las defunciones por paludismo en la República Mexicana: Desde el punto de vista de su diagnóstico médico y su clasificación estadística.* Mexico City: Dirección General de Bioestadística, 1956.

Armstrong, Orland Kay. "All Out Attack on Malaria." *Reader's Digest,* July 1958, 188–91.

Armus, Diego, ed. *Disease in the History of Modern Latin America: From Malaria to AIDS.* Durham, N.C.: Duke University Press, 2003.

Arnold, David. *Colonizing the Body: State, Medicine and Epidemic Disease in Nineteenth Century India.* Berkeley: University of California Press, 1993.

———, ed. *Warm Climates and Western Medicine: The Emergence of Tropical Medicine, 1500–1900.* Amsterdam: Rodopi, 1996.

Arreola Cortés, Raúl. *Manuel Martínez Báez, científico y humanista.* Morelia: Universidad Michoacana de San Nicolás de Hidalgo, 1994.

Ávila Cisneros, Ignacio. "El Dr. Manuel Martínez Báez." *Revista de Investigaciones de Salud Pública* 29, no. 3 (1969): 173–78.

Ayala Blanco, Jorge. *La aventura del cine mexicano en la época de oro y después.* Mexico City: Grijalbo, 1993.

Babb, Sarah. *Managing Mexico: Economists from Nationalism to Neoliberalism.* Princeton, N.J.: Princeton University Press, 2001.

Babione, R. W. "Special Technical Problems in Malaria Eradication in Latin America, 6 February 1964." World Health Organization. http://whqlibdoc.who.int/malaria/WHO_Mal_430.pdf.

Backman, Jules. *Chemicals in the National Economy.* Washington, D.C.: Manufacturing Chemists' Association, 1964.

Baily, Samuel L. *The United States and the Development of South America: 1945–1975.* New York: Franklin Watts, 1976.

Barlow, R. "The Economic Effects of Malaria Eradication." *American Economic Review* 57, no. 2 (1968): 130–48.

Barnet, Richard. *The Giants: Russia and America.* New York: Simon & Schuster, 1977.

Barret, Bruce. "Identity, Ideology and Inequality, Methodologies in Medical Anthropology, Guatemala 1950–1955." *Social Science and Medicine* 44, no. 5 (1997): 579–87.

Beaton, Kendall. *Enterprise in Oil: A History of Shell in the United States.* New York: Appleton-Century-Crofts, 1957.

Beaulac, Williard L. "Technical Cooperation as an Instrument of Foreign Policy." *Department of State Bulletin* 35 (1955): 964–70.

Bedwell, Mary Elizabeth. "A Bio-Bibliography of Dr. Fred L. Soper (1893–), Director Emeritus of the Pan-American Sanitary Bureau." Master's thesis, Catholic University of America, Washington, 1963.

Beltrán, Enrique, and Eduardo Aguirre Pequeño. *Lecciones de paludología.* Monterrey: Universidad de Nuevo León, 1948.

Beltrán, Enrique, and Luís Vargas. "El paludismo en el Distrito Federal: Características de una cepa de *Plasmodium vivax* aislada en Xochimilco." *Revista del Instituto de Salubridad y Enfermedades Tropicales* 9, no. 1 (1948): 21–26.

Bell, Betty, ed. *Indian Mexico: Past and Present, Symposium Papers, 1965.* Los Angeles: University of California, 1967.

Benchimol, Jaime. *Dos micróbios aos mosquitos: Febre amarela e a revolução pasteuriana no Brasil.* Río de Janeiro: Editora Fiocruz, 1999.

Berger, Mark T. "Managing Latin America: U.S. Power, North American Knowledge and the Cold War." *Journal of Iberian and Latin American Studies* 2, (1996): 41–63.

Berle, Adolf A. "Alliance for Progress versus Communism." *Department of State Bulletin* 43 (1961): 763.

Birn, Anne-Emmanuelle. "Eradication, Control or Neither? Hookworm versus Malaria Strategies and Rockefeller Public Health in México." *Parassitologia* 40, no. 1–2 (1998): 137–47.

———. *Marriage of Convenience: Rockefeller International Health and Revolutionary Mexico.* Rochester: Rochester University Press, 2006.

———. "A Revolution in Rural Health? The Struggle over Local Health units in Mexico, 1928–1940." *Journal of the History of Medicine and Allied Sciences* 53, no. 1 (1998): 43–76.

———. "Wa(i)ves of Influence: Rockefeller Public Health in Mexico, 1920–50." *Studies in the History and Philosophy of Biological and Biomedical Sciences* 31, no. 3 (2000): 381–95.

Black, Maggie. *The Children and the Nations: The Story of UNICEF.* Sydney: UNICEF, 1986.

Bobadilla, José Luis. "La mortalidad en Mexico." In *Vida y muerte del mexicano,* vol. 1, ed. Federico Ortiz Quesada. Mexico City: Folios Ediciones, 1982.

Bonfil Batalla, Guillermo. *México profundo: Una civilización negada.* Mexico City: Secretaría de Educación Pública, 1987.

Bordas, E., and W. G. Downs. "Ecología de *Anopheles aztecus* en la región de Xochimilco." *Revista del Instituto de Salubridad y Enfermedades Tropicales* 11 (1951): 48–56.

Bowerman, W., J. Giesy, D. Best, and V. Kramer. "A Review of Factors Affecting Productivity of Bald Eagles in the Great Lakes Region: Implications for Recovery." *Environmental Health Perspectives* 103, supplement 4 (1995): 51–59.

Bowles, Chester. "Foreign Aid: The Great Decision of the Sixties." *Department of State Bulletin* 43 (1961): 703–9.

———. "Why Foreign Aid?" *Department of State Bulletin* 48 (1963): 777–84.

Brain, W. R. "Science and Antiscience." *Science* 148 (1965): 192–98.

Branderburg, Frank. *The Making of Modern Mexico.* Englewood Cliffs, N.J.: Prentice-Hall, 1964.

Bravo-Becherelle, M. A., and Luis Mazotti. "Distribución geográfica de la mortalidad por picadura de alacrán en México." *Revista del Instituto de Salubridad y Enfermedades Tropicales* 21, nos. 3–4 (1961): 129–40.

———. "Escorpionismo en la República Mexicana." *Revista del Instituto de Salubridad y Enfermedades Tropicales* 21, nos. 1–2 (1961): 3–19.

Briggs, Charles L., and Clara Mantini-Briggs. *Stories in the Time of Cholera: Racial Profiling during a Medical Nightmare.* Berkeley: University of California Press, 2003.

Brown, Anthony William A. *Insecticide Resistance in Arthropods.* Geneva: World Health Organization, 1958).

Brown, C. V., and Gustav J. Nossal. "Malaria: Yesterday, Today, and Tomorrow." *Perspectives in Biology and Medicine* 20, no. 1 (1986): 65–76.

Brown, Theodore M., Marcos Cueto, and Elizabeth Fee. "The World Health Organization and the Transition from 'International' to 'Global' Public Health." *American Journal of Public Health* 96, no. 1 (2006): 62–71.

Bruce-Chwatt, L. J. "Malaria Eradication at the Crossroads." *Bulletin of the New York Academy of Medicine* 45, no. 10 (1969): 999–1012.

———. "Malaria Research and Eradication in the USSR. A Review of Soviet Achievements in the Field of Malariology." *Bulletin of the World Health Organization* 21 (1959): 737–72.

———. "Man against Malaria: Conquest or Defeat." *Transactions of the Royal Society of Tropical Medicine* 73, no. 6 (1979): 605–16.

———. "Need for New Weapons." *World Health Forum* 1 (1980): 23–24.

———. "Transfusion Malaria." *Bulletin of the World Health Organization* 50 (1970): 337–46.

Bull, David. *Growing Problem: Pesticides and the Third World.* Oxford and Birmingham: Oxfam and Third World Publications, 1982.

Bustamante, Miguel E. "Hechos sobresalientes en la historia de la Secretaría de Salubridad y Asistencia." *Salud Pública de México* 25, no. 5 (1983): 465–82.

———. "La lucha antipalúdica en el mundo y en México." *Gaceta Médica de México* 110, no. 6 (1975): 389–91.

Bynum, William F., and Roy Porter, eds. *Companion Encyclopedia of the History of Medicine.* London: Routledge, 1993.

Cade, Tom J., Jeffrey L. Lincer, Clayton M. White, David G. Roseneau, and L. G. Swartz. "DDE Residues and Eggshell Changes in Alaskan Falcons and Hawks." *Science* 172, no. 3986 (1971): 955–57.

Cahn, M., E. Levy. "The Tolerance to Large Weekly Doses of Primaquine and Amodiaquine in Primaquine-Sensitive and Non-Sensitive Subjects." *American Journal of Tropical Medicine and Hygiene* 11 (1962): 605–6.

Cámara, Fernando. "Contemporary Mexican Indian Cultures: The Problems of Integration." In *Indian México: Past and Present, Symposium Papers, 1965,* ed. Betty Bell. Los Angeles: University of California, 1967.

Camp, Roderic. *Mexican Political Biographies: 1935–1975.* Tucson: University of Arizona Press, 1976.

Campbell, Eugene P. "The Role of the International Cooperation Administration in International Health." *Archives of Environmental Health* 1, no. 6 (1960): 502–11.

Cañedo, Luis. "Rural Health Care in Mexico." *Science* 185: 4157 (September 27, 1974): 1131–37.

Carson, Rachel. *Primavera silenciosa.* Barcelona: Luis de Caralt, 1964.

———. *Silent Spring.* Boston: Houghton Mifflin, 1962.

Casman, Elizabeth A., and Hadi Dowlatabadi, eds. *Contextual Determinants of Malaria.* Washington, D.C.: Resources for the Future, 2002.

Caso, Alfonso, Silvio Zavala, and José Miranda, eds. *Memorias del Instituto Nacional Indigenista,* vol 6. Mexico City: Instituto Nacional Indigenista, 1954.

Center for Policy Studies of the Population Council. "Population Brief: Latin America." *Population and Development Review* 6, no. 1 (1980): 126–52.

"Ceremony at Mexican Border Marks Settlement of Chamizal Dispute." *Department of State Bulletin* 51 (1964): 545–52.

Cervantes, Domingo G. *Breve reseña de la lucha antipalúdica en México.* Mexico City: Secretaría de Salubridad y Asistencia, 1979.

Chandler, Alfred D., Jr. *Shaping the Industrial Century: The Remarkable Story of the Evolution of the Modern Chemical and Pharmaceutical Industries.* Cambridge, Mass.: Harvard University Press, 2005.

Chargoy Martínez, J. "La cinematografía y la educación higiénica." *Salud Pública de México* 2 (1960): 81–84.

Charnow, John. *Maurice Pate: UNICEF Executive Director, 1947–1965.* Geneva: UNICEF, 1989.

Chávez, Ignacio. *México en la cultura médica.* Mexico City: FCE, 1947.

Cleveland, Harlan, Gerard J. Mangone, and John Clarke Adams. *The Overseas Americans.* New York: McGraw-Hill, 1960.

Cleaver, Harry. "Malaria and the Political Economy of Public Health." *International Journal of Health Services* 7, no. 4 (1977): 557–79.

II Congreso Nacional de Paludismo: Programa de sesiones, convocado por la Secretaría de Salubridad y Asistencia de los Estados Unidos Mexicanos en la ciudad de México durante los días 12, 13 y 14 de abril, 1951. Mexico City: Secretaría de Salubridad y Asistencia, 1952.

Cook, Robert C. "Latin America: A Decade of Decision." *Population Bulletin* 17, no. 2 (1961): 17–38.

Cockburn, Aidan. "Eradication of Infectious Diseases." *Science* 133 (1961): 1050–58.

———, ed. *Infectious Diseases: Their Evolution and Eradication.* Springfield, Ill.: Charles C. Thomas, 1967.

Coerr, Wymberley DeR. "Forces of Change in Latin America." *Department of State Bulletin* 44 (1961): 251–55.

Colombia, Servicio Nacional de Erradicación de la Malaria. *Plan de erradicación de la malaria.* Bogotá: Servicio Nacional de Erradicación de la Malaria, 1957.

Comité de Expertos en Paludismo de la Agencia de Desarrollo Internacional. *El paludismo: Métodos para su erradicación.* Mexico City: Limusa/Wiley, 1963.

Cook, Scott, and Jong-Taick Joo. "Ethnicity and Economy in Rural Mexico: A Critique of the Indigenista Approach." *Latin American Research Review* 30, no. 2 (1995): 33–59.

Cooter, Joseph. "The Rockefeller Foundation's Mexican Agricultural Project: A Cross-Cultural Encounter, 1943–1949." In *Missionaries of Science: The Rockefeller Foundation and Latin America,* ed. Marcos Cueto. Bloomington: Indiana University Press, 1994.

"El costo de la erradicación del paludismo en las Américas." *Chronicle of the World Health Organization* 12, no. 1 (1958): 337–41.

Critchlow, Donald T. "Birth Control, Population Control and Family Planning: An Overview." *Journal of Health Policy* 7, no. 1 (1995): 1–21.

Cueto, Marcos. "The Origins of Primary Health Care and Selective Primary Care." *American Journal of Public Health* 94, no. 11 (2004): 1864–74.

———. *The Return of Epidemics: Health and Society in Peru during the 20th Century.* Aldershot, U.K.: Ashgate, 2001.

———. "Sanitation from Above: Yellow Fever and Foreign Intervention in Peru, 1919–1922." *Hispanic American Historical Review* 72, no. 1 (1992): 1–22.

———. *El valor de la salud: Historia de la Organización Panamericana de la Salud.* Washington, D.C.: Pan-American Health Organization, 2004.

Cueto, Marcos, ed. *Missionaries of Science: The Rockefeller Foundation and Latin America.* Bloomington: Indiana University Press, 1994.

———. *Salud, cultura y sociedad en América Latina.* Lima: Instituto de Estudios Peruanos, 1996.

Cunningham, Andrew, and Bridie Andrews, eds. *Western Medicine as Contested Knowledge.* Manchester: Manchester University Press, 1997.

Da Silva, Oswaldo José. "Malaria Eradication in the Americas." In *Infectious Diseases: Their Evolution and Eradication,* ed. Aidan Cockburn. Springfield, Ill.: Charles C. Thomas, 1967.

Dame, David. A. "Donald James Pletsch: Six Decades of International Commitment." *Journal of the American Mosquito Control Association* 21, no. 3 (2005): 331–36.

Daniels, Walter M. *Latin America in the Cold War.* New York: H. W. Wilson Company, 1952.

Davidson, G. "Studies on Insecticide Resistance in *Anopheline* Mosquitoes." *WHO Bulletin* 18 (1958): 579–621.

De la Fuente, Julio. "El Centro Coordinador Tzeltal-Tzotzil." *América Indígena* 13, no. 1 (1953): 55–64.

———. "Creencias indígenas sobre la Onchocercosis, el paludismo y otras enfermedades." *América Indígena* 1, no. 1 (1941): 43–46.

De la Peña, Sergio, and Marcel Morales Ibarra. *Historia de la cuestión agraria mexicana: El agrarismo y la industrialización de México, 1940–1950.* Mexico City: Siglo XXI, 1990.

De la Riva Rodríguez, Xavier. "Salubridad y asistencia medico social." In *México: Cincuenta años de revolución, la vida social,* ed. Julio Durán Ochoa. Mexico City: Fondo de Cultura Económica, 1961.

"Decreto que crea la Secretaría de Salubridad y Asistencia, 18 Octubre 1943." *Gaceta Médica de México* 73 (1943): 435–37.

"The Department of State, 1930–1955: Expanding Functions and Responsibilities." *Department of State Bulletin* 32 (1955): 470–77.

Desowit, Robert S. "The Malaria Vaccine: Seventy Years of the Great Immune Hope." *Parassitologia* 42 (2000): 173–82.

Diccionario enciclopédico de la medicina tradicional mexicana. Mexico City: Instituto Nacional Indigenista, 1994.

Dion, Michelle. "The Political Origins of Social Security in Mexico during the Cárdenas and Avila Camacho Administrations." *Mexican Studies / Estudios Mexicanos* 21, no. 1 (2005): 59–95.

Dirección General de Higiene Escolar y Servicios Médicos. *Magisterio nacional y paludismo.* Mexico City: Secretaría de Educación Pública, 1957.

Dobson, M., M. Malowany, and R. Snow. "Malaria Control in East Africa: The Kampala Conference and the Pare-Taveta Scheme: A Meeting of Common and High Ground." *Parassitologia* 42, nos. 1–2 (2000):149–66.

Dobson, M. J., M. Malowany, and D. H. Stapleton. "Dealing with Malaria in the Last Sixty Years: Aims, Methods and Results." *Parassitologia* 42, nos. 1–2 (2000): 3–7.

Doremus, Anne. "Indigenism, Mestizaje and National Identity in Mexico during the 1940s and 1950s." *Mexican Studies / Estudios Mexicanos* 17, no. 2 (2001): 375–402.

Dowdle, Walter, and Donald R. Hopkins, eds. *The Eradication of Infectious Diseases.* New York: John Wiley & Sons, 1998.

Downs, Wilburg. "Actividades de la Oficina de Especialización Sanitaria." *Medicina, Revista Mexicana* 31, no. 629 (1951): 213–14.

———. "History of Epidemiological Aspects of Yellow Fever." *Yale Journal of Biology and Medicine* 55 (1982): 179–85.

Downs, Wilburg, E. Bordas, and A. Enriquez Chávez. "El control del paludismo en la región de Xochimilco, D.F." *Revista del Instituto de Salubridad y Enfermedades Tropicales* 11, nos. 1–3 (1950): 99–103.

Downs, Wilburg, Heliodoro Celis, and James B. Gahan. "Control of *Anopheles Pseudopunctipennis* in Mexico with DDT Residual Sprays Applied in Buildings, Part III: Malariological Observations after Five Years of Annual Spraying." *American Journal of Hygiene* 52, no. 3 (1950): 348–52.

"Dr. Ignacio Morones Prieto, President of the Eight World Health Assembly." *Chronicle of the World Health Organization* 9, no. 6 (1955): 208.

"Dr. M. G. Candau and WHO." *British Medical Journal* 58, no. 64 (1973): 433.

Duffy, P. E., and T. K. Mutabingwa. "Artemisinin Combination Therapies." *The Lancet* 367, no. 9528 (2006): 2037–39.

Dunlap, Thomas R. *DDT, Scientists, Citizens, and Public Policy.* Princeton, N.J.: Princeton University Press, 1981.

Duran Ochoa, Julio, ed. *México: Cincuenta años de revolución, la vida social.* Mexico City: Fondo de Cultura Económica, 1961.

Dyer, Davis, and David B. Sicilia. *Labor of a Modern Hercules: The Evolution of a Chemical Company.* Boston: Harvard Business School Press, 1990.

"E. Pampana: 40 Years against Malaria." *World Health* 13, no. 2 (1960): 26–29.

Earle, David P., Jr., and Robert W. Berliner. "Chloroquine." In *Fourth International Congress on Tropical Medicine and Malaria, Washington D.C., May 10–18, 1948.* Washington, D.C.: U.S. Government Printing Office, 1948.

"Editorial. A Vaccine against Malaria." *Boletín Indigenista* 14, no. 4 (1954): 231.

Egbert, Jean P. "Experiences in Mexico." *Nursing Outlook* (1964): 38–42.

Ehrlich, Paul R. *The Population Bomb.* New York: Ballantine Books, 1971.

Eisenhower, Dwight D. "Toward Mutual Understanding among the Americas." *Department of State Bulletin* 42 (1960): 471–86.

Eisenhower, Milton. *The Wine Is Bitter: The United States and Latin America.* New York: Doubleday, 1963.

"La enfermedad más cara del mundo, nueva estrategia antipalúdica." *Chronicle of the World Health Organization* 13, nos. 9–10 (1959): 355–62.

"The Epidemiology of a Disappearing Disease: Malaria." *American Journal of Tropical Medicine and Hygiene* 8 (1960): 357–66.

"Epitaph for Global Malaria Eradication?" *The Lancet,* July 5, 1975, 15–16.

Escobar, C. Sergio. "La Erradicación del paludismo: Producto del esfuerzo conjunto nacional." *Salud Pública de México* 5 (1963): 727–31.

Expert Committee on Malaria, World Health Organization. *Eighth Report.* Technical Report 205. Geneva: World Health Organization, 1961

———. *Malaria Terminology: Report of a Drafting Committee Appointed by WHO.* Geneva: World Health Organization, 1953.

———. *Sixth Report.* Geneva: World Health Organization, 1957.

Expert Panel on Malaria, International Cooperation Administration. "Report and Recommendations on Malaria: A Summary." *American Journal of Public Health* 10, no. 4 (1961): 451–502.

Fabrega, Horacio, Jr., and Daniel Silver. *Illness and Shamanistic Curing in Zinacatan.* Stanford, Calif.: Stanford University Press, 1973.

Fadrique, Jesús Gracia, ed. *Estado y fertilizantes, 1760–1985.* Mexico City: Universidad Nacional Autónoma de México / FCE, 1988.

Farmer, Paul. *AIDS and Accusation: Haiti and the Geography of Blame.* Berkeley: University of California Press, 1992.

Favre, Henri. *Cambio y continuidad entre los Mayas de México.* Mexico City: Siglo XXI, 1972.

Fernández de Castro, J. "El paludismo en México y la lucha para su control." In *A cien años del descubrimiento de Ross: El paludismo en México,* ed. Jesús Kumate and Adolfo Martínez Palomo. Mexico City: Colegio Nacional, 1998.

"Fifth International Congress on Malaria and Tropical Medicine." *Journal of Tropical Medicine and Hygiene* 56, no. 10 (1953): 225–42.

Fitzgerald, Deborah. "Exporting American Agriculture: The Rockefeller Foundation in Mexico, 1943–1953." In *Missionaries of Science: The Rockefeller Foundation and Latin America,* ed. Marcos Cueto. Bloomington: Indiana University Press, 1994.

Foster, George M. *Applied Anthropology.* Boston: Little, Brown, 1969.

———. "Bureaucratic Aspects of International Health Agencies." *Social Science and Medicine* 25 (1987): 1039–48.

———. "The Institute of Social Anthropology of the Smithsonian Institution, 1943–1952." *Anuario Indigenista* 27 (1967): 173–92.

———. "Medical Anthropology and International Health Planning." *Medical Anthropology Newsletter* 7, no. 3 (1976): 12–18.

———. "Relationship between Theoretical and Applied Anthropology: A Public Health Program Analysis." *Human Organization* 11, no. 3 (1952): 5–16.

———. "Use of Anthropological Methods and Data in Planning and Operation." *Public Health Reports* 69, no. 9 (1953): 841–57.

Foreign Relations of the United States, 1958–1960, American Republics, vol. 5. Washington, D.C.: U.S. Government Printing Office, 1991.

Forrestal, Dan J. *Faith, Hope and $5,000: The Story of Monsanto—The Trials and Triumphs of the First 75 Years.* New York: Simon & Schuster, 1977.

Freebairn, Donald K. "Agricultural Interactions between Mexico and the United States." *Journal of Interamerican Studies* 25, no. 3 (1983): 275–98.

Friedman, Max Paul. "Retiring the Puppets, Bringing Latin America Back In: Recent Scholarship on United States–Latin American Relations." *Diplomatic History* 27, no. 5 (2003): 611–36.

Gabaldón, Arnoldo. "Difficulties Confronting Malaria Eradication." *American Journal of Tropical Medicine and Hygiene* 21, no. 5 (1972): 634–39.

———. "Global Malaria Erradication: Changes of Strategy and Future Outlook." *American Journal of Tropical Medicine and Higiene* 18, no. 5 (1969): 641–56.

———. "Influencia del Rociamiento Intradomiciliario con DDT sobre las tasas específicas de mortalidad general en Venezuela." *Boletín de la Oficina Sanitaria Panamericana* 40, no 35 (1956): 93–106.

Gaddis, John Lewis. *The Cold War: A New History.* New York: Penguin Press, 2005.

———. "The Emerging Post-Revisionist Thesis on the Origins of the Cold War." *Diplomatic History* 7 (1983): 171–90.

Gahan, J. B., and G. C. Payne. "Control of *Anopheles Pseudopunctipennis* in Mexico with DDT Residual Sprays Applied in Buildings." *American Journal of Hygiene* 45 (1947): 123–32.

Galo Soberón y Parra, 1896–1956. Mexico City: Fundación Mexicana para la Salud, 1998.

García, Hernán, Antonio Sierra, and Gilberto Balám. *Wind in the Blood: Maya Healing and Chinese Medicine.* Berkeley, Calif.: North Atlantic Books, 1999.

García Cruz, Miguel. "Los problemas demográficos de México." *Suplemento de Medicina* 1964: 9–14.

Garret, Mildred. "The United States–Mexico Border Public Health Association." *Nursing Outlook* 7, no. 5 (1959): 295–97.

Gereffi, Gary. *The Pharmaceutical Industry and Dependency in the Third World.* Princeton, N.J.: Princeton University Press, 1983.

Giglioli, George. "Eradication of *Anopheles Darlingi* from the Inhabited Areas of British Guiana by DDT Residual Spraying." *Journal of the National Malaria Society* 10, no. 2 (1951): 142–61.

———. "Malaria Control in British Guiana." *Bulletin of the World Health Organization* 11, nos. 4–5 (1954): 849–53.

———. "Residual Effect of DDT in a Controlled Area of British Guiana Tested by the Continued Release of *Anopheles Darlingi* and *Aedes Aegypti:* A Practical Guide for the Standardized Evaluation of Overall Residual Efficiency under Field Conditions." *Transactions of the Royal Society of Tropical Medicine and Hygiene* 48, no. 6 (1954): 506–21.

Gilles, Herbert M., and David A. Warrell, eds. *Bruce-Chwatt's Essential Malariology,* 3rd ed. London: Arnold, 1993.

Gilman, Nils. *Mandarins of the Future: Modernization Theory in Cold War America.* Baltimore: Johns Hopkins University Press, 2003.

Gladwell, Malcom. "The Mosquito Killer: Millions of People Owe Their Lives to Fred Soper, Why Isn't He a Hero?" *New Yorker,* July 2, 2001, 42–51.

Glennon, John P., ed. *Foreign Relations of the United Status, 1955–1957: American Republics; Multilateral; Mexico; Caribbean.* Washington, D.C.: U.S. Government Printing Office, 1987.

Global Fund to Fight Aids, Tuberculosis, and Malaria. *The Framework Document of the Global Fund.* http://www.theglobalfund.org/en/files/publicdoc/Framework_uk.pdf.

"Global Malaria War." *World of Medicine, Medical Magazine* 1, no. 9 (1957): 325.

Global Partnership to Roll Back Malaria. *Roll Back Malaria Country Strategies & Resource Requirements.* Geneva: World Health Organization, 2001.

Gómez-Dantes, H., and Anne E. Birn. "Malaria and Social Movements in México: The Last 60 Years." *Parassitologia* 42, nos. 1–2 (2000): 69–85.

González, Yólolt, ed. *Homenaje a Isabel Kelly.* Mexico City: Instituto Nacional de Antropología e Historia, 1989.

González Casanova, Pablo. *La democracia en México.* Mexico City: Era, 1967.

González Rivera, Manuel. "Diez años de trabajo en el Instituto de Salubridad y Enfermedades Tropicales." *Revista del Instituto de Salubridad y Enfermedades Tropicales* 10, no. 1 (1949): 3–16.

———. *Las enfermedades transmisibles en el medio agrario: Cartilla para uso de los maestros rurales.* Mexico City: Dirección General de Educación Higiénica, Secretaría de Salubridad y Asistencia, 1946.

Graham, Richard, ed. *The Idea of Race in Latin America.* Austin: University of Texas Press, 1990.

Gramicia, G. "Health Education in Malaria Control: Why Has it Failed?" *World Health Forum* 2, no. 3 (1981): 385–89.

Gray, Virginia M. *Love Is Not Enough: Recollections of a Capitol Hill Lobbyist for UNICEF.* Washington, D.C.: Klinge Press, 1984.

Greenough, Paul. "Intimidation, Coercion and Resistance in the Final Stages of the South Asian Smallpox Eradication Campaign, 1973–1975." *Social Science and Medicine* 41, no. 5 (1995): 633–45.

Grier, J. "Ban of DDT and Subsequent Recovery of Reproduction in Bald Eagles." *Science* 218, no. 4578 (1982): 1232–35.

Guerrero, I., B. Weniger, and M. Schultz. "Transfusion Malaria in the United States, 1972–1981." *Annals of Internal Medicine* 99, no. 2 (1983): 221–26.

Guhin, Michael A. *John Foster Dulles: A Statesman and His Times.* New York: Columbia University Press, 1972.

Gutiérrez, Ana Teresa. *Tiempos de guerra y paz: Arnoldo Gabaldón y la investigación sobre malaria en Venezuela (1936–1990).* Caracas: Cendes, 1998.

Guzmán Clark, Ernesto. "Participación de la autoridades municipales en la solución de los problemas de salud pública." *Boletín de la Sociedad Oaxaqueña de Salud Pública* 6, no. 3 (1971): 36–40.

Hackett, Lewis W. *Malaria in Europe: An Ecological Study.* London: Oxford University Press, 1937.

Halperin Frisch, David C., and Homero De León Montenegro. *México-Guatemala: Salud en la frontera Guatemala-México.* San Cristóbal de las Casas: Colegio de la Frontera Sur, 1996.

Handler, Philip. "The Federal Government and the Scientific Community." *Science* 171, no. 3967 (1971): 144–51.

Harrison, Gordon. *Mosquitoes, Malaria, and Man: A History of the Hostilities since 1880.* New York: Dutton, 1978.

Hays, C. W. "The United States Army and Malaria Control in World War II." *Parassitologia* 42, nos. 1–2 (2000): 47–52.

Herber, Lewis. *Our Synthetic Environment.* New York: Alfred A. Knopf, 1962.

Hernández Llamas, Héctor. "Historia de la participación del estado en las instituciones de atención medica en México, 1935–1980." In *Vida y muerte del mexicano,* vol. 2, ed. Federico Ortiz Quesada. Mexico City: Folios Ediciones, 1982.

Hernández Llamas, Héctor, ed. *La atención médica rural en México, 1930–1980.* Mexico City: Instituto Mexicano del Seguro Social, 1984.

Hewitt de Alcántara, Cynthia. *Anthropological Perspectives on Rural Mexico.* London: Routledge & Kegan Paul, 1984.

———. *Modernizing Mexican Agriculture: Socio-economic Implications of Technological Change, 1940–1970.* Geneva: United Nations Research Institute for Social Development, 1976.

Hochman, Gilberto, and Diego Armus, eds. *Cuidar, Controlar, Curar: Ensaios históricos sobre saúde e doença na América Latina e Caribe.* Rio de Janeiro: Editora Fiocruz, 2004.

Hoopes, Townsend, and Douglas Brinkley. *FDR and the Creation of the U.N.* New Haven, Conn.: Yale University Press, 1997.

Hopkins, Donald R. "Yaws in the Americas, 1950–1975." *Journal of Infectious Diseases* 4, no. 136 (1977): 548–54.

Hounshell, David A. "Epilogue: Rethinking the Cold War; Rethinking Science and Technology in the Cold War; Rethinking the Social Study of Science and Technology." *Social Studies of Science* 31, no. 2 (2001): 289–97.

Huisman, Frank, and John Harley Warner, eds. *Locating Medical History: The Stories and Their Meanings.* Baltimore: Johns Hopkins Univesity Press, 2004.

Humphreys, Margaret. *Malaria: Poverty, Race, and Public Health in the United States.* Baltimore: Johns Hopkins University Press, 2001.

Ianska, Alicja. "The Mexican Indian: Image and Identity." *Journal of Interamerican Studies* 6, no. 4 (1964): 529–36.

Immerman, Richard H., ed. *John Foster Dulles and the Diplomacy of the Cold War.* Princeton, N.J.: Princeton University Press; 1990.

Imperialismo y medios masivos de comunicación, vol. 2. Lima: N.p., 1973.

Industrial Council for Tropical Health. *Industry and Tropical Health: Proceedings of the First Tropical Health Conference Sponsored by the Harvard School of Public Health, 8–10 December 1950.* Boston: Harvard School of Public Health and International Council for Tropical Health, 1950.

———. *Industry and Tropical Health: Proceedings of the Third Tropical Health Conference Sponsored by the Harvard School of Public Health.* Boston: Harvard School of Public Health and International Council for Tropical Health, 1960.

Ingham. John M. "Human Sacrifices at Tenochitlan." *Comparative Studies in Society and History* 16 (1984): 379–400.

Institute of Inter-American Affairs. *Cooperative Health Programs of the U.S. and Latin America.* Washington, D.C.: Health and Sanitation Division, Institute of Inter-American Affairs, 1948.

Instituto Nacional Indigenista. *¿Qué es el INI?* Mexico City: Instituto Nacional Indigenista, 1955.

Inter-American Affairs Office. *Mexico: Next Door Neighbor.* Washington, D.C.: U.S. Government Printing Office, 1943.

"Inter-American Committee Completes Work." *Department of State Bulletin* 36 (1957): 1014–16.

International Cooperation Administration. *Technical Cooperation in Health.* Washington, D.C.: International Cooperation Administration, 1956.

———. *Technical Cooperation in Health.* Washington D.C.: International Cooperation Administration, 1961.

"International Organizations: Aid to World Trade and Prosperity." *Department of State Bulletin* 37 (1957): 749–54.

"Intervention of International Communism in the Americas." *Department of State Bulletin* 30 (1954): 419–26.

Isserman, Maurice, and Michael Kazin. *America Divided: The Civil War of the 1960s.* New York: Oxford University Press, 2004.

Jeffery, Geoffrey M. "Malaria Control in the Twentieth Century." *American Journal of Tropical Medicine and Hygiene* 25, no. 3 (1976): 361–71.

Johnson, Donald R. "Recent Developments in Mosquito-Borne Diseases: Malaria." *Mosquito News* 33, no. 3 (1973): 341–48.

Johnson, Donald R., and Roy Fritz. "Status Report on Malaria Eradication." *Mosquito News* 22, no. 2 (1962): 80–81.

Jones, Joseph M. *Does Overpopulation Mean Poverty? The Facts about Population Growth and Economic Development.* Washington, D.C.: Center for International Economic Growth, 1962.

Joy, R. J. "Malaria in American Troops in the South and Southwest Pacific in World War II." *Medical History* 43, no. 2 (1999): 192–207.

Kapelusz-Poppi, Ana María. "Physician Activists and the Development of Rural Health in Postrevolutionary Mexico." *Radical History Review* 80 (2001): 35–50.

———. "Rural Health and State Construction in Post-Revolutionary Mexico: The Nicolaita Project for Rural Medical Services" *The Americas* 58, no. 2 (2001): 261–83.

Karaim, Reed. "Not So Fast with the DDT: Rachel Carson's Warnings Still Apply." *American Scholar* 74, no. 3 (2005): 53–59.

Kelly, Isabel. "El adiestramiento de parteras en México desde el punto de vista antropológico." *América Indígena* 15, no. 2 (1955): 109–17.

———. *Folk Practices in North Mexico: Birth Customs, Folklore, Medicine and Spiritualism in the Laguna Zone.* Austin: University of Texas Press, 1965.

———. "Preliminary Report on the Laguna Housing Project, Ejido El Cuije, near Torreón, Cohauila." Institute of Inter-American Affairs, Mexico City, 1953.

Kelly, Isabel, and Héctor García Manzanedo. "Santiago Tuxtla, Veracruz: Cultura y salud." Instituto de Asuntos Interamericanos, Mexico City, 1956.

Kennel, A. J., ed. *Malaria.* London: Wellcome Trust, 1991.

Key, David McK. "World Security and the World Health Organization." *Department of State Bulletin* 31 (1954): 616–18.

Kitron, Uriel. "Malaria, Agriculture and Development: Lessons from Past Campaigns." *International Journal of Health Services* 17, no. 2 (1987): 295–326.

Knight, Alan. "Peasant into Patriots: Thoughts on the Making of the Mexican Nation." *Mexican Studies/Estudios Mexicanos* 10, no. 1 (1994): 135–61.

———. "Racism, Revolution and *Indigenismo*: México, 1910–1940." In *The Idea of Race in Latin America*, ed. Richard Graham. Austin: University of Texas Press, 1990.

Knipe, F. W. "Nozzles of Insecticide Sprayers: Comments from the Point of View of Malaria Control." *Bulletin of the World Health Organization* 12, no. 3 (1955): 401–9.

Kohn Loncarica, Alfredo G., and Abel L. Agüero. "Carlos Alberto Alvarado y los planes de salud rural: Las condiciones del éxito y del fracaso en técnica médica." *Saber y Tiempo* 4, no. 1 (1997): 489–96.

Kort, Michael. *The Columbia Guide to the Cold War.* New York: Columbia University Press, 1998.

Kumate, Jesús. "Las enfermedades infecciosas en México." In *Vida y muerte del mexicano,* vol. 1, ed. Federico Ortiz Quesada. Mexico City: Folios Ediciones, 1982.

Kumate, Jesús, and Adolfo Martínez Palomo, eds. *A cien años del descubrimiento de Ross: El paludismo en México.* Mexico City: Colegio Nacional, 1998.

Kuznick, Peter J., and James Gilbert. *Rethinking Cold War Culture.* Washington, D.C.: Smithsonian Institution Press, 2001.

Lasman, Thomas C. "Government Science in Postwar America: Henry A. Wallace, Edward U. Condon and the Transformation of the National Bureau of Standards, 1945–1951." *Isis* 96 (2005): 25–51.

Lasso Echevarría, Fernando. *Historia de los servicios de salud en el Estado de Guerrero.* Mexico City: N.p., 2003.

Lathman, Michael E. "Ideology, Social Science and Destiny: Modernization and the Kennedy-Era Alliance for Progress." *Diplomatic History* 22, no. 2 (1998): 199–229.

Laurell, Asa Cristina. "Crisis, Neoliberal Health Policy, and Political Processes in Mexico." *International Journal of Health Services* 21, no. 3 (1991): 457–70.

Lee, Sung. "WHO and the Developing World: The Contest for Ideology." In *Western Medicine as Contested Knowledge,* ed. Andrew Cunningham and Bridie Andrews. Manchester: Manchester University Press, 1997.

Leeds, Roger S. "The Origins of the Alliance for Progress: Continuity and Change in the U.S. Policy toward Latin America." Ph.D. dissertation, Johns Hopkins University, Baltimore, 1976.

Leffler, Melvyn P. "The Cold War: What Do 'We Now Know'?" *American Historical Review* 104, no. 2 (1999): 501–24.

León Portilla, Miguel. "México." *Indianist Yearbook* 22 (1962): 65–82.

————. "Panorama de la población indígena de México." *América Indígena* 19 (1959): 43–68.

Levinson, Jerome, and Juan de Onis. *The Alliance That Lost Its Way: A Critical Report on the Alliance for Progress.* Chicago: Quadrangle Books, 1970.

Lippmann, Walter. *The Cold War: A Study in U.S. Foreign Policy.* New York: Harper & Brothers, 1947.

Litsios, Socrates. "Criticism of WHO's Revised Malaria Eradication Strategy." *Parassitologia* 42 (2000): 167–72.

————. "Malaria Control, the Cold War, and the Postwar Reorganization of International Assistance." *Medical Anthropology* 17:3 (1997): 255–278.

————. "Rene J. Dubos and Fred L. Soper: Their Contrasting Views on Vector and Disease Eradication." *Perspectives in Biology and Medicine* 141, no. 1 (1997): 138–49.

————. *The Tomorrow of Malaria.* Karori, N.Z.: Pacific Press, 1997.

Loaeza, Antonio. *Breve resumen de los estudios acera del paludismo en los Estados Unidos Mexicanos.* Mexico City: Tipográfica de la Viuda, 1911.

Lodge, Henry Cabot. "12th Anniversary of United Nations." *Department of State Bulletin* 37 (1957): 768.

Lommintz, Claudio. *Death and the Idea of Mexico.* New York: Zone Books, 2005.

López Carrillo, L., L. Torres-Arreola, L. Torres-Sánchez, F. Espinosa-Torres, C. Jiménez, M. Cebrian, S. Waliszeski, and O. Saldate. "Is DDT Use a Public Health Problem in Mexico?" *Environmental Health Perspectives* 104, no. 6 (1996): 584–87.

Lorey, David E., ed. *United States–Mexico Border Statistics, since 1900.* Los Angeles: UCLA Latin American Center Publications, 1990.

"A Lottery That Helped to Build a Nation." *WLA Magazine,* March 2005: 20–21. http://www.world-lotteries.org/documents/magazine/wla16/wla16_mexico.pdf.

Lucas, Scott. *Freedom's War: The American Crusade against the Soviet Union.* New York: New York University Press, 1999.

Maclaurin, John. *The United Nations and Power Politics.* New York: Harper & Brothers, 1951.

Madsen, Claudia. *A Study in Mexican Folk Medicine.* New Orleans: Middle American Research Institute, Tulane University, 1965.

Magner, Lois N., ed. *Doctors, Nurses and Medical Practitioners: A Biographical Source Book.* Westport, Conn.: Greenwood Press, 1977.

"Malaria." *Journal of Tropical Medicine and Hygiene* (London) 61 (1958): 53–54.

"Malaria Division." *Journal of Tropical Medicine and Hygiene* (London) 61 (1958): 251.

"Malaria and Ecosystems: Historical Aspects—Proceedings of a Rockefeller Foundation Conference, Como, Italy, 18–22 October 1993." *Parassitologia* 36, nos. 1–2 (1994): 1–227.

"Malaria Eradication in 1966." *WHO Chronicle* 21, no. 9 (1967): 373–88.

Manfredi, C. "Can the Resurgence of Malaria Be Partially Attributed to Structural Adjustment Programmes?" *Parassitologia* 41 (1999): 389–90.

Manrique Paz, Rafael. *Informe médico-sanitario del pueblo de Chicomuselo, Chiapas y breves consideraciones sobre el paludismo.* Tesis Facultad de Medicina para examen profesional de médico cirujano. Mexico City: Tipográfica Ortega, 1955.

"Marcolino Gomez Candau." *Revista de Malariologia e Doenças Tropicais* 34 (1982): 119–22.

Martell Ramírez, Ricardo. "La cultura trique." *Boletín de la Sociedad Oaxaqueña de Salud Pública* 7, no. 1 (1972): 11–18.

Martínez Báez, Manuel. "Consecuencias sociales y económicas del paludismo de México." *Gaceta Médica de México* 87 (1957): 11–17.

―――. "El Instituto de Salubridad y Enfermedades Tropicales." *Anales de la Sociedad Mexicana de Historia de la Ciencia y de la Tecnología* 1 (1969): 143–62.

―――. *Manual de parasitología médica.* Mexico City: La Prensa Médica Mexicana, 1953.

Martínez Palomo, Adolfo, ed. *Obras.* Mexico City: Colegio Nacional, 1994.

McClarnand, Elaine, and Steve Goodson, eds. *Impact of the Cold War on American Popular Culture.* Carrollton: State University of West Georgia, 1999.

McDermott, Walsh. "Pharmaceuticals: Their Role in Developing Societies." *Science* 89 (1980): 240–45.

McGregor Giacinti, Felipe. *Mosquitos y paludismo.* Mexico City: Oficina Central del Servicio de Puertos y Fronteras, 1940.

Meany, George. "Cooperation in Science, Culture and Education." *Department of State Bulletin* 37 (1957): 764–68.

Medhurst, Martin J., ed. *Cold War Rhetoric: Strategy, Metaphor and Ideology.* East Lansing: Michigan State University Press, 1997.

Medina Aguilar, Rolando. *El banco de sangre: Organización, funcionamiento, legislación.* Mexico City: Prensa Médica Mexicana, 1963.

Memoria de la Secretaría de Salubridad y Asistencia Pública, Sexenio 1952–1958. Mexico City: Secretaría de Salubridad y Asistencia Pública, 1959.

"Memoria del CNEP." *Boletín del CNEP* 11, no. 4 (1958): 3–55.

"In Memory of Dr. M. G. Candau." *WHO Chronicle* 37, no. 4 (1983): 144–47.

México, Dirección General de Estadística. *Anuario estadístico compendiado de los Estados Unidos Mexicanos, 1968.* Mexico City: Dirección General de Estadística, 1969.

México, Poder Ejecutivo Federal. *Acción educativa del Gobierno Federal del 1 de Septiembre de 1954 al 31 de Agosto de 1955.* Mexico City: Secretaría de Educación Pública, 1955.

México, Secretaría de Salubridad y Asistencia. Dirección General de la Campaña Nacional contra el Paludismo. *Trabajos realizados en la Zona Norte de Petróleos Mexicanos.* Mexico City: Secretaría de Salubridad y Asistencia, 1949.

Meyer, Michael C., and William H. Beezley. *The Oxford History of Mexico.* New York: Oxford University Press, 2000.

Meyer, Michael C., and William L. Sherman. *The Course of Mexican History.* New York: Oxford University Press, 1979.

Miller, Robert R. *Mexico: A History.* Norman: University of Oklahoma Press, 1985.

Mitter, Rana, and Patrick Major, eds. *Across the Blocs: Cold War Cultural and Social History.* London: Frank Cass, 2004.

Mohyeddin, Farid A. "The Malaria Programme: Euphoria to Anarchy." *World Health Forum* 1 (1980): 8–33.

Moreno Valle, Rafael, and Guillermo Suárez Torres. "La erradicación del paludismo en México: Informe de actividades en 1964." *Salud Pública de México* 8, no. 1 (1966): 83–97.

―――. "Evolución del paludismo en la frontera mexicano-guatemalteca en 1964 y plan de acción para 1965." *Salud Pública de México* 7, no. 1 (1963): 33–38.

Morgan, Murray C. *Doctors to the World.* New York: Viking Press, 1958.

Mungai, Mary, Gary Tegtmeier, Mary Chamberland, and Monica Parise. "Transfusion-

Transmitted Malaria in the United States from 1963 through 1999." *New England Journal of Medicine* 26, no. 344 (2001): 1973–78.

Murray, Douglas. *Cultivating Crisis: The Human Cost of Pesticides in Latin America.* Austin: University of Texas Press, 1994.

Musgrove, Philip. "The Impact of the Economic Crisis on Health and Health Care in Latin America and the Caribbean." *WHO Chronicle* 40, no. 40 (1986): 152–57.

Nabarro, D., and K. Mendis. "Roll Back Malaria Is Unarguably both Necessary and Possible." *Bulletin of the World Health Organization* 78, no. 12 (2000): 1454–55.

Nájera, José A. "Malaria and the Work of WHO." *Bulletin of the World Health Organization* 67, no. 3 (1989): 229–43.

National Institutes of Health. *Manual for the Microscopical Diagnosis of Malaria in Man.* Bulletin 180. Washington, D.C.: U.S. Public Health Service, 1942.

Newell, Kenneth. "Selective Primary Health Care: The Counter Revolution." *Social Science and Medicine* 26, no. 9 (1988): 903–6.

Niblo, Stepen A. "Allied Policy towards Axis Interests in Mexico during World War II." *Mexican Studies/Estudios Mexicanos* 17, no. 2 (2001): 351–73.

———. *War, Diplomacy and Development: The United States and Mexico, 1938–1954.* Wilmington, Del.: Scholarly Resources, 1995.

Novell, Gordon, Paul F. Russell, and N. H. Swellengrebel. *Malaria Terminology: Report of a Drafting Committee Appointed by the World Health Organization.* Geneva: World Health Organization, 1953.

Oaxaca. 1ª Convención Regional para la Campaña Nacional contra el Paludismo, 21–27 marzo 1938. Oaxaca: Fundación Cultural Bustamante Vasconcelos, 1938.

Obregón, Diana. *Batallas contra la lepra: Estado, medicina y ciencia en Colombia.* Medellín: Banco de la República de Colombia, 2002.

"Octava Asamblea Mundial de la Salud." *Chronicle of the World Health Organization* 9, no. 7 (1955): 217–23.

Olszyna-Marzys, A. E. "Residuos de plaguicidas clorados en la leche humana en Guatemala." *Boletín de la Oficina Sanitaria Panamericana* 74, no. 2 (1973): 93–107.

Organización Sanitaria Panamericana. *Actas de la Decimocuarta Conferencia Sanitaria Panamericana: Sexta Reunión del Comité Regional de la Organización Mundial de la Salud para las Américas, Santiago, Chile, 7–22 Octubre 1954, Documentos Oficiales N. 14.* Washington, D.C.: Oficina Sanitaria Panamericana, 1955.

———. *La Malaria en las Américas: Bosquejo de la batalla que libra el hemisferio para terminar con un viejo enemigo.* Washington, D.C.: Organización Panamericana de la Salud, 1963.

———. *Situación de la lucha antimalarica en las Américas: V informe.* Washington, D.C.: Oficina Sanitaria Panamericana, 1956.

Ortiz Quesada, Federico, ed. *Vida y muerte del mexicano.* 2 vols. Mexico City: Folios Ediciones, 1982.

Osakwe, Christopher. *The Participation of the Soviet Union in Universal International Organization: A Political and Legal Analysis of Soviet Strategies and Aspirations Inside ILO, UNESCO and WHO.* Leiden: A. J. Sijthoff, 1972.

Osgood, Kenneth A. "Total Cold War: U.S. Propaganda in the 'Free World,' 1953–1960." Ph.D. dissertation, University of California, Santa Barbara, 2001.

Owen, Marguerite. *The Tennessee Valley Authority.* New York: Praeger, 1973.

Packard, Randall M. "Malaria Dreams: Postwar Visions of Health and Development in the Third World." *Medical Anthropology* 17, no. 3 (1997): 279–96.

————. "No Other Logical Choice: Global Malaria Eradication and the Politics of International Health in the Post-War Era." *Parassitologia* 40, nos. 1–2 (1998): 217–29.

Packard, Randall M., and Peter J. Brown. "Rethinking Health, Development and Malaria: Historicizing a Cultural Model in International Health." *Medical Anthropology* 17, no. 3 (1997): 181–94.

Packard, Randall M., and Paulo Gadelha. "A Land Filled with Mosquitoes: Fred L. Soper, the Rockefeller Foundation and the *Anopheles Gambiae* Invasion of Brazil." *Parassitologia* 36 (1994): 197–213.

Packenham, Robert A. *The Dependency Movement: Scholarship and Politics in Development Studies.* Cambridge, Mass.: Harvard University Press, 1992.

Page Pliego, Jaime Tomás. *Política sanitaria dirigida a los pueblos indígenas de México y Chiapas 1857–1995.* Mexico City: Universidad Nacional Autonoma de México, 2002.

Palmer, Steven. *From Popular Medicine to Medical Populism: Doctors, Healers, and Public Power in Costa Rica, 1800–1940.* Durham, N.C.: Duke University Press, 2003.

"Paludismo: Problema mundial." *Chronicle of the World Health Organization* 9, no. 2 (1955): 35–104.

Pampana, Emilio J. "Changing Strategy in Malaria Control." *Bulletin of the World Health Organization* 11 (1954): 513–20.

————. *Erradicación de la Malaria.* Mexico City: Limusa/Wiley, 1966.

————. *A Textbook of Malaria Eradication.* London: Oxford University Press, 1963.

————. *A Textbook of Malaria Eradication.* 2nd ed. London: Oxford University Press, 1969.

Pan-American Health Organization. *Informe de los Seminarios sobre la Misión de los Servicios Generales de Salud en la Erradicación de la Malaria, Pocos de Caldas, Brasil, 26 de junio–4 de julio de 1964/Cuernavaca, México 4–13 Marzo, 1965.* Washington, D.C.: Pan-American Health Organization, 1965.

————. *Manual for the Microscopic Diagnosis of Malaria.* 2nd ed. Washington, D.C.: Pan-American Health Organization, 1963.

————. *Status Report on Malaria Programs in the Americas.* Report of 26th Pan-American Sanitary Conference, 54th Session of the Regional Committee. Washington, D.C.: Pan-American Health Organization, 2002.

Parker, Richard, ed. *A AIDS no Brasil, 1982–1992.* Rio de Janeiro: ABIA, 1994.

Parker, Thomas. *America's Foreign Policy 1945–1976: Its Creators and Critics.* New York: Facts on File, 1980.

Parsons, Elsie Clews. "Curanderos in Oaxaca, Mexico." *Scientific Monthly* 32, no. 1 (1931): 60–68.

"Partida de la Doctora Isabel Kelly." *Boletín Indigenista* 17, no. 4 (1957): 294.

Paul, Benjamin D. *Health, Culture and Community.* New York: Russell Sage Foundation, 1955.

Pearce, Kimber C. *Rostow, Kennedy and the Rhetoric of Foreign Aid.* East Lansing: Michigan State University Press, 2001.

Peard, Julyan G. *Race, Place, and Medicine: The Idea of the Tropics in Nineteenth-Century Brazilian Medicine.* Durham, N.C.: Duke University Press, 1999.

Perdiguero Gil, Enrique, Josep Bernabeu Mestre, Rafael Huertas García, and Esteban Rodríguez Ocaña. "History of Health, a Valuable Tool in Public Health." *Journal of Epidemiological Community Health* 55, no. 9 (2001): 667–73.

Pérez García, Rosendo. *La Sierra Juárez: Apuntes sobre arqueología, orografía, hidro-*

grafía, historia, estadística, economía, sociología, lingüística, biología, etc. de los pueblos del distrito de Ixtlán de Juárez. Mexico City: Gráfica Cervantina, 1956.

Pesquiera, Manuel E. "Programa de Erradicación del Paludismo en México." *Boletín de la Oficina Sanitaria Panamericana* 42, no. 6 (1957): 537–47.

Pesticides in South America and Mexico. New York: Frost and Sullivan, 1981.

Peters, Wallace. *Chemotherapy and Drug Resistance in Malaria.* London: Academic Press, 1970.

Pine, L. G., ed. *The International Yearbook and Statesmen's WHO's Who 1958.* London: Burke's Peerage Limited, 1958.

Pinotti, Mario. "The Nation-Wide Malaria Eradication Program in Brazil." *Journal of the National Malaria Society* 10, no. 2 (1951): 162–82.

Pletsh, Donald. "Malaria Control and Economics." *Science* 149, no. 3687 (1965): 926.

———. "Progress toward Malaria Eradication in the Americas with special reference to Mexico." *American Journal of Public Health* 48 (1958): 713–16.

Potter, Joseph E. "Population and Development in Mexico since 1940: An Interpretation." *Population and Development Review* 12, no. 1 (1986): 47–75.

"President Johnson and President López Mateos of Mexico Hold Talks in California." *Department of State Bulletin* 50 (1964): 396–403.

"Problemas actuales del control y erradicación de la malaria en América Latina." *Boletín de la Dirección de Malariología y Saneamiento Ambiental* 28, nos. 1–2 (1988): 1–12.

Prothero, Mansell R. "Malaria in Latin America: Environmental and Human Factors." *Bulletin of Latin American Research* 14, no. 3 (1995): 357–65.

Rabe, Stephen G. *Eisenhower and Latin America: The Foreign Policy of Anticommunism.* Chapel Hill: University of North Carolina Press, 1988.

"Rehabilitation of the Eradication Concept in Prevention of Communicable Diseases." *Public Health Reports* 80 (1965): 855–69.

Redfield, Robert. *A Village That Chose Progress: Chan Kom Revisited.* Chicago: University of Chicago Press, 1950.

Reeves, William C. "Can the War to Contain Infectious Disease Be Lost?" *American Journal of Tropical Medicine and Hygiene* 21, no. 3 (1972): 251–59.

Rehwagen, C. "WHO Recommends DDT to Control Malaria." *British Medical Journal* 333, no. 7569 (2006): 622.

"Resistance of Insects to Insecticides." *Chronicle of the World Health Organization* 8, no. 3 (1954): 397–400.

Restrepo, Iván. *Naturaleza muerta: Los plaguicidas en México.* Mexico City: Oceano, 1988.

Reyna, José Luis, and Raúl Trejo Delarbre. *De Adolfo Ruíz Cortines a Adolfo López Mateos (1952–1964).* Mexico City: Siglo Veintiuno, 1981.

Reynolds, Donna J. "The Demarara Doctor." *Perspectives, Pan-American Health Organization* 1, no. 2 (1996). http://www.paho.org/English/DPI/Number2_article1.htm.

Roberts, D. R., S. Magin, and J. Mouchet. "DDT House Spraying and Re-emerging Malaria." *The Lancet* 356, no. 9226 (2000): 330–32.

Rodman, Peter W. *More Precious Than Peace: The Cold War and the Struggle for the Third World.* New York: Charles Scribner's Sons, 1994.

Rodríguez de Romo, Ana Cecilia, and Martha Eugenia Rodríguez. "Historia de la salud pública en México: Siglos XIX y XX." *História, Ciências, Saúde—Manguinhos* 5, no. 2 (1998): 293–310.

Rodríguez Prats, Juan José. *El Poder Presidencial: Adolfo Ruíz Cortines.* Mexico City: Miguel Ángel Porrua, Grupo Editorial, 1992.

Roemer, Milton I. *Medical Care in Latin America.* Washington, D.C.: Organization of American States, 1963.

"Rolling Back Malaria: Action or Rhetoric." *Bulletin of the World Health Organization* 78, nos. 1–2 (2000): 1450–54.

Román y Carrillo, G. "El paludismo en México." *Gaceta Médica de México* 110, no. 6 (1975): 401–10.

Romano Delgado, Agustín. *Historia evaluativa del Centro Coordinador Indigenista Tzeltal-Tzotzil.* 2 vols. Mexico City: Instituto Nacional Indigenista, 2002.

Romero-Álvarez, Humberto. "Contaminación ambiental y salud." In *La Evolución de la Medicina en México durante las últimas cuatro décadas,* ed. Ramón de la Fuente. Mexico City: Colegio Nacional, 1984.

———. "Estrategia y tácticas de la erradicación." *Gaceta Médica de México* 110, no. 6 (1975): 410–19.

———. *Health without Boundaries: Notes for the History of the United States–Mexico Border Public Health Association, on the Celebration of Its 30 years of Active Life, 1943–1973.* Mexico: United States–Mexico Border Public Health Association, 1975.

———. "Comisión Nacional para la Erradicación del Paludismo." *Salud Pública de México* 6, no. 6 (1964): 1123–52.

———. *La Campaña Nacional para la Erradicación del Paludismo: Su importancia para la salud pública.* Mexico City: Talleres Gráficos de la Nación, 1973.

Ros Romero, María del Consuelo. *La imagen del Indio en el discurso del Instituto Nacional Indigenista.* Mexico City: Centro de Investigaciones y Estudios Superiores en Antropología Social, 1992.

Ross, John B. *The Economic System of Mexico.* Stanford, Calif.: California Institute of International Studies, 1971.

Rostow, Walt W. "The Alliance for Progress." *Department of State Bulletin* 50 (1964): 496–500.

———. "Guerrilla Warfare in the Underdeveloped Areas." *Department of State Bulletin,* August 7, 1961, 233–38.

———. *The Stages of Economic Growth: A Non-Communist Manifesto.* Cambridge, Mass.: Cambridge University Press, 1960.

Rozeboom, L. E. "DDT: The Life-Saving Poison." *Johns Hopkins Magazine* 22 (1971): 29–32.

Rubottom, Roy R. "Communism in the Americas." *Department of State Bulletin* 38 (1958): 180–85.

———. "Economic Interdependence in the Americas." *Department of State Bulletin* 36 (1957): 732–35.

———. "Economic Relations between the U.S. and Latin America," *The Department of State Bulletin* 37 (1957): 536-540.

———. "The Goals of United States Policy in Latin America." *Annals of the American Academy of Political and Social Sciences* 342 (1962): 30–41.

———. "The Significance of Latin America in the Free World." *Department of State Bulletin* 37 (1957): 923–29.

Rusk, Dean. "The Alliance for Progress in the Context of World Affairs." *Department of State Bulletin* 46 (1962): 787–94.

Russell, Edmund. *War and Nature: Fighting Humans and Insects with Chemicals from World War I to Silent Spring.* Cambridge: Cambridge University Press, 2001.

Russell, Paul F. *Man's Mastery of Malaria.* Oxford: Oxford University Press, 1955.

———. "Obituary: Fred Lowe Soper." *Transactions of the Royal Society of Tropical Medicine and Hygiene* 71, no. 3 (1977): 272–73.

———. *Paludismo: Compendio de principios básicos.* Mexico City: La Prensa Médica Mexicana, 1953.

———. "Symposium Nation-Wide Malaria Eradication Projects in the Americas: Introductory Remarks by the President." *Journal of the National Malaria Society* 10, no. 2 (1951): 98–99.

———. "The United States and Malaria: Debits and Credits." *Bulletin of the New York Academy of Medicine* 44, no. 6 (June 1968): 623–53.

———. "The World Wide Malaria Eradication." *Industrial Medicine and Surgery* 27, no. 8 (1958): 378–83.

Russell, Paul F., Lloyd E. Roszenboom, and Alan Stone. *Keys to the Anopheline Mosquitoes of the World, with Notes on their Identification, Distribution, Biology, and Relation to Malaria.* Philadelphia, American Entomological Society, 1943.

"Rural Health Services in Latin America." *WHO Chronicle* 22, no. 6 (1968): 249–53.

Sachs, Jeffrey D., and Pia Malaney. "The Economic and Social Burden of Malaria." *Nature* 415 (2002): 680–85.

Sadik, Nafis, ed. *United Nations Fund for Population Activities: An Agenda for people: The UNFPA through Three Decades.* New York: New York University Press, 2002.

La salud en Oaxaca: Su evolución hacia el siglo XXI, 1998–2004. Oaxaca: Servicios de Salud de Oaxaca, 2004.

Sánchez Rosado, Manuel. "Horizontalización de la lucha contra el paludismo en México." *Boletín de la Oficina Sanitaria Panamericana* 106, no. 2 (1959):163–67.

Sánchez Vargas, Gustavo. *Orígenes y Evolucín de la Seguridad Social en México.* (Mexico City: Universidad Nacional Autonoma de México, 1963).

Saull, Richard. *Rethinking Theory and History in the Cold War: The State, Military Power, and Social Revolution.* London: F. Cass, 2001.

Schell, Patience A. "Nationalizing Children through Schools and Hygiene: Porfirian and Revolutionary Mexico City." *The Americas* 60, no. 4 (2004): 559–87.

Scheman, Ronald, ed. *The Alliance for Progress: A Retrospective.* New York: Praeger, 1988.

Schuler, Alexandrina. *Malaria: Meeting the Global Challenge.* Boston: Oelgeschlager, Gunn & Hain, 1985.

Schulman, Bruce J. *Lyndon B. Johnson and American Liberalism: A Brief Biography with Documents.* New York: St. Martin's Press, 1995).

Secretaría de Educación Pública. *Ciencia y tecnología en México en el siglo XX: Biografías de personajes ilustres.* Vol. 3. Mexico City: Academia Mexicana de Ciencias, 2003.

———. *Higiene Escolar Mexicana.* Report by Dirección General de Higiene Escolar y Servicios Médicos. Mexico City: Secretaría de Educación Pública, 1959.

———. *Legislación y Reglamentación, 1921–1958.* Mexico City: Secretaría de Educación Pública, 1958.

———. *Manual de técnicas y procedimientos, zonas médico escolares.* Mexico City: Secretaría de Educación Pública, 1958.

Secretaría de Industria y Comercio. "Viviendas urbanas y rurales en el país por entidades federativas, según el número de cuartos, 1960." In *Anuario Estadístico Compendiado de los Estados Unidos Mexicanos, 1968.* Mexico City: Dirección General de Estadística, 1969).

Secretaría de Relaciones Exteriores. *Testimonios de 40 años de presencia de México en las Naciones Unidas.* Mexico City: Secretaría de Relaciones Exteriores, 1985.

Secretaría de Salubridad y Asistencia. *Memoria, 1947–1950.* Mexico City: Secretaría de Salubridad y Asistencia, 1951.

Secretaría de Salud. *Guía del fondo de salubridad pública.* Report by Centro de Documentación y Archivo Histórico. Mexico City: Secretaría de Salud, 1991.

———. *Guía de la Sección Sub-Secretaría de Salubridad y Asistencia Fondo Secretaría de Salubridad y Asistencia Oficialía Mayor, Centro de Documentación Institucional Departamento de Archivo Histórico.* Mexico City: Secretaría de Salud, 1994.

Secretaría de Salud del Estado de Oaxaca. "Información epidemiológica de morbilidad, Estado de Oaxaca, 1988." Secretaría de Salud del Estado de Oaxaca, Oaxaca, 1988.

———. "Situación actual y perspectivas de la salud en el Estado de Oaxaca, 1986." Secretaría de Salud del Estado de Oaxaca, Oaxaca, 1986.

El Señor José E. Larumbe, descubridor de la causa eficiente de la ceguera onchocercosica: La microfilaria de los tejidos oculares. Mexico City: N.p., 1960.

Servicios Coordinados de Salud Pública de Campeche. "Consideraciones sobre factores humanos para la erradicación del paludismo." *Salud Pública de México* 8:3 (1966): 379-382.

Sharpless, John. "World Population Growth, Family Planning and American Foreign Policy." *Journal of Policy History* 7, no. 1 (1995): 72–102.

Shell Oil Company. *Annual Report 1956.* New York: Shell Oil Company, 1956.

Shlesinger, Stephen C. *Bitter Fruit: The Untold Story of the American Coup in Guatemala.* New York: Doubleday, 1982.

Siddiqi, Javed. *World Health and World Politics: The World Health Organization and the UN System.* London: Hurst and Co., 1995.

Sieglin, Verónica. *Modernización y devastación de la cultura tradicional campesina.* Mexico City: Plaza y Valdez, 2004.

"Situación de la Malaria en las Américas." *Boletín Epidemiológico de la Organización Panamericana de la Salud* 17, no. 4 (1996): 1–3.

Skidmore, Thomas E., and Peter H. Smith. *Modern Latin America.* New York: Oxford University Press, 2001.

Smedley, Max J. "Mexican–United States Relations and the Cold War, 1945–1954." Ph.D. thesis, University of Southern California, Los Angeles, 1981.

Smith, J. H., Jr. "The Mutual Security Program: A Fight for Peace." *Department of State Bulletin* 39, no. 1002 (1958): 380–84.

Smith, Peter H. *Talons of the Eagle: Dynamics of U.S.–Latin American Relations.* New York: Oxford University Press, 2000.

Soper, Fred L. "El concepto de la erradicación de las enfermedades transmisibles." *Boletín de la Oficina Sanitaria Panamericana* 42, no. 1 (1957): 1–5.

———. "YAWS: Its Eradication in the Americas." Washington, D.C., 1956. http://profiles .nlm.nih.gov/VV/B/B/D/H/.

Sowell, David. *The Tale of Healer Miguel Perdomo Neira: Medicine, Ideologies, and Power in the Nineteenth-Century Andes.* Wilmington, Del.: SR Books, 2001.

Spielman, Andrew, and Michael D'Antonio. *Mosquito, A Natural History of Our Most Persistent and Deadly Foe.* New York: Hyperion, 2001.

"The Spirit of Inter-American Unit, Address by Secretary Dulles, Made at Caracas, 4 March 1954." *Department of State Bulletin* 30 (1954): 379-383.

Stapleton, Darwin H. "Lessons of History? Anti-Malaria Strategies of the International Health Board and the Rockefeller Foundation from the 1920s to the Era of DDT." *Public Health Reports* 119, no. 2 (2004): 206–15.

———. "A Lost Chapter in the Early History of DDT: The Development of Anti-Typhus Technologies by the Rockefeller Foundation's Louse Laboratory, 1942–1944." *Technology and Culture* 46, no. 3 (2005): 513–40.

Starr, Douglas. *Blood: An Epic History of Medicine and Commerce.* New York: Alfred A. Knopf, 1998.

Stavenhagen, Rodolfo. *El campesinado y las estrategias del desarrollo rural.* Mexico City: Colegio de México, 1977.

Stepan, Nancy Leys. *"The Hour of Eugenics": Race, Gender, and Nation in Latin America.* Ithaca, N.Y.: Cornell University Press, 1991.

Stevens, James. "Welcoming Address." In *Industry and Tropical Health: Proceedings of the First Tropical Health Conference Sponsored by the Harvard School of Public Health, 8–0 December 1950,* ed. Industrial Council for Tropical Health. Boston: Harvard School of Public Health and International Council for Tropical Health, 1950.

Stoll, David. *Fishers of Men or Founders of Empire? The Wycliffe Bible Translators in Latin America.* London: Zed Press, 1982.

"Strategies against Malaria: Eradication or Control? Proceedings of a Conference, Annecy, France, April 17–26, 1996." *Parassitologia* 40, nos. 1–2 (1998): 1–246.

Stycos, J. Mayone. "Population Control in Latin America." *World Politics* 20, no. 1 (1967): 66–82.

Suárez Torres, Guillermo. *La Campaña Nacional para la Erradicación del Paludismo y su importancia para la salud pública* (Mexico City: Secretaría de Salubridad y Asistencia, 1973).

———. "Incremento de la lucha antipalúdica en el Estado de Oaxaca." *Boletín de la Sociedad Oaxaqueña de Salud Pública* 5, no. 1 (1970): 22.

———. "El Programa de Erradicación del Paludismo, plan de seis años." *Salud Pública de México* 12, no. 6 (1970): 751–73.

Summer Institute of Linguistics. *Veinticinco años del Instituto Lingüístico de Verano en México, 1935–1960.* Mexico City: Summer Institute of Linguistics, 1960.

Symonds, R., and M. Carder. *The United Nations and the Population Question, 1945–1970.* New York: McGraw-Hill, 1973.

Taliaferro, William H., ed. *Medicine and the War.* Chicago: University of Chicago Press, 1944.

Temin, P. *Taking Your Medicine: Drug Regulation in the United States.* Cambridge, Mass.: Harvard University Press, 1980.

Thibodeaux, Ben H. "The Role of Economic Cooperation and Technical Assistance in Our Foreign Policy." *Department of State Bulletin* 35 (1956): 808–12.

"33,000,000 Pounds of DDT Shipped Overseas in Malaria Program." *Department of State Bulletin* 39 (1958): 290–91.

Tipps, Dean C. "Modernization Theory and the Comparative Study of Societies: A Critical Perspective." *Comparative Studies in Society and History* 15, no. 2 (1973): 199–226.

Trout, Ben Thomas. "Political Legitimation and the Cold War." *International Studies Quarterly* 19, no. 3 (1975): 57–60.

Tudda, Chris. "Reenacting the Story of Tantalus, Eisenhower, Dulles and the Failed Rhetoric of Liberation." *Journal of Cold War Studies* 7, no. 4 (2005): 3–35.

Tulchin, Joseph S. "The United States and Latin America in the 1960s." *Journal of Interamerican Studies and World Affairs* 30, no. 1 (1988): 1–36.

Tuthill, J. W. "Malathion Poisoning." *New England Journal of Medicine* 258, no. 20 (1958): 1018–19.

"The United States and Mexico: Partners in a Common Task." *Department of State Bulletin* 46 (1962): 919–21.

U.S. Department of Commerce. *Investment in Mexico: Conditions and Outlook for United States Investors.* Washington, D.C. U.S. Government Printing Office, 1956.

U.S. Department of Health and Human Services. *Malaria.* Washington, D.C.: National Institute of Allergy and Infectious Diseases, National Institutes of Health, 2002.

U.S. Department of State. *American Foreign Policy: Current Document, 1956.* Washington, D.C.: U.S. Government Printing Office, 1959.

U.S. Environmental Protection Agency. *Health Effects Support Document for Aldrin/Dieldrin.* Washington, D.C.: U.S. Environmental Protection Agency, 2003.

U.S. House of Representatives. *HIV/AIDS, TB, and Malaria: Combating a Global Pandemic, Hearing before the Subcommittee on Health of the Committee on Energy and Commerce, House of Representatives, 108th Congress, First Session, 20 March 2003.* Washington, D.C.: U.S. Government Printing Office, 2003.

———. *The United States and International Health, Hearings before a Subcommittee of the Committee on Interstate and Foreign Commerce, House of Representatives, 84th Congress, February 8 and 9, 1956.* Washington, D.C.: U.S. Government Printing Office, 1956.

"U.S. Contribution to Help Fight Malaria in American Republics." *Department of State Bulletin* 36 (1957): 56–66.

Ulloa, M. "Malaria Eradication in Chile." *Parasitology Today* 5, no. 2 (1989): 31.

United Nations Children's Fund (UNICEF). *Children of the Developing Countries: A Report.* Cleveland: World Publishing, 1963.

United Nations Environment Program. *The United Nations Environment Program: A Brief Introduction.* Nairobi: United Nations Environment Program, 1975.

"United States Gives $7 Million to Malaria Eradication Campaign." *Department of State Bulletin* 37 (1957): 1000–3.

"United States–Mexico Border Public Health Association." *Public Health Reports* 73, no. 12 (1958): 1133–40.

Uribe González, Antonio. *Campeche: Ciudad del Carmen—historia, paludismo, inundaciones, petróleo.* Campeche: N.p., 1992.

U.S. Department of State. *American Policy, Current Document, 1956.* Washington, D.C.: U.S. Government Printing Office, 1959.

———. *Foreign Relations of the United States, 1958–1960, American Republics,* vol. 5. Washington, D.C.: U.S. Government Printing Office, 1991.

———. *Health and Sanitation, Cooperative Program in Mexico: Agreement between the United States of America and Mexico, Effected by Exchange of Notes Signed at Mexico September 20 and November 23, 1950, Entered into Force January 22, 1951; Operative Retroactively from June 30, 1950.* Washington: U.S. Government Printing Office, 1951).

———. *Principal Officers of the Department of State and United States Chiefs of Mission, 1778–1990.* Washington D.C.: U.S. Government Printing Office, 1991.

Valdespino Gómez, José Luis, Aurora del Rio Zolezzi, Alejandro Escobar Gutiérrez, and José Luis Mora Galindo, eds. *Una Institución Académica Mexicana y dieciséis investigadores distinguidos.* Mexico City: Secretaría de Salud, 1994.

Vargas, Lázaro. "Importancia de la Coordinación en Salud Pública y sus perspectivas." *Boletín de la Sociedad Oaxaqueña de Salud Pública* 5:2 (1970): 28-31.

Vargas, Luís. "Aspectos socioeconómicos de las zonas rurales mexicanas en relación con la erradicación del paludismo." *Revista del Instituto de Salubridad y Enfermedades Tropicales* 18, nos. 3–4 (1958): 145–86.

———. "Las casas y la transmisión del paludismo." *Boletín Epidemiológico* 20 (1956): 160–66.

———. "Consideraciones generales sobre la epidemiología de la malaria evanescente de México." *Gaceta Médica de México* 88, no. 9 (1958): 613–33.

———. "Fundamentos evolutivos de la teoría del estado y sus alcances en la erradicación el paludismo en México." *Salud Pública de México* 2 (1960): 489–99.

———. "La interpretación epidemiológica del paludismo, con énfasis en campañas de erradicación." *Revista Venezolana de Sanidad y Asistencia Social* 28, no. 4 (1963): 339–509.

———. "Malaria along the Mexico–United States Border." *Bulletin of the World Health Organization* 2, no. 4 (1950): 611–20.

———. "Notas sobre la transfusión sanguínea y el paludismo inducido en México." *Salud Pública de México* 14 (1972): 353–63.

———. "Problemas de identificación de vectores del paludismo y su biología, en las principales zonas endémicas de México." *Boletín de Sanidad Militar* 9 (1951): 435–39.

———. "Realizaciones del programa de Erradicación." *Salud Pública de México* 7 (1965): 737–40.

———. "El Tamaño de la localidad como factor epidemiológico en malariología." *Revista del Instituto de Salubridad y Enfermedades Tropicales* 20, no. 1 (1960): 193–211.

Vargas, Luís, and A. Almaraz Ugalde. "La erradicación del paludismo en México durante el segundo año de cobertura integral." *Revista del Instituto de Salubridad y Enfermedades Tropicales* 20, no. 3 (1960): 193–221.

———. "Evaluación epidemiológica de la erradicación del paludismo en 1959, tercer año de cobertura integral." *Salud Pública de México* 5 (1963): 257–69.

Vargas, Luís, and Amado Martínez Palacios. *Anofelinos mexicanos, taxonomía y distribución.* Mexico City: Secretaría de Salubridad y Asistencia, 1950.

———. "Distribución de los Anofelinos Mexicanos." *Revista del Instituto de Salubridad y Enfermedades Tropicales* 15, no. 2 (1955): 81–123.

———. *Estudio taxonómico de los mosquitos anofelicos de México.* Mexico City: Secretaría de Salubridad y Asistencia, 1950.

Vargas, Luís, G. Román y Carillo, and A. Almaraz y Ugalde. "Organization and Evaluation of the Malaria Eradication Campaign in Mexico during the First Year of Complete Coverage." *Bulletin of the World Health Organization* 19, no. 4 (1958): 621–35.

Vargas Lozano, René. "Dirección de servicios médicos rurales cooperativos." *Salud Pública de México* 6, no. 6 (1964): 967–78.

Villalobos Revilla, José L. "Informe médico de la población de Jalpa, Zacatecas, Indice de Ross: Tratamiento de la ulcera gastroduodenal por la uroenterona (Kutrol)." Tesis para sustentar examen profesional de médico cirujano y partero, Universidad Nacional Autonoma de México, Mexico City, 1954.

Villaseñor, F. "Los medios audiovisuales en la enseñanza." *Salud Pública de México* 2 (1960): 77–80.

Vries, Lini de. *The People of the Mountains: Health Education among Indian Communities in Oaxaca, Mexico.* Cuernavaca: Centro Intercultural de Documentación, 1969.

Walgate, Robert. "Global Fund for AIDS, TB and Malaria Opens Shop." *Bulletin of the World Health Organization* 80, no. 3 (2002): 259–59.

Wang, Jessica. *American Science in the Age of Anxiety: Scientists, Anticommunism and the Cold War.* Chapel Hill: University of Carolina Press, 1999.

Warrell, David A., and Herbert M. Gilles, eds. *Essential Malariology,* 4th ed. London: Arnold, 2002.

Weir, David, and Mark Schapiro. *Circle of Poison: Pesticides in a Hungry World.* San Francisco: Institute for Food and Development Policy, 1981.

Werner, Michael S., ed. *Encyclopaedia of Mexico, History, Society and Culture,* vol. 2. London: Fitzroy Dearborn, 1997.

Westad, Odd Arne, ed. *Reviewing the Cold War: Approaches, Interpretations, and Theory.* London: F. Cass, 2000.

"WHA22.39 Re-examination of the Global Strategy of Malaria Eradication." Twenty-Second World Health Assembly, July 24, 1969, Boston. http://policy.who.int/cgibin/om_isapi.dll?infobase=WHA&softpage=Browse_Frame_Pg42

White, L. *Speaking with Vampires: Rumor and History in Colonial Africa.* Berkeley: University of California Press, 2000.

Whiteford, Michael B. "Homeopathic Medicine in the City of Oaxaca, Mexico: Patients' Perspectives and Observations." *Medical Anthropology Quarterly* 13, no. 1 (1999): 69–78.

White House. *U.S. Participation in the UN: Report by the President to the Congress for the Year 1959.* Washington, D.C.: U.S. Government Printing Office, 1959.

Whorton, James. *Before Silent Spring: Pesticides and Public Health in Pre-DDT America.* Princeton, N.J.: Princeton University Press, 1975.

Wilcox, Aimee. *Manual for the Microscopical Diagnosis of Malaria in Man.* Washington, D.C.: U.S. Government Printing Office, 1950.

Wilcox, Francis O. "The First Ten Years of the World Health Organization." *Department of State Bulletin* 38 (1958): 987–88.

———. "International Organizations: Aid to World Trade and Prosperity." *Department of State Bulletin* 37 (1957): 749–54.

———. "World Population and Economic Development." *Department of State Bulletin* 42 (1960): 860–67.

Williams, Glen. "WHO: The Days of the Mass Campaigns." *World Health Forum* 9 (1988): 7–23.

Williams, Louis, Jr. "The Entomologist and the International Health Program." *Journal of Economic Entomology* 42, no. 4 (1949): 710–12.

———. "Malaria Eradication: Growth of the Concept and Its Application." *American Journal of Tropical Medicine and Hygiene* 7, no. 3 (1958): 259–67.

Worboys, Michael. "Tropical Diseases." In *Companion Encyclopedia of the History of Medicine,* vol. 1, ed. William F. Bynum and Roy Porter. London: Routledge, 1993.

World Health Organization. *Implementation of the Global Malaria Control Strategy: Report of a WHO Study Group on the Implementation of the Global Plan of Action for Malaria Control 1993–2000.* Geneva: World Health Organization, 1993.

————. *Malaria Control as Part of Primary Health Care: Report of WHO Study Group.* Geneva: World Health Organization, 1984.

————. *A Plea for Health.* Geneva: World Health Organization, 1958.

————. *Resolutions and Decisions: Plenary Meetings, Verbatim Records, Committees, Minutes and Annexes—Official Records of the WHO, No. 63.* Geneva: World Health Organization, 1955.

————. *The Work of WHO 1956.* Geneva: World Health Organization, 1957.

————. *The Work of WHO 1992–1993: Biannual Report of the Director General to the World Health Assembly and to the United Nations.* Geneva: World Health Organization, 1994.

————. *Twenty-Second World Health Assembly, Boston, Massachusetts, 8–25 July 1969, Part II, Plenary Meetings, Committees, Summary Records and Reports.* Geneva: World Health Organization, 1969.

————. *World Directory of Medical Schools.* Geneva: World Health Organization, 1957.

Woodbridge, George. *UNRRA: The History of the United Nations Relief and Rehabilitation Administration.* 3 vols. New York: Columbia University Press, 1950.

Wright, Angus. *The Death of Ramón González: The Modern Agricultural Dilemma.* Austin: University of Texas Press, 1997.

————. "Rethinking the Circle of Poison: The Politics of Pesticide Poisoning among Mexican Farm Workers." *Latin American Perspectives* 13, no. 4 (1986): 26–59.

Yekutiel, Perez. "Lessons from the Big Eradication Campaigns." *World Health Forum* 2 (1981): 465–90.

Yoder, Andres J. "Lessons from Stockholm: Evaluating the Global Convention on Persistent Organic Pollutants." *Indiana Journal of Global Legal Studies* 10, no. 2 (2003): 113–56.

Zeiler, Thomas W. *Dean Rusk: Defending the American Mission Abroad.* Wilmington, Del.: Scholarly Books, 2000.

Zimmerman, Oswald T., and Irvin Lavine. *DDT: Killer of Killers.* Dover, N.H.: Industrial Research Service, 1946.

Zulueta, J. de, and C. Garret-Jones. "An Investigation of the Persistence of Malaria Transmission in Mexico." *American Journal of Tropical Medicine and Hygiene* 14, no. 1 (1965): 63–77.

Index

Acapulco, 75, 114
Act of International Development
(1951), 31
Africa: eradication as unachievable, 44;
excluded from programs, 44–45,
180n125; incidence in, 163
agreement for malaria eradication
(Mexico), 86–88
Agricultural Act (1933), 3
agriculture, 57–58; costs of malaria,
58–59, 71–72; Mexico, 71, 156
Aguascalientes, 115, 133
Aguirre Beltrán, Gonzalo, 120
AHEH (hygienic education honorary
auxiliaries), 109–11
AIDS, 11, 162–63
Aldrin, 61
Alemán, Miguel, 74
Alliance for Progress, 6, 27–28, 152–53,
174n47
Alvarado, Carlos, 39, 45, 46, 52–53; on
educational work, 115; on malaria
eradication, 177n85; at Santiago
meeting, 34, 35–36
Álvarez Amézquita, José, 80
Americanization, 28–30
*American Journal of Tropical Medicine
and Hygiene,* 67

American Republic Affairs Office, 19
anemia, 133
Anopheles mosquito, 1–2, 15, 17, 140,
153, 177n84
anthropological critique of malaria
eradication, 120–28
anticommunism: code terms validating,
7; Dulles on, 19; health and disease,
16; Mexico, 80–81; modernization
model, 22
antimalaria vaccines, 162
antipesticide activists, 134
applied medical anthropology, 123, 135
Argentina, 18, 34, 45, 97
Artemisinin Combination Therapies, 162
Artesimin, 154
assimilation, 119, 135
Atabrine, 5, 49
atomic energy: in medicine, 40; in
Mexico, 75
attack phase, 46–47
audiovisual materials, 201n168
authoritarian regimes, 9, 12
Ávila Camacho, Manuel, 72, 74, 78

Baz, Gustavo, 73
bedbugs, 136–39
Belgium, 43–44

bilateral agencies, multilateral agencies vs., 52–53
bilateral cooperation, 18; first U.S., 31; technical aid, 23, 25; UN cost-sharing, 20–21
Bill and Melinda Gates Foundation, 162
bioethical dimensions, 131
blood smears: AHEHs taking, 111; blood samples, 116*f;* diagnostic tool, 48, 99; fears of, 126; indigenous reaction to, 13, 120, 125–27, 210*n*72; morbidity trends, 98
Board of Health (Mexico), 72
Board of Rural Hygiene and Social Medicine, 83
border areas, Mexico-U.S., 56, 77, 192*n*41
Brazil: Campbell in, 50; Candau and, 40–41; Cloroquinated salt, 45; incidence, 163; Kubitschek, 26; malaria control, 18, 97, 145; reactions to public health interventions, 11; Rockefeller Foundation and, 77; Soper and, 3
British Guiana, 4, 45
Bruce-Chwatt, Leonard, 150
bulletins, CNEP, 105–9, 111
Bureau of Inter-American Affairs, 20; organization of, 171*n*13
Bureau of International Organization Affairs, 19–20
Bustamante, Miguel, 80

campaign, use of term, 8, 16
Campbell, Eugene P., 50–53; background, 50–51, 182*n*146; as key player, 33; malaria eradication hearings, 55–60; report, 67
cancer, 134
Candau, Marcelino, 60, 66; background, 40–41; as key player, 33; retirement, 150; at Santiago meeting, 34
Cárdenas, Lázaro, 117, 129

Catholic Church: development and, 10; malaria eradication, 86; pro-natalism, 58
Centers for Disease Control and Prevention (CDC), 50–51, 87
Central America, pesticide poisoning, 150, 161
Ceylon, 57, 144
Chiapas, 105, 106–7, 115, 117, 126, 132, 140–41, 160–61, 206*n*20, 207*n*32, 209*n*64
Chile, 97
China, 18, 197*n*104
chinches, 136–37
Chloroquine, 4–5, 15; effects of, 48–49; as leading drug, 61; origins, 182*n*141
circle of poison, 150, 218*n*190
Ciudad Juárez, 77, 84
CNEP (National Commission for the Eradication of Paludism): achievements, 97; assumptions, 164; bulletins, 105–9, 111; cause for failure, 144–45; creation, 88; day-to-day operations, 89; decline of campaign, 139–46; five-year plan (1963), 143–44; four-stage design, 96; goals modified, 96; health education eforts, 112–20; health workers blamed, 142; "human bait" for mosquitos, 131; inauguration, 70; individual treatment adopted, 158; Mexicanization of campaign, 100–111; as model, 97; new perspective, 158; non-Spanish materials, 101–2; organization, 88–91; perceived as eliminating the poor, 133–34, 137; persistence of program, 154–55; pilot programs, 95–96, 141–42; problem areas, 99, 139–40, 142; propaganda, 101–9, 138; relaunch effort, 145; response to criticisms, 135, 157; rural schoolteachers, 100–101, 111; salaries, 95; staff growth, 94–95,

98; on traditional medicine, 119; unions, 155; as vertical health program, 158, 159; Villalobos's criticisms of, 130–33; Villalobos's initial ties, 130; zones, 91, 92*t*–93*t*
code terms, 7
Cold War: aid and national security, 5; as all-encompassing culture, 7; contradictions noted, 13; foreign aid, 17–33; health agencies and, 28–30; metaphors, 42, 64–65, 103; Mexico on, 82; Rio Treaty, 23; role in scientific research, 7; *Sputnik* significance, 65; U.S. foreign policy, 5–6; vanishing, 152
Colegio de México, 155
Collective Plan of Antimalaria Treatment (PTCA), 141
Colombia, 11, 35, 97
commercial agriculture: anticommunism and, 7–8; Mexico, 72, 75–76, 98; model of development, 9–10, 12; pesticides, 62; rural peoples and, 13; toxic chemicals, 140
Committee on Foreign Relations, 2, 26
communism: in Latin America, 25–26, 174*n*41; malaria-related, 34; U.S. efforts to contain, 5–6, 7; as virus, 8
communists, in Mexico, 16, 80
community-supported or horizontal approaches, 164
Congress, U.S.: appearances in, 51–52; bill authorizing, 63; foreign aid questioned, 50; funding, 60; ICA in, 54; malaria eradication hearing, 54; reservations of, 39
congressional committees, 54–55
consolidation phase, 47, 140
Constitution of 1917, 72
containment policy, 171*n*11; double political discourse, 45; Dulles on, 19; significance of term, 8

control phase, 47
Correa, Manuel, 137
corridos, 107
Corsica, 4
Costa Rica, 11, 44, 97
cost-sharing concept, 57, 59
costs of malaria, Mexico, 71, 87
costs of malaria eradication: estimated, 44; hearings in Congress, 58, 63; in Latin America, 186*n*198; in Mexico, 86–87, 99, 143–44; report on, 67; spraying, 53
Cuba, 16, 43, 52, 82, 97
Cuban revolution, 6, 27
cultural diffusion, 68, 118
cultural hegemony, 28–30
culture of survival, 8–9, 158, 165, 166

DDT (dichloro-diphenyl-trichloroethane): assumptions about, 15; as atomic bomb of insect world, 17; background, 61; as carcinogenic in humans, 134; concerns about, 12; debate on, 148–49; discovery of, 4; environmental impact, 131, 148–49, 161; exports dumped, 149–50; in Mexico, 83–85, 145; phaseout, 161; produced by Mexican government, 146; recent advocates, 161; recent use, 161; U.S. ban on, 149; and World War II, 17
DDT resistance: Candau on, 41–42; Russell on, 43, 44; WHO on, 214*n*128
DDT sprayers, 91, 92*t*–93*t*, 94–96; bedbug proliferation, 136–39; as *matagatos,* 132, 211*n*95; risks, 131; suspicions about quality, 138
DDT spraying: acculturation centers, 118; costs, 53; described, 15, 69; impact reported, 194*n*73; indigenous dwellings, 119–20, 124; Santiago proposal, 34; *Sixth Report,* 46–47

death, attitudes toward, 108
Democratic Party, 16, 54
demonstration campaigns, 8, 57
Department of State Bulletin, 19–20, 22, 26, 28
Department of State. *See* State Department
détente foreign policy, 6
diagnostic techniques, 47–48, 98
dictatorial regimes, 9, 65–66
Dieldrin, 61, 62, 95, 214*n*128; amounts used in Mexico, 132; resistance, 140
Dieldrin Study Project, 113
Dirección General de Epidemiología y Campañas Sanitarias, 83, 84, 88
disease, research on, 11
disease eradication, 170*n*36
Does Overpopulation Mean Poverty? (Black), 146
Dominican Republic, 65–66, 97
Downs, W. G., 83–84
drugs: costs of, 185*n*195; PAHO on, 199*n*135; Santiago proposal, 34; Western and indigenous medicine compared, 127
drugs and medical supplies, 29
Dulles, John Foster, 19, 25, 31, 45, 55, 65, 80, 187*n*220
DuPont, 62

Echeverría, Luís, 135, 155–56
economic benefits, 59
economic miracle, Mexican, 74, 156
economic policies, 79
economic take-off theory, 28
Ecuador, 97, 180*n*120
Education, Secretariat of, 100
education: teaching Indians Spanish, 118; as tool for political legitimacy, 10
Educational Action Groups, 109
Ehrlich, Paul, 147
Eighth World Health Assembly (Mexico City), 40, 42–43, 86

Eisenhower, Dwight: double political discourse, 45; Dulles and, 19; Latin America policy, 27; Mexican relations, 79, 82; nonmilitary aid, 24–25; Operation Pan-America, 26; on population control, 58; reelection, 50; rhetorical diplomacy, 25; on world health, 22
Eisenhower, Milton S., 54, 183–84*n*164
ejidos, 75–76
elites, local professional, 68
El Paso, Texas, 77, 84
El Salvador, 35, 97
enslaving, use of term, 16, 26, 64–65
environmental pollution, 131–32
environmental sanitation, 3
environmental studies, 148–49
eradicationist perspective, 14
Europe, economic aid to, 21, 174*n*45
European influences, 28, 29
European involvement in malaria eradication, 66
executive agencies, 54
experts: panel, 66; role of, 8, 68

family-planning and birth control programs, 151
Fertilizations Mexicanos (Fertimex), 146, 147
films, 102
Finlay, Carlos, 2
Food and Agriculture Organization (FAO), 149
foreign aid: as business subsidy, 61; Cold War, 17–33; cultural hegemony and, 28; debates in Congress, 55–56; development and medical science, 64; funding, 50; goals questioned, 50; humanitarian, 37; nonmilitary, 24–25, 26; participation, 49
Foreign Operations Administration, 183*n*163
foreign policy: Cold War, 5–6, 171*n*11;

return to unilateralism, 153; social reform, 27; State Department, 18, 22; UN participation, 20–21
Foster, George, 120–21
France, 37, 43
"free world," as symbolic term, 8
Fulbright program, 28–29

G-8 (Group of Eight), 162
Gabaldón, Arnoldo, 45–46, 148, 150, 155, 177n81
García Manzanedo, Héctor, 123–28
General Law of Population (1947), 78
German Bayer Company, 4
Giglioli, George, 45, 181n133
Global Fund to Fight AIDS, Tuberculosis, and Malaria, 13, 162–63
global health concept, xii
Global Malaria Control Strategy, 162
global treaty banning pesticides, 161
González, Carlos Luís, 86
Gorgas, William, 2
grants, 56
Green Revolution, 76–77
Guanos y Fertilizantes de México (Guanomex), 146
Guatemala, 50, 82, 97, 140–41, 161, 174n43
Guerrero, 106, 113, 133, 137–38, 144, 160, 206n20, 212n100

Haiti, 11, 38, 43, 97, 219n199
health agencies, Cold War motivations, 28–30
health education: mass media in, 12; in Mexico, 17
health interventions, significance of, 10
health systems, xii
health workers, 105–9; conspiracy against poor peasants, 137; coordination among health services, 151–52; hegemonic trend, 12; local reception, 114

Hercules, 62
Hexachlorocyclohexane (HCH), 145–46
historical knowledge: about public health issues, xi; need for, 165
Hoffman, Carlos C., 197n115
Hollister, John B., 31–32
homes. *See* indigenous dwellings
Honduras, 97
hookworm, 18
Horwitz, Abraham, 144
host governments, 38–39, 40, 51, 57, 59
Hudson Manufacturers, 62
human body, indigenous view of, 125
humanitarian dimension, 63
Hyde, Henry van Zile, 51, 121

ICA (International Cooperation Agency), 31–33; DDT purchased, 62; expert panel, 66; funding, 188n234; International Development Advisory Board, 49–50; origins, 183n163; public health activities, 32; Rockefeller Foundation compared, 32–33; role, 52; status, 60; technical staff, 32
ideology: in Cold War, 7; USSR bloc on WHO, 21–22
imperialism, U.S., 26
indigenous dwellings, DDT spraying, 119–20, 124, 130
indigenous languages: anthropologists on, 122; campaign ignoring, 123–24; CNEP health education, 112–20; health communication problems, 115, 117; non-Spanish materials, 101–2; resistance to malaria eradication, 136; teaching Indians Spanish, 118
indigenous medicine, 109–10, 114, 119; anthropologists on, 120; differing concepts, 125; doctors on, 123; less antagonistic view, 207n32; persistence of, 127; types of fever, 209n68; views on drugs compared, 127

indigenous peoples, 11; assumptions about, 112–13; attitude to aid, 75; as disease carriers, 118; Mexicanization of, 118; resistance to malaria eradication programs, 128, 136–39, 157; stereotypes, 118, 120
indigenous revolt, 13
Industry and Tropical Health meetings, 6–7
infectious diseases, 61
insecticide resistance: Candau on, 41–42; dilemma of eradication, 179n114; Frankenstein mites, 139; Villalobos on, 132
insecticides: bilateral agency purchases, 62–63; contamination from, 125, 131–32, 135, 213n108; costs of, 185n195; criticisms of, 131–35; environmental effects, 136–39; FAO on, 149; indigenous resistance to use, 119–20; on mud walls, 113; uneven application, 35; U.S. as source, 60–61
insecticide sprayers, 51
Institute of Inter-American Affairs, 31, 175n57
Institute for Social Anthropology, 121
Institutional Revolutionary Party (PRI), 73, 78, 156
Instituto Nacional Indigenista, 117, 135
Integral Planned Acculturation Program, 117
interagency coordination, 53
Inter-American Conference (Caracas), 26
Inter-American Treaty of Reciprocal Assistance, 23
intercultural perspective, lacking, 13
international congresses on malaria and tropical medicine, 33–34, 176n78
International Development Advisory Board, 49–50

International Educational Exchange Services (IEES), 28–29, 30
international health cooperation, xii, 6, 33–49
international health programs, political ends and, 7
international public health, 6
investment: in Latin America, 23–24, 172–73n27; in Mexico, 79
Iron Curtain, 18
islands of eradication, 57
isolationism, 56

jaundice, 133
Johnson, Lyndon, 27, 55, 151, 153

Kelly, Isabel, 121–28
Kennan, George, 19
Kennedy, John F., 27
Khrushchev, Nikita, 25
Korean War, 24

laboratory techniques, 47–48
labor unions, 155
Labouisse, Henry R., 150
Lacandona people, 106–7
The Lancet, 151
land reform, 75–76, 100
Laredo, Texas, 79
Latin America: Americans residing in, 22–23; CNEP model, 97; Cold War politics in, 9; costs to, 59–60; economic interest in, 22; eradication record, 164; malaria control projects, 182n146; population growth, 57–58; postwar ties, 23–24; prestige of programs, 68; role of experts, 68; urgency of malaria situation, 180n120
League of Nations, 20
León Portilla, Miguel, 124
"liberating," use of term, 16
Lombardo Toledano, Vicente, 81

López Mateos, Adolfo, 80
López Portillo, 221*n*223
loyalty oaths, 122

McCarthy, Joseph, 55, 122
magic bullets, 14, 17, 152, 157
malaria: associated maladies, 39; effects of, 41; hopes raised for definitive solution, 13; incidence, 34, 163; incidence in Mexico, 71, 163; as king of diseases, 1; main vectors in Mexico, 90; racialized version, 118; reestablished in Mexico, 141; shift from control to eradication, 39–40; as source of lethargy, 63–64; Spanish and indigenous terms for, 117, 206*n*19; symptoms, 1; types in Latin America, 2
malaria control: malaria eradication programs compared, 47*t;* methods, 17; in Mexico, 82–86; origins and development, 2–7
malaria eradication: assumptions about, 15; as belief system, 164; bill authorizing, 63; biological and political aspects, 16; CNEP program compared, 96; as containment strategy, 45; critics, 43–44; decline of, 146–51; division of labor, 40; driving force, 15; educational goal of, 114–15; engineering virtuosity required, 177*n*85; feasibility, 34–36; goal of, 8; lessons of, 163–66; local responses, 12–13, 112–20, 156; Mexican experience summarized, 1; numbers of programs, 41; organization in Mexico, 86–99; postwar campaigns, 5; requirements for success, 12
malaria eradication, resistance to: by anthropologists, 120–28; by indigenous peoples, 128, 136–39; by provincial doctor, 128–36

malaria eradication: reversal of position on, 144; Russell on, 43, 44; social aspects, 57–58; as state building and political centralization, 10; U.S. Cold War goals related, 6; U.S. commitment, 49–50; vertical campaigns, 41
malaria eradication determinism, 44
Malathion, 51, 145–46
Malthus, Thomas, 147
Maracay Malaria School, 45, 87, 94, 97, 177*n*81
March to the Seas program, 76
Márquez Escobedo, Manuel B., 89–90
Marshall Plan, 21
Martínez Báez, Manuel, 73
medical acculturation, 119–20
medicalization, process of, 88
medical schools, 160
medical technologies, magic bullets and, 14
mefloquine, 153
Merck, 62
metaphors: Cold War, 42, 64–65, 103, 148; master, 16; medical, 28; military, 16, 43, 49, 68, 70, 102–3, 145. *See also* propaganda
Mexican Agricultural Program, 76–77
Mexican-American Cultural Institute, 29
Mexican Communist Party, 80
Mexicanization, 70; of campaign, 100–111; of indigenous peoples, 118; with lay volunteers, 109–11
Mexican Revolution of 1910, 72, 78
Mexico: contributions, 190–91*n*27; DDT in, 83–85; first location for program, 68; malaria control, 82–86; persistence of malaria eradication, 154–55; productivity losses, 58–59; recent experience with malaria, 159–63; Russell's methods in, 42; stereotypes, 63–64; tourism, 24

Mexico City, 147; world health
conference, 40, 42–43, 86
Mexico-U.S. relations, 78–82, 193*n*55
military, Mexican, 89
military metaphors, 16, 43, 49, 68, 70,
102–3, 145
model agreement for health delivery,
38–39
modernization: malaria eradication as
tool, 53–54; use of term, 10
modernization model, 6, 9–10;
anticommunism and, 22; critics,
152–53; foreign aid, 18, 21; Mexican,
74–75, 104; Mexican anthropologists
on, 152; Rostow on, 28
Monsanto, 62
Montrose Chemical Corporation, 62
Morelos, 142
Morones Prieto, Ignacio, 73, 86, 99
mortality: annual, 1; in Mexico, 71,
97–98, 189*n*6, 206*n*20, 209*nn*59, 64
mosquitoes: species in Mexico,
195–96*n*90; view of indigenous people,
125. *See also Anopheles* mosquito
mosquito resistance to DDT, 35, 132
Muller, Paul, 4
multilateral agencies: bilateral agencies
vs., 52–53; developing nation
preference for, 21; emergence, 18
mutual defense pacts, 23
Mutual Security legislation, 31

National Commission of Malaria, 85
National Coordinated Services, 125
National Institute of Allergy and
Infectious Diseases, 162
nationalism, among host countries, 51
nationalism, Mexican: among health
workers, 12; health education and,
100; mild postwar, 103; offical, 10,
103–4; pro-natalism and, 78, 104; and
U.S. relations, 79–82

National Lottery, 102
National Museum of Anthropology, 104
National Nuclear Energy Commission, 75
National Peasant Conferederation
(CNC), 73
national security, 5, 7, 22
Nation-Wide Malaria Eradication
Projects in the Americas symposium,
33
The Natural History of Mosquitoes
(Bates), 49
Neghme, Amador, 35
New Century Scholars Program, xiii
newspaper articles, 133
Nicaragua, 35, 97
Nixon, Richard, 26
North American Institute, 114
Norway, 43
notification posts, 109–11
nuclear arms, 24

Oaxaca, 71, 83, 85, 91, 101, 114,
117–18, 123, 126, 127, 130, 136–37,
141, 152, 156, 157, 159–60, 187*n*215,
206*n*20, 209*n*59
Oficina de Especialización Sanitaria, 83
oil expropriation, 78
Operation Pan-America, 26
Organization of American States (OAS),
23, 153
organization of this book, 7–11
overpopulation, 57–58, 104, 146–48,
151, 155–56, 217*n*169

paludismo, use of term, 115–17
Pampana, Emilio, 35, 39, 177*n*84, 198*n*118
Panama, 2, 16, 97
Pan-American Health Organization
(PAHO): on drug use, 199*n*135;
Global Malaria Control Strategy, 162;
on malaria eradication, 144; Special
Malaria Fund, 151

Pan-American Union, 23
Paraguay, 97, 144
Paris green, 17
Partido Popular, 81
PASB (Pan-American Sanitary Bureau):
  division of labor, 40; fourteenth
  conference (Santiago), 34–36;
  funding, 32, 37, 66, 75; limited
  programs, 45; Mexican study project,
  113; Mexico's contribution, 191n27;
  role, 52; shift from control to
  eradication, 39; Special Office of
  Malaria Eradication, 36; as technical
  institution, 39; Tripartite Plan in
  Mexico, 86–87; U.S. aid, 65,
  183n164
Patarroyo, Manuel, 162
Pate, Maurice, 33, 37–38, 39, 150
Pérez Jiménez, Marco, 66
perfection, 46
Peru, 3, 26, 97
pesticide poisoning, 218n192;
  antipesticide activists, 134; Central
  America, 150; Lagunera, 161
Petróleos Mexicanos (PEMEX), 84
pharmaceutical purchases from U.S.
  suppliers, 29, 60–61, 79
physicians: compulsory rural year, 129;
  rate among population, 129;
  unemployment in Mexico, 160
pilot project, Mexican, 87; field-spraying
  operations, 95–96
Pinotti, Mario, 45
Plan of Individual Responsibility
  (PRIAL), 141–42
plan of this book, 11–14
Plasmodium, 2, 15, 125, 126–27, 139,
  153, 154, 160, 162
Pletsch, Donald J., 88–89, 133, 148,
  197n105
poems, 107–9, 203n203

Poland, 21
Policy Planning Council, 28
political rhetoric, language used, 16–17
politicians, in Mexico, 78–81
politics of Mexico, 71–82
poor people: view of experts, 8–9; view
  of public health work, 165
population control, 57–58, 146–48,
  221n223
population explosion, 146–48
posters, 102–3
poverty, disease and, 9
primaquine, 49, 141, 142
Primary Health Care, 157–58
primitivism, 51
PRI. *See* Institutional Revolutionary
  Party (PRI)
privileges of poverty, 165, 166
pro-natalism, 58, 78, 104, 148, 156
propaganda: anticommunist, 8; CNEP,
  101–9, 138; limitations, 115; pro-U.S.
  psychological warfare, 30; Soviet
  shortwave, 25; stereotypes, 63–64.
  See also metaphors
Protestants, 114
public health: community-supported or
  horizontal approaches, 164; main
  issues, xi; Mexico, 72, 75; tradition of
  discontinuity, 142–43; understanding
  of nature and aims, 165
Public Health Division, 32
public health education, xi, 165; critics
  of, 124–25
public health programs, 121;
  fragmentation of, 143; recent capacity
  in Mexico, 160
pyrimethamine, 49

qinghaosu, 154
quinine, 4, 83, 167n10
Quiotepec, Oaxaca, 136–37

racial prejudice, 118
radio, 102, 104
Rajchman, Ludwig, 37
Reader's Digest, 68–69, 134
Red Scare, 48, 122
regional security, 22
Republican Party, 16
research, need for, 165
Resochin, 4–5, 182*n*141
Rio Treaty, 23
Rockefeller, Nelson, 31, 36
Rockefeller Foundation: agreements with
    host governments, 38–39; agricultural
    development, 19; Americanization, 29;
    cultural hegemony, 29; DDT testing,
    194*n*72; demonstration system, 57;
    Green Revolution, 76–77; as health
    leader, 33; ICA compared, 32–33; in
    interwar period, 18; and malaria in
    Mexico, 77, 83; military-style
    campaigns, 2–3; role in organizing
    public health systems, 11; Rusk at, 28;
    and Russell, 42; U.S. foreign policy,
    18–19
Roll Back Malaria program, 13, 162
Romero Álvarez, Humberto, 90
Rostow, Walt W., 28
Rubottom, Roy R., 171–72*n*13
Ruíz Cortines, Adolfo, 70, 74–75, 79, 87
rural medicine, 129
rural peoples: demographics, 124; health
    care for, 143, 157; "incorporating,"
    117; Mexico, 75, 112
rural sanitation, 3
rural schools, 100
rural schoolteachers, 100–101, 111
Rusk, Dean, 27–28, 36
Russell, Paul F.: background, 42;
    blueprint, 46; and expert panel, 66; on
    feasibility and advantages, 53, 54; and
    funding, 50; influence in Mexico, 90;
    malaria eradication hearings, 55–60;

in Mexico, 86; Mexico City
    conference, 42–43; retirement, 150;
    vocabulary for health workers, 117

sanitary perspectives, xi, 3, 12;
    acculturation centers, 117–18;
    indigenous reaction, 138
San Luís Potosí, 115
school textbooks, 104
Science, 148, 149
science and technology, attitudes about,
    60
scorpion bites, 132
Secretaría de Salubridad y Asistencia, xv,
    72–73
Secretaría de Salud (Secretariat of
    Health), xv, 82–83, 100
Shell Chemical Corporation, 61, 62, 113
Silent Spring (Carson), 148, 150
Sixth Report (1956), 46–48
Soberón y Parra, Galo, 84–85, 195*n*86
social consequences of malaria
    eradication, 57–58
socialist education, 100
social reform, 27
Social Security program (IMSS), 73–74
Sonora, 134
Soper, Fred L.: anticommunist remarks
    in Mexico, 81; at Santiago meeting,
    34, 35–36; background, 34, 40–41;
    eradication plea, 39; and expert panel,
    66; on funding, 52, 53; as key player,
    33; and malaria control in Brazil, 3,
    18; Mexican campaign, 88; Mexican
    research, 91; rationale followed, 50;
    research dismissed, 144; retirement,
    150
Southeast Asia, 53
southern United States, 3
Soviet Union, former: de-Stalinization,
    25; donations, 188*n*226; fears about
    Latin America, 24; malaria eradication

plans, 67–68; Mexican relations, 81; peaceful coexistence era, 145; post-colonial era, 19; propaganda, 25; on UN and WHO, 21; in U.S. propaganda, 8
space race, 145
Spanish-American War, 16
spraying equipment, 62, 95. *See also* DDT spraying
Sputnik significance, 65
Stalin, Joseph, 25
State Department: on foreign technical aid, 6; and funding, 54; as key actor, 18; on Mexico, 82; on military aid, 23; on multilateral health agencies, 32; organizational changes, 19–20; reorganization, 30–31; under Dulles, 19–20
Stavenhagen, Rodolfo, 152
stereotypes: indigenous peoples, 118, 120; in malaria propaganda, 63–64
Summer Institute of Linguistics, 114, 205*n*11

Taft, Robert A., 31
technical cooperation, institutionalizing, 31
Technical Cooperation Administration, 31
Tennessee Valley Authority (TVA), 3, 163–64, 184*n*168
thick blood film technique, 48
Tlateloco massacre, 156
Torres Bondet, Jaime, 80
tourism, 24
trade, 23–24
Training Center for Malaria Eradication Field Officers, 87
transfusion malaria, 143
translators/interpreters, 113, 114
Tripartite Agreement, 88, 99
Tripartite Plan, 86–87, 143, 190*n*14
Trique Indians, 127

tropical health care, 11
tropical medicine, 3
Truman, Harry, 31, 197*n*104
tuberculosis, 162–63
typhus, 4
Tzeltal-Tzotzil Center, 117

underdeveloped countries, 7, 60
underpopulation, 148
undocumented workers, 79
United Fruit Company, 19
United Kingdom, 43
United Nations: important agencies in, 172*n*15; Latin American votes, 24; Population Division, 148; U.S. contributions, 179*n*110, 186*n*212; U.S. policy, 19, 20
United Nations Children's Fund (UNICEF): change in emphasis, 37–38; division of labor, 40; donations, 39, 75, 99, 179*n*104; eradication crusade, 36–37; eradication equipment in Mexico, 95; eradication investment, 217*n*166; Executive Board, 40, 41; funding, 32, 37; funds spent in Latin America, 38; limited programs, 45; in malaria control, 39; Mexico programs, 87, 196*n*95; program abandoned, 146; public image, 38; Roll Back Malaria, 162; as technical institution, 39; Tripartite Plan in Mexico, 86–87
United Nations Development Program, 162
United Nations Relief and Rehabilitation Administration, 4, 168*n*12
United States: international health cooperation, xii; malaria eradication accomplished, 97, 163–64; post-colonial era, 19; reemergence of malaria, 153–54; World War II era, 3–5

United States–Mexico Border Public Health Association, 77, 135
United States Public Health Service, 20
University of California–Berkeley, 122
UN Security Council, 21
urbanization, 147
U.S. Agency for International Development (USAID), 31, 148, 151, 186n211, 219n199
U.S. Army Malaria Drug Development Program, 4
U.S. Environmental Protection Agency, 149
U.S. Information Agency (USIA), 29–30
U.S. National Malaria Society, 33
U.S. Public Health Service, 33

Vargas, Luís, 42, 90–91, 139, 148, 197n115
Vasconcelos, José, 103
Venezuela, 4, 11, 26, 44, 45–46, 163; celebration, 68; Pérez Jiménez, 66. *See also* Maracay Malaria School
vertical health program, 163–66; CNEP as, 158, 159
Vietnam veterans, 153–54
Villalobos, José, 128–36, 213n108
viral mutations due to environmental changes, 134, 135
Virgin of Guadalupe, 86
Voice of America, 30
volunteers, 109–11, 204n209

war in Vietnam, 153–54, 162
Welfare Secretariat, 72
Western medicine: anthropologists on, 120; malaria eradication as tool for expansion of, 119; propaganda, 114; responses to, 10–11, 121; socio-economic factors and medicalization, 142, 207n31; traditional indigenous medicine vs., 109–10, 114, 119–20; views on drugs compared, 127
WHO-UNICEF Joint Committee on Health Policy, 38, 39
WHO (World Health Organization): assessment and surveillance, 151; bilateral campaigns, 5; Candau role, 40–41; critics at, 181n126; decline of program, 151; design and direction from, 38; Division of Malaria Eradication, 46; Foster at, 121; four-stage design, 96; funding, 32, 37, 41, 65, 66; Global Malaria Control Strategy, 162; goals of, 6; limited programs, 45; Malaria Expert Committee, 45–46; malaria unit, 35; Mexico City conference, 40; on Primary Health Care, 158; on program failure, 145; role, 42; "safe" use in poor rural areas, 161; U.S. support, 19, 20, 65, 179n110
Wilcox, Francis O., 20, 172n13
Williams, Louis L., Jr., 66, 184n168; malaria eradication hearings, 55–60
Winthrop Steams, 5
women, seen as mothers, 104
World Bank, 146, 162
World War II, 3–5, 16, 17; DDT, 17; Mexican relations, 78–79

yaws, 38
yellow fever, 2, 8, 18, 97
Yucatán, 111, 145

Zacatecas, 128–36
Zozaya, José, 89, 91